Imaging of Headache

Editor

SANGAM KANEKAR

NEUROLOGIC CLINICS

www.neurologic.theclinics.com

Consulting Editor
RANDOLPH W. EVANS

August 2022 • Volume 40 • Number 3

ELSEVIER

1600 John F. Kennedy Boulevard • Suite 1800 • Philadelphia, Pennsylvania, 19103-2899

http://www.theclinics.com

NEUROLOGIC CLINICS Volume 40, Number 3
August 2022 ISSN 0733-8619, ISBN-13: 978-0-323-89750-1

Editor: Stacy Eastman
Developmental Editor: Hannah Almira Lopez

Neurologic Clinics (ISSN 0733-8619) is published quarterly by Elsevier Inc., 360 Park Avenue South, New York, NY 10010–1710. Months of issue are February, May, August, and November. Periodicals postage paid at New York, NY, and additional mailing offices. Subscription prices are $343.00 per year for US individuals, $916.00 per year for US institutions, $100.00 per year for US students, $420.00 per year for Canadian individuals, $953.00 per year for Canadian institutions, $475.00 per year for international individuals, $953.00 per year for international institutions, $210.00 for foreign students/residents, and $100.00 for Canadian students/residents. To receive student/resident rate, orders must be accompanied by name of affiliated institution, date of term, and the *signature* of program/residency coordinator on institution letterhead. Orders will be billed at individual rate until proof of status is received. Foreign air speed delivery is included in all *Clinics* subscription prices. All prices are subject to change without notice. **POSTMASTER:** Send address changes to *Neurologic Clinics*, Elsevier Health Sciences Division, Subscription Customer Service, 3251 Riverport Lane, Maryland Heights, MO 63043. **Customer Service: Telephone: 1-800-654-2452 (U.S. and Canada); 314-447-8871 (outside U.S. and Canada). Fax: 314-447-8029. E-mail: journalscustomerservice-usa@elsevier.com (for print support); journalsonlinesupport-usa@elsevier.com (for online support).**

Reprints. For copies of 100 or more of articles in this publication, please contact the Commercial Reprints Department, Elsevier Inc., 360 Park Avenue South, New York, New York, 10010-1710; Tel.: +1-212-633-3874; Fax: +1-212-633-3820, and E-mail: reprints@elsevier.com.

Neurologic Clinics is also published in Spanish by Nueva Editorial Interamericana S.A., Mexico City, Mexico.

Neurologic Clinics is covered in *Current Contents/Clinical Medicine, MEDLINE/PubMed (Index Medicus), EMBASE/Excerpta Medica, and PsycINFO, and ISI/BIOMED.*

Contributors

CONSULTING EDITOR

RANDOLPH W. EVANS, MD
Clinical Professor, Department of Neurology, Baylor College of Medicine, Houston, Texas

EDITOR

SANGAM KANEKAR, MD, DNB
Professor of Radiology and Neurology, Vice Chair, Radiology Research, Chief, Division of Neuroradiology, Milton S. Hershey Medical Center, Penn State Health, Penn State College of Medicine, Hershey, Pennsylvania

AUTHORS

AMIT AGARWAL, MD
Senior Associate Consultant, Department of Radiology, Mayo Clinic, Jacksonville, Florida

SHADI ASADOLLAHI, MD
Research Fellow, Russell H. Morgan Department of Radiology and Radiological Sciences, The Johns Hopkins Hospital, Baltimore, Maryland

ALINE CAMARGO, MD
Department of Radiology, Penn State Health, Penn State College of Medicine, Hershey, Pennsylvania

MAURICIO CASTILLO, MD, FACR
Matthew A. Mauro Distinguished Professor, Division of Neuroradiology, Department of Radiology, The University of North Carolina at Chapel Hill, University of North Carolina School of Medicine, Chapel Hill, North Carolina

CHRISTINE M. GLASTONBURY, MBBS
Professor of Radiology and Biomedical Imaging, Otolaryngology–Head and Neck Surgery and Radiation Oncology, Department of Radiology and Biomedical Imaging, University of California, San Francisco, San Francisco, California

SAMIKA KANEKAR, MS
Medical Student, The Warren Alpert Medical School, Brown University, Providence, Rhode Island

SANGAM KANEKAR, MD, DNB
Professor of Radiology and Neurology, Vice Chair, Radiology Research, Chief, Division of Neuroradiology, Milton S. Hershey Medical Center, Penn State Health, Penn State College of Medicine, Hershey, Pennsylvania

JONATHON MAFFIE, MD, PhD
Assistant Professor, Department of Radiology, Division of Neuroradiology, Penn State Health Milton S. Hershey Medical Center, Hershey, Pennsylvania

ABDELKADER MAHAMMEDI, MD
Department of Radiology, University of Cincinnati Medical Center, Cincinnati, Ohio

IAN T. MARK, MD
Clinical Instructor of Neuroradiology, Department of Radiology and Biomedical Imaging, University of California, San Francisco, San Francisco, California

KASSIE MCCULLAGH, MD
Clinical Assistant Professor, Division of Neuroradiology, Department of Radiology, The University of North Carolina at Chapel Hill, Chapel Hill, North Carolina

ROHINI NADGIR, MD
Assistant Professor, Neuroradiology Division, Russell H. Morgan Department of Radiology and Radiological Sciences, The Johns Hopkins Hospital, Baltimore, Maryland

MANAL SAIF, DO
Radiology Resident, Department of Radiology, Penn State Health, Penn State College of Medicine, Hershey, Pennsylvania

ERIC SOBIESKI, BS
Pennsylvania State College of Medicine, Hershey, Pennsylvania

ACHALA S. VAGAL, MD, MS
Department of Radiology, University of Cincinnati Medical Center, Cincinnati, Ohio

LILY L. WANG, MBBS, MPH
Department of Radiology, University of Cincinnati Medical Center, Cincinnati, Ohio

ALLISON WEYER, MD
Assistant Professor of Radiology, Division of Neuroradiology, University of Pittsburgh Medical Center, Pittsburgh, Pennsylvania

BLAIR A. WINEGAR, MD
Associate Professor of Radiology, University of Utah School of Medicine, Salt Lake City, Utah

DAVID M. YOUSEM, MD, MBA
Professor, Neuroradiology Division, Russell H. Morgan Department of Radiology and Radiological Sciences, The Johns Hopkins Hospital, Baltimore, Maryland

CARLOS ZAMORA, MD, PhD
The Division Chief of Neuroradiology, Clinical Associate Professor, Division of Neuroradiology, Department of Radiology, The University of North Carolina at Chapel Hill, University of North Carolina School of Medicine, Chapel Hill, North Carolina

Contents

Headache is a common presenting symptom in the ambulatory setting that often prompts imaging. The increased use and associated health care money spent in the setting of headache have raised questions about the cost-effectiveness of neuroimaging in this setting. Neuroimaging for headache in most cases is unlikely to reveal significant abnormality or impact patient management. In this article, reasons behind an observed increase in neuroimaging and its impact on health care expenditures are discussed. The typical imaging modalities available and various imaging guidelines for common clinical headache scenarios are presented, including recommendations from the American College of Radiology.

Headache disorders rank third among the worldwide causes of disability, measured in years of life lost to disability. Primary headaches, such as migraine-type headache (MTH) and tension-type headache (TTH), are the most prevalent type of headache disorders. According to the Global Burden of Disease Study 2010 (GBD2010), TTH and migraine were reported as the second (20.1%) and third (14.7%) most prevalent disorders in the world, respectively, (after dental caries first). The global prevalence of TTH is 40% and migraine 10%.

Imaging is essential in the diagnosis of vascular causes of headaches. With advances in technology, there are increasing options of imaging modalities to choose from, each with its own advantages and disadvantages. This article will focus on imaging pearls and pitfalls of vascular causes of headaches. These include aneurysms, vasculitides, vascular malformations, and cerebral venous thrombosis.

Evaluation of headaches warrants a careful history and neurologic assessment to determine the need for further workup and imaging. Identifying patients who are at risk for underlying pathology is important and this includes individuals with known or suspected malignancy and those who are immunocompromised and at increased risk for intracranial infection. While CT is helpful in the acute setting and to screen for intracranial hypertension, MRI is the modality of choice for the evaluation of underlying pathologies. Imaging in substance abuse may show injury related to direct toxicity or secondary to vascular complications.

Changes in intracranial pressure are a potentially serious etiology of headache. Headache secondary to changes in intracranial pressure frequently present with characteristic clinical features. Imaging plays a key role in the diagnosis and management of this category of headache. In this article, we will review the physiology, clinical presentation, and key imaging findings of major etiologies of changes in intracranial pressure resulting in headache including obstructive and nonobstructive hydrocephalous, idiopathic intracranial hypertension (IIH), and cerebrospinal fluid (CSF) leak.

The article describes the approach to imaging that clinicians should adopt in cases of headaches suspected to be secondary to cranial vault or skull-base disorder. As a rule, computed tomography (CT) is superior to MRI for most of the osseous lesions, and lesions of the middle and external ear. MRI provides a complimentary role to CT and is the modality of choice in a few conditions such as extraosseous neoplasms of the skull base.

Cranial neuralgia (CN) can cause significant debilitating pain within a nerve dermatome. Accurate diagnosis requires detailed clinical history and examination, understanding of pathophysiology and appropriate neuroimaging to develop an optimal treatment plan. The objective of this article is to review and discuss some of the more common CNs including trigeminal neuralgia and its associated painful neuropathies, occipital neuralgia, and less common glossopharyngeal neuralgia (GPN). The neuroanatomy, pathophysiology, diagnostic imaging, and treatment of each of these pathologies are reviewed with emphasis on the role of CT and MR imaging findings in guiding diagnosis. Although CT is often used to initially identify an underlying cause such as neoplasm, infection, or vascular malformation, MRI is optimal. Clinical history and examination findings along with MRI constructive interference steady state/fast imaging employing steady-state acquisition sequences and MRA of the brain can be used to distinguish between primary and secondary cranial neuropathies and to discern the best treatment option. Pharmacologic and noninvasive therapy is the first-line of treatment of these cranial and cervical neuralgias. If symptoms persist, stereotactic radiosurgery is an option for some patients, although microvascular decompression surgery is the most curative option for both trigeminal and GPN. Refractory occipital neuralgia can be treated with a nerve block, an ablative procedure such as neurectomy or ganglionectomy, or more recently occipital nerve stimulation.

Headaches following head trauma or craniotomy have multiple causes, each of which has characteristic imaging features. Posttraumatic headaches may relate to intracranial hemorrhage, fracture, shear injury, mass effect, or vascular injury. Various complications of craniotomy and craniectomy may manifest with headache. CT and MRI of the brain play important roles in diagnosing these causes of headache.

When brain imaging is performed as a first-line investigation for headaches and no intracranial abnormality is found, attention should always be paid to potential non-CNS causes of headache including paranasal sinus inflammatory, infectious, and occasionally malignant disease, and also to odontogenic sinusitis. Non-enhanced CT (NECT) head offers an initial evaluation of these areas which may be an unexpected source of symptomatology. Further imaging may then be required with either dedicated sinus NECT [particularly if surgical intervention is necessary for paranasal sinus disease], a contrast-enhanced (CECT) head and sinus CT, or an MRI if intracranial complications of sinonasal disease or acute invasive fungal sinusitis is suspected.

Cross-sectional imaging with computed tomography (CT) and MRI are diagnostic examinations useful in the diagnosis of painful ophthalmologic disorders and their potential complications. CT is a first-line imaging study for suspected orbital infections, particularly useful in differentiating preseptal cellulitis and orbital cellulitis and detecting complications such as orbital abscess. When compared with CT, MRI is better for orbital soft tissue evaluation, particularly useful for optic neuritis, ocular diseases such as endophthalmitis, and invasive fungal rhinosinusitis with orbital involvement. CT angiography is the preferred noninvasive imaging modality for the detection and classification of carotid cavernous fistula.

Approximately 35% of acute headaches in pregnant women are secondary to an underlying condition. Headaches are also common in the postpartum period where they occur in 30% to 40% of patients. The majority of secondary headaches are due to hypertensive disorders: preeclampsia-eclampsia, posterior reversible encephalopathy syndrome, and acute arterial hypertension. Other causes include reversible cerebral vasoconstriction syndrome and pituitary apoplexy, as well as life-threatening conditions such as cerebral venous thrombosis. In this article, we review general recommendations for imaging the pregnant patients and discuss the imaging findings of common causes of headaches in pregnancy and the postpartum period.

Aline Camargo and Sangam Kanekar

Headache represents one of the most common disorders in childhood and leads to nearly half a million visits to the physician's office or emergency department every year. Although the estimated prevalence is around 58.4%, the actual incidence of headache in the pediatric population might be underestimated, given only a percentage of cases seek medical attention. The first step in the evaluation of pediatric headache is a detailed clinical history and relevant clinical examinations. AAN and ACR do not recommend neuroimaging for patients with primary headache. However, neuroimaging becomes mandatory in presence of red flags to rule out the underlying cause.

NEUROLOGIC CLINICS

Preface

Imaging of Headache

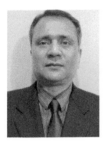

Sangam Kanekar, MD, DNB
Editor

Headache is one of the most common presenting symptoms in clinical practice. As per World Health Organization criteria, it is one of the 10 most debilitating conditions in the world with respect to days lost from employment. The use of neuroimaging in patients with headaches is growing. Imaging in headaches has increased from 17.5% to 33.3% per visit from 1996 to 2014. The overuse of imaging modalities for the evaluation of patients with headaches has posed a potential risk to the patient and to society in a resource-limited health care system. Almost $78 billion is spent on direct and indirect expenses of headaches in the United States.

The first step in evaluating headaches is a detailed clinical history and relevant clinical examination to differentiate between primary and secondary headaches. The main goal of the clinical examination and history is to identify the presence of "red flags," which will favor neuroimaging. The American Academy of Neurology and the American College of Radiology do not recommend neuroimaging for patients with primary headaches unless there are associated other clinical findings. The main goal of this issue is to give a comprehensive review and appropriate selection of imaging techniques in primary and secondary headache patients. This issue has 12 articles focusing on imaging of primary and secondary causes of headaches.

I thank all the authors for their excellent contributions that make this issue a great review for imaging in headaches. I take this opportunity to thank Elsevier for giving me a chance to present this topic to a wider audience. I thank my wife, Revati, and my children, Samika and Rachita, for their love and support.

Happy reading!!

Sangam Kanekar, MD, DNB
Division of Neuroradiology
Hershey Medical Center
Penn State Health
Penn State College of Medicine
Mail code H066; 500 University Drive
Hershey, PA 17033, USA

E-mail address:
skanekar@pennstatehealth.psu.edu

Neuroimaging of Headache

Indications and Controversies

Shadi Asadollahi, MD[1], David M. Yousem, MD, MBA[2], Rohini Nadgir, MD*,[3]

KEYWORDS

- Headache • Computed tomography • MRI • Brain • Neuroimaging

KEY POINTS

- Over the past several decades, the increased use and associated health care money spent have raised questions about the cost-effectiveness of neuroimaging among patients presenting with headache.
- For most patients presenting with a primary headache syndrome, there is no need for neuroimaging.
- Neuroimaging should be reserved for patients with any red flag signs or alterations in chronic headache pattern.

INTRODUCTION

Headache is a common presenting symptom in patients in the emergency department (ED) and accounts for 1% to 4% of all emergency visits. Each year in the United States, 18 million outpatients are treated for headaches.[1,2] Based on World Health Organization (WHO) criteria, it is among the 10 most debilitating conditions in the world with respect to days lost from employment. The life-long prevalence of experiencing any type of headache is 31% to 96%. The diagnostic work-up begins with a complete history and physical examination including a comprehensive neurologic evaluation to classify the type of headache disorder.[3–5]

Headache disorders are usually categorized as either primary or secondary:

- Migraine, cluster headache, and tension headache are examples of primary headaches, which are not caused by other medical conditions and whose diagnoses are derived through a detailed history and symptom pattern identification. Approximately 90% of headaches seen in practice are of the primary category.[6,7]

Russell H. Morgan Department of Radiology and Radiological Sciences, The Johns Hopkins Hospital
[1] 600 N. Wolfe Street, Phipps B-199A, Baltimore, MD 21287.
[2] 600 N. Wolfe Street, Phipps B-112D, Baltimore, MD 21287.
[3] 600 N. Wolfe Street, Phipps B-100, Baltimore, MD 21287.
* Corresponding author.
E-mail address: rnadgir1@jhmi.edu

Neurol Clin 40 (2022) 471–489
https://doi.org/10.1016/j.ncl.2022.02.001
0733-8619/22/© 2022 Elsevier Inc. All rights reserved.

neurologic.theclinics.com

- Secondary headaches are caused by organic diseases such as stroke, brain tumors, head trauma, and vascular disorders.

For most patients presenting with a primary headache syndrome, there is no need for neuroimaging, as it is unlikely to change the management of care or reveal any abnormalities. However, a considerable proportion of ED patients with headaches are imaged, nonetheless, to rule out serious pathologic abnormalities. Because of the medicolegal risk that ED physicians face, some may feel obliged to scan patients with headaches who have no specific neurologic symptoms.[8,9] Furthermore:

- Primary headaches may sometimes present in an atypical manner without meeting the diagnostic criteria
- Secondary headaches may present in the same way as primary headaches
- Both primary and secondary headaches may coexist in rare cases[10]

These variations in the presentation can make headache diagnosis difficult.

COST OF IMAGING

Headache imaging specifically has increased from 17.5% to 33.3% per visit from 1996 to 2014.[2] Although clinical guidelines, appropriateness criteria, and practical parameters have been promulgated, the use of neuroimaging in patients with headaches is growing.[11] Overuse of imaging modalities and a continuous rise in annual ED visits for headaches pose potential risks to the patient and society in a resource-limited health care system. This has sparked alarm among health care professionals and policymakers.[3,12]

In recent years, considerable emphasis has been placed on the cost-effectiveness of imaging in patients with primary headache disorders, especially those with chronic headache and nonfocal neurologic examinations whose imaging studies often show negative results. Cost-effectiveness should be assessed based on the category of headache, symptoms, and signs as well as the applied imaging technique.[13–15] Almost $78 billion is spent on direct and indirect expenses of headaches in the United States. Apart from treatment, direct costs include the imaging services provided in the outpatient and ED setting.[16–18]

Computed tomography (CT) scanning in the ED is the most common study ordered and has led to growing national concern of the substantial economic consequences. Head CT and MRI of the brain nationally cost, on average, $340 and $660 per scan, respectively.[19,20] Several studies have highlighted the poor cost-effectiveness of CT imaging in patients without neurologic abnormalities. Accordingly, reducing unnecessary imaging and rising health care costs remain top national priorities given the growing awareness and realities of limited health care resources.

In an attempt to control health care costs in the United States, the Centers for Medicare & Medicaid Services (CMS) have implemented the "Appropriate Use Criteria Program," which at the time of this writing is intended to go into full effect for all providers starting January 1, 2023, and headache imaging is considered one of the priority clinical areas of focus. Once this program is initiated, claims will be denied if ordering providers do not confirm with a Clinical Decision Support Mechanism (CDSM, an interactive electronic method of communication) that a requested imaging study is appropriate based on specific appropriate use criteria. Several CDSMs are currently being evaluated by CMS for this future implementation.[21]

To calculate the costs associated with diagnostic imaging services, 2 components are generally considered, a technical component (TC) and a professional component (PC). The TC and PC may be provided together as a global service. The Medicare fee schedule for diagnostic assessment of headache is summarized in **Table 1** for each component.[21]

AVAILABLE MODALITIES

In the clinical setting of frequent headaches, imaging is aimed to rule out an underlying lesion.[22] Although CT scans are not the ideal tests for many headache conditions, they are the recommended tests for evaluating patients with acute thunderclap headache, suspected infection of the paranasal sinuses, trauma, brain edema, bone abnormalities, and in situations where MRI is contraindicated.[10] CT is often used as the most appropriate first investigation in the diagnostic work-up of patients with acute headaches because of its high sensitivity to acute hemorrhage and specifically subarachnoid hemorrhage (SAH). When current-generation CT images are acquired within 6 hours of symptoms, CT has a 99.9% negative predictive value for SAH detection.[23–25] Noncontrast-enhanced CT is typically ordered; intravenous (IV) contrast is only utilized when noncontrast studies show masses or uncharacterized lesions.

Many efforts have been made to restrict CT misuse; however, its utilization grew by 330% from 2008 to 2012, with over 70 million CT scans performed annually in the United States.[26,27] Several factors have contributed to the increase in CT use, including ready availability, fast scanning techniques, consistent high quality, and known accuracy in excluding lethal cerebral bleeding, masses, and sinusitis in headache patients.

There are some disadvantages in the routine use of CT, including patients' exposure to ionizing radiation, which progressively increases the risk of future malignancy, particularly in young patients who may require repeated scans.[28,29]

In contrast, MRI techniques can provide improved soft tissue resolution without exposure to ionizing radiation. However, MRI is an expensive imaging tool requiring a more elaborate screening protocol to ensure the patient does not have a contraindication to MRI. MRI requires longer examination times compared with CT, and patients who are claustrophobic or in physical discomfort may be unable to undergo a prolonged MRI examination. The presence of artifacts from metal hardware and lack of 24-hour availability are other limitations of MRI.[15]

Generally, MRI is the preferred technique for studying a patient with a change in headache severity and frequency or chronic headache with new neurologic examination findings.[8] An MRI scan is more helpful than a CT scan and is the preferred modality for headache patients, especially when there are red flags. MRI (with and without contrast) is more useful than CT in the detection of the following intracranial conditions; cerebrospinal fluid (CSF) leak, idiopathic intracranial hypertension, demyelinating lesions, primary tumors and metastases, meningeal infections, brain abscesses, venous thrombosis, and other space-occupying lesions. MRI is also safe and effective in excluding secondary headaches in pregnancy.[10]

Table 1			
Medicare fee schedule for evaluations of headache patients			
Procedure	**Technical Fee**	**Professional Fee**	**Total (Technical and Professional)**
30-min office visit	Not applicable (NA)	NA	$132.55 (bundled)
Noncontrast brain CT	$98.47	$46.96	$145.43
Noncontrast brain MRI	$148.30	$72.23	$220.53
Lumbar puncture	NA	NA	$164.34 (bundled)

Role of Appropriateness Criteria

Although no imaging is needed for primary headaches without complications, headaches with critical features need additional imaging evaluation to rule out life-threatening intracranial pathology. The purpose of obtaining neuroimaging studies for patients is to recognize more harmful conditions, such as tumors, vascular malformations, aneurysms, cerebral venous sinus thrombosis, subdural and epidural hematomas, infections, stroke, and hydrocephalus.[30,31] Recommendations regarding when to perform imaging for headaches have been released by the American College of Radiology (ACR) in its Appropriateness Criteria (ACR-AC).[8] ACR-AC are evidence-based guidelines to rate the appropriateness of imaging and treatment methods for 211 diagnostic imaging areas with more than 1000 variants and nearly 1900 clinical scenarios. The criteria were established in the 1990s and are evaluated annually, based on an analysis of current medical literature and a well-established consensus methodology.

The ACR-AC address different clinical scenarios for adult patients with headache, including chronic headache presenting with new features, new headache in a person with immunosuppression or during pregnancy, and headaches in patients with cancer.

The expert panel of the ACR-AC rates the appropriateness of different imaging methods (eg, CT, MRI, or angiography) for each particular clinical scenario from "usually not appropriate," "may be appropriate," to "usually appropriate." For instance, the criteria suggest that a patient with new classic migraine or tension-type primary headache should not get head CT without contrast ("usually not appropriate"); however, a patient with a thunderclap headache has a high appropriateness rating ("usually appropriate") to undergo head CT without contrast (**Table 2**).[8,32]

Table 2
American College of Radiology-Appropriateness Criteria variants and initial imaging

	Variant	Computed Tomography of Head without Intravenous Contrast	MRI of Head With or Without Intravenous Contrast
1	Sudden, severe headache or WHOL	Usually appropriate	Usually not appropriate
2	New headache with optic disc edema	Usually appropriate	Usually appropriate
3	New or progressively worsening headache with one or more of the red flags[a]	Usually appropriate	Usually appropriate
4	New headache, classic migraine or tension-type primary headache, normal neurologic examination	Usually not appropriate	Usually not appropriate
5	New primary headache of suspected trigeminal autonomic origin	Usually not appropriate	Usually appropriate
6	Chronic headache, no new features, no neurologic deficit	Usually not appropriate	Usually not appropriate
7	Chronic headache, new features or increasing frequency	May be appropriate	Usually appropriate

[a] Red flags include subacute head trauma, related activity or event (eg, sexual activity, exertion, or position), neurologic deficit, known or suspected cancer, immunosuppressed or immunocompromised state, currently pregnant, or 50 y of age or older.

(*Adapted from* Whitehead MT, Cardenas AM, Corey AS, et al. ACR appropriateness Criteria® headache. J Am Coll Radiol 2019;16:S364–77; with permission.)

SPECIFIC CLINICAL SCENARIOS
Worst Headache of Life

Specific consideration is given to a sudden, severe headache (thunderclap headache or "the worst headache of life [WHOL]"), which is characterized as an extreme pain (pain score of 7/10 or higher) that reaches its peak in less than 1 minute.[33,34] These headaches have a higher imaging yield in the ED because of the high probability of serious intracranial hemorrhages. Such thunderclap or WHOL headaches are substantially more likely to result from SAH or reversible cerebral vasoconstriction syndrome (RCVS). The most serious cases of SAH are caused by ruptured cerebral aneurysms.[35] Approximately 80% of all SAH cases in the United States are caused by aneurysmal rupture, with severe disability or mortality occurring in 50% to 70% of those suffering this calamity.[36,37]

In addition to the headache, patients with SAH often show other neurologic manifestations (impaired consciousness, neck stiffness, photophobia, aneurysm-induced cranial neuropathies, and local weakness) that suggest the specific diagnosis. However, in individuals with headache as the only presentation of SAH, a correct diagnosis can be missed ,with the estimated range of 12% to 51%.[38–40] It is critical not to overlook the diagnosis in patients with normal mental state, because the initial misdiagnosis causes high rates of mortality because of rebleeding, severe short- and long-term disability, and poor quality of life.[41,42]

SAH is estimated to be found on noncontrast head CT in 29% to 71% of adult patients presenting with sudden-onset thunderclap headache or WHOL.[30,43–46] As such, the standard protocol for assessing SAH is a noncontrast head CT, followed by a lumbar puncture (LP) if the CT reveals no abnormalities. The sensitivity of noncontrast head CT to detect acute SAH is 92% to 95% during the first 12 to 24 hours after the aneurysm rupture, and 82% to 84% afterward.[30,44] Failure to correctly diagnose SAH at a patient's initial contact with a medical professional may be as high as 50%.[47] The most common diagnostic error is failure to obtain a head CT, accounting for 73% of cases of SAH misdiagnosis.[45,47]

There are several factors reducing the sensitivity of CT scans for the detection of SAH, including reduction in sensitivity over time, technical inability of older-generation scanners to find small hemorrhages in regions concealed by artifact or bone, diverse levels of readers' proficiency, and decreased sensitivity for blood in the setting of anemia.[30]

Once SAH has been confirmed, CT angiography (CTA) and/or catheter angiography should be used to determine the location and characteristics of the aneurysm with greater accuracy to facilitate endovascular or surgical repair.[48,49]

Migraine

Many guidelines and literature reviews recommend that neuroimaging is not generally necessary for patients with migraine headaches who have a normal neurologic examination and no abnormalities or red flags. If there are no new or additional symptoms, or new and identifiable worrying characteristics (such as fever, seizure, or trauma), imaging is not required in the absence of substantial changes in the existing pattern of a persistent headache.[50]

There are several reasons contributing to doctors' decision to acquire head imaging for suspected migraine, including

- Excluding secondary diseases resembling migraine[51]
- Discomfort with migraine as a clinical diagnosis[52]
- Ordering tests as a shortcut in busy practice settings

- Considering patients' and families' expectations and anxieties, which may be expressed in negative online patient reviews or patient satisfaction surveys[53]
- Cognitive bias (ie, failure to perceive or properly interpret an abnormality)[54]
- Considering the concerns and expectations by headache specialists of referring physicians
- Medicolegal concerns[55]

The critical conditions that may mimic a migraine include conditions where a delay in diagnosis may result in significant morbidity and death. For instance, serious non-ischemic cerebrovascular illnesses (eg, intracranial hemorrhage, posterior reversible encephalopathy syndrome [PRES]) can manifest in the form of isolated headaches and are sometimes misinterpreted as migraine or other headache disorders.[42,56] Migraine with aura is a well-known risk factor for stroke, and aura symptoms may resemble focal neurologic impairments. Migraine can also lead to cerebral infarction through vasospasm.[57,58] On the other hand, acute ischemic stroke may initiate a migraine episode or produce a secondary headache.[59] The judicious use of neuroimaging, especially brain MRI, is indicated in such circumstances.

Meningitis

Patients with meningitis may sometimes be confused with those who have migraines, because they often share symptoms of photophobia, phonophobia, and neck stiffness.[60,61] Noncontrast CT in individuals with uncomplicated (viral) meningitis typically does not reveal abnormalities. According to the Infectious Diseases Society of America, a nonenhanced CT scan should be performed before LP to exclude cerebral edema or mass effect so that an LP can be conducted without risk of herniation.[62] In later stages of meningitis, brain MRI with and without contrast may show meningeal enhancement, but is not required for medical therapy given confirmatory CSF findings unless complications such as epidural, subdural or parenchymal abscess, encephalitis, or vascular compromise are suspected.[62]

Head Trauma

Head trauma is a major public health issue imposing a substantial financial and social burden on society in the form of medical expenses, lost productivity, and disability affecting both children and the young adult population.[63] Traumatic brain injury (TBI) causes more than 2.5 million ED visits each year in the United States.[64,65] The most common mechanisms of TBI include falls, motor vehicle accidents, interpersonal violence, and sports injuries.

In the acute phase, blunt TBI has been generally categorized as mild, moderate, or severe according to the Glasgow Coma Scale (GCS) score (**Table 3**), while penetrating head injury is less prevalent and is always classified as severe.[66,67] Most TBIs are of mild severity, accounting for 70% to 90% of all head traumas.

Table 3
Severity of traumatic brain injury according to Glasgow Coma Score

	Mild	Moderate	Severe
Glasgow Coma Scale (GCS) score[a]	13–15	9–12	≤8

[a] The scale GCS is determined based on 3 components: eye opening (4: opening spontaneously, 3: opening to verbal command, 2: opening to pain, and 1: no eye opening), verbal (5: oriented, 4: disoriented, 3: inappropriate words, 2: incomprehensible sounds, and 1: no verbal response), and motor response (6: obeys, 5: localizes pain, 4: withdrawal, 3: abnormal flexion, 2: abnormal extension, and 1: no motor response).

Headache is the most commonly reported symptom of mild TBI, present in almost 90% of patients.[68,69] Post-traumatic headaches are more incapacitating than nontraumatic headaches.[70] These headaches are characterized as a new headache or a severe exacerbation of a previous kind of headache that occurred within 7 days after the injury and may mimic a primary headache. According to the International Classification of Headache Disorders 3rd edition criteria (ICHD-3), post-traumatic headaches are classified based on the duration (acute, <3 months or persistent, >3 months), and severity of the injury (mild, moderate, or severe).[71]

Neuroimaging in the ED is warranted in post-traumatic headache if there is localized neurologic abnormalities or symptom progression.[72] However, common experience is that CT scans of the brain are routinely performed in patients with MVCs and falls even without symptoms, particularly in the setting of

- Dementia
- Altered mental state from drugs or alcoholism
- Loss of consciousness at the time of the event
- Traumatic amnesia
- Elderly patients susceptible to delayed complications
- Anticoagulation
- Distracting injuries

Approximately 30% of post-traumatic patients with a normal neurologic evaluation have intracerebral abnormalities related to the injury.[44] It is crucial to identify those individuals with post-traumatic brain lesions such as intracranial bleeding, skull fractures, cerebral edema, and high intracranial pressure that require urgent surgical intervention.[73,74] Nonsurgical patients with hemorrhages and skull fractures should have repeat imaging after the initial injury, especially within the first 72 hours if they have deteriorating clinical symptoms, increasing headache, or a change in headache pattern.[72,75]

The most important imaging technique for determining delayed consequences of brain trauma is MRI. Conventional brain MRIs are used for acute severe head trauma and when clinical deficits are at a greater degree of severity than CT findings. The ACR-AC recommends performing MRI without contrast for acute TBI with a new or progressive neurologic deficit and for subacute or chronic TBI with unexplained cognitive or neurologic deficit. TBI with suspected acute intracranial arterial or venous injury due to clinical risk factors or positive findings on prior imaging should be evaluated by CTA of head and neck with IV contrast.[72,76,77]

Headache with Red Flags

Neuroimaging should be considered for patients with any red flag signs or symptoms to assess for underlying conditions that can potentiate headaches. It has been suggested that the appearance of red flag characteristics or the presence of other underlying conditions increases the specificity of imaging in new or worsening headaches (**Box 1**).[5,78] Additional red flag symptoms reported by studies include systemic symptoms (eg, fever, weight loss, or neck stiffness), red eye and visual halos around lights, and recent travel history.[79–82] Over 10 years ago, the widely used SNOOP mnemonic was developed to assist providers to recall these red flag signs (**Table 4**).[83] Since then, different guidelines have included more criteria to check for secondary causes of headaches and led to the present SNNOOP10.[84]

Headaches associated with any of the aforementioned warning signs require a particular imaging strategy, as they may indicate increased intracranial pressure. There are various causes of high intracranial pressure (ICP), which can be related to

Box 1
Headache Red Flag Symptoms and Signs

First or worst headache of life

Severe headache with sudden onset (thunderclap)

New-onset headache at age $\geq$50 years

Change in typical headache pattern or frequency

Current pregnancy

Known or suspected cancer

Immunosuppressed or immunocompromised state

Abnormal neurologic examination

Headache triggered by Valsalva or exertion

Headache with seizure or alteration of consciousness

- Intracranial masses and edema
- Intracranial hemorrhage
- Obstruction of CSF flow and reabsorption
- Pseudotumor cerebri syndrome related to primary idiopathic intracranial hypertension (IIH)
- Cerebral venous thrombosis

In such cases, head MRI (with and without contrast) is the preferred imaging study.[85,86] MR venography (MRV) may also be performed to evaluate for the presence of venous thrombosis or venous sinus stenosis.[87] In case of an MRI contraindication or

Table 4
Red flags according to SNNOOP10 list

Mnemonic	Red Flag
S	Systemic symptoms (fever, chills, or weight loss)
N	Neurologic signs or symptoms (confusion, change in mental status, asymmetric reflexes or other abnormalities on examination)
N	Neoplasm of brain in history
O	Onset (acute, sudden or split-second thunderclap)
O	Older age (after 50 y)
P	Pattern change or recent onset of headache
P	Precipitated by sneezing, coughing, or exercise
P	Papilledema
P	Progressive headache and atypical presentation
P	Pregnancy
P	Painful eye with autonomic features
P	Post-traumatic onset of headache
P	Pathology of the immune system (such as HIV)
P	Painkiller overuse or new drug
P	Positional Headache

(*Modified from* Do TP, Remmers A, Schytz HW, et al. Red and orange flags for secondary headaches in clinical practice: SNNOOP10 list. Neurology. 2019;92(3):134–144; with permission.)

unavailability, the second alternative is head CT with contrast. CT venogram is a reliable alternative to MRV.

In case of headache with sudden development of a focal neurologic deficit, a vascular ischemic event (transient ischemic attack [TIA] or stroke) should be considered in the differential diagnosis. The incidence of headache accompanying TIAs or strokes varies from 15% to 65% between studies (average 30%). Headache appears to be more prevalent in patients with posterior circulation ischemia.[88] Noncontrast head CT is the initial imaging approach to evaluate for intracranial hemorrhage in patients presenting with acute ischemic or hemorrhagic stroke. Head CT with contrast is not typically used in this setting.[89]

Noncontrast brain MRI provides a practical alternative method, particularly for the evaluation of individuals with a hyperacute ischemic stroke (<6 hours). The main value of MRI is for diffusion-weighted images determining the extent of the infarcted tissue.[89,90] Magnetic resonance perfusion and CT perfusion can also be performed in the hyperacute setting and can show the cerebral ischemic penumbra in the hyperacute phase of ischemic stroke.[91,92]

Immunocompromised individuals are more vulnerable to intracranial infectious diseases, neoplastic disorders, and their complications. For example, patients with human immunodeficiency virus (HIV) infection and headache had a yield of 35% on neuroimaging, but it may be as high as 82%.[93] An immediate neuroimaging scan should be considered for immunocompromised individuals who have developed a new or progressively worsening headache,[94,95] and either a head CT without contrast or MRI with and without contrast can be performed.

Compared with the general population, patients presenting with new, progressive, or changes in chronic headache patterns during pregnancy are more likely to have intracranial pathologies.[96,97] Several secondary causes of headaches have a high incidence in this population. A pregnant patient has a fivefold increased risk of developing SAH compared with a nonpregnant patient. Moreover, headache can present as an accompanying symptom of several conditions during pregnancy, necessitating special imaging evaluation:

- Hypertensive encephalopathy following preeclampsia/eclampsia
- Pseudotumor cerebri
- Primary brain tumors and brain metastases
- Embolic stroke caused by amniotic fluid embolism to the brain vasculature[98]

An MRI brain scan without gadolinium is the preferred modality to evaluate for these conditions. A head CT without contrast is recommended for excluding life-threatening conditions such as new subarachnoid or parenchymal hemorrhage, significant mass effect, or hydrocephalus. There is no evidence to support the use of CT head with contrast or CTA as the initial imaging procedure in this setting. If there is a high suspicion for venous/sinus thrombosis, magnetic resonance venography should be considered.[8]

It is crucial to consider radiation dose and contrast usage during imaging procedures in pregnancy. The ACR and the American College of Obstetricians and Gynecologists (ACOG) have provided similar guidance in this area.[99–101] The estimated radiation exposure is low for CT when the fetus is outside the field of view. Therefore, head CT can be safely performed during any trimester of pregnancy.[102,103] An IV administration of iodinated or gadolinium-based contrast media to pregnant patients thus far has not been associated with either mutagenic or teratogenic effects on human fetuses.[104,105] However, some studies have raised concerns for neonatal hypothyroidism in using iodinated contrast media.[106] Because the long-term effects of gadolinium-based contrast agents in utero are unknown, these agents should be administered with caution to pregnant or potentially pregnant patients.[101]

In unilateral severe headaches with short-term duration, the diagnosis of trigeminal neuralgia (TN) should be considered in presenting patients. TN is characterized by excruciating attacks of electric shock-like facial pain and has been described as one of the most severe pains one can experience. The initial diagnosis of TN is made according to history and clinical assessment. Atypical history and clinical findings including long-standing persistent pain, resistance to medical therapy, or cranial nerve abnormalities may prompt the physician to suspect an underlying structural lesion.[107,108] So far, high-resolution brain MRI and magnetic resonance angiography (MRA) have shown to be the most effective method for identifying an intracranial etiology.[109–111] These techniques are also helpful noninvasive methods for reviewing the anatomy of potentially compressing vascular loops encroaching on the trigeminal nerve root entry zone. Head CT is helpful for assessing the skull base foramina if an invasive process is suspected, but it is usually performed in conjunction with MRI.[48]

Chronic Headache with New Features or Neurologic Deficit

Chronic headache is defined clinically as any headache experienced for at least 15 days per month, for at least 3 consecutive months. The commonly proposed mechanism by which headaches become chronic is that an existing episodic primary headache increases in frequency over time, such that the headache becomes continuous—a process often referred to as headache transformation.[112] The chronic headache may also be secondary to another disease process.

Two common types of primary headaches that may become chronic are chronic migraine and chronic tension-type headache. Increased headache frequency or intensity is a red flag.[113,114] Additional evaluation using neuroimaging is warranted when characters of headache change in the setting of a prior history of benign headaches. Head CT without contrast can be used to detect new intracranial bleeding, significant mass effect, or high and low ICP disorders. Head CT with contrast should be avoided as the primary imaging technique in the acute situation because the IV contrast may conceal hemorrhage.[96,115]

As an alternative to CT, MRI is a more thorough imaging technique and should be used as the first imaging method when a patient is in a stable situation. According to the American Headache Society guideline, head CT is not recommended when MRI is available, except in emergency situations.[116] When there is a suspicion of an intracranial mass or infection, a brain MRI with and without IV contrast should be performed.

Neuroimaging in Children

Many of the diagnostic neuroimaging approaches recommended in the ACR-AC guidelines involve exposure of patients to ionizing radiation. It is critical to consider the potential health risks related to radiation exposure when choosing the proper imaging technique.

Among children, radiation exposure is a major concern.[117] The risk of cancer induction and mortality associated with radiation exposure in children is about 10 and 4 times greater than the risk in adults, respectively.[118,119] The pediatric population has a longer life expectancy and higher organ sensitivity; therefore, children have a greater potential for manifesting possible detrimental outcomes of radiation.

The concept of ALARA (As Low As Reasonably Achievable) was introduced in 2001 to encourage the use of alternatives to CT scans and use CT only when necessary with the lowest possible dose of radiation.[120,121] Moreover, ACR-AC recommended relative radiation levels (RRLs) for most imaging examinations determining radiation exposures related to different diagnostic procedures.[122,123] The RRLs are a method of rating effective doses, expressed in units of millisievert (mSv). It measures the radiation sensitivity of different organs and tissues in the human body. The RRL dosage estimation ranges for pediatric examinations are lower than those for adults because of their smaller size. It is important to consider radiation exposure levels when selecting appropriate imaging examinations for children because of their greater sensitivity to radiation exposure.[124,125]

For this reason, MRI is preferred over CT for most of the cross-sectional imaging workup in children.[115] However, an important limitation of MRI in this population is the long acquisition time, which requires patients to remain motionless for prolonged

Table 5
Common headache conditions and recommended neuroimaging modalities by different guidelines

	Conditions	Guidelines	Initial Imaging	Additional Imaging
1	Sudden severe headache or WHOL	ACR	Head CT without contrast	CTA[a]
		ACEP	Head CT without contrast	CTA or LP
2	Classic migraine headache with normal neurologic examination	ACR	None	None
		AHS	None	None
		ANN	None	None
		USHC	None	None
3	Tension-type headache with normal neurologic examination	ACR	None	None
		USHC	None	None
4	Headache with abnormal neurologic examination	ACR	Head CT without IV contrast (emergency situation) Head MRI without and with IV contrast (stable patient)	None
		USHC	CT or MRI (not specified)	None
5	Headache worsened by Valsalva maneuver, headache causing awakening from sleep, new headache in the older population, or progressively worsening headache	ACR	Head CT without IV contrast (emergency situation) Head MRI without and with IV contrast (stable patient)	None
		USHC	None[b]	None
6	New or progressively worsening headache in immunosuppressed or immunocompromised state	ACR	Head CT without contrast	MRI head without/with IV contrast LP (if infection suspected)

[a] CTA is a useful method in conjunction with a noncontrast head CT if there are 2 or more first-degree family members with aneurysmal subarachnoid hemorrhages.
[b] According to USHC, evidence is insufficient to make specific recommendations regarding neuroimaging in this group.

periods. Thus, it usually necessitates patient sedation. Sedation limits MRI clinical feasibility because of the increased cost of imaging, longer examination and recovery times, limited anesthesia availability, and a higher risk for complications of the sedative and anesthetic agents.[126–128] Consequently, fast MRI protocols were developed to overcome the limitations of patient movement during conventional MRI.[129]

CONSENSUS AND UNCERTAINTY IN COMMON HEADACHE SCENARIOS

The Choosing Wisely recommendations of the American Headache Society (AHS) indicated that MRI is preferred over CT for headache evaluation, except in emergency settings. For stable patients, MRI is more comprehensive than CT, and generally the imaging technique of choice. Brain MRI without and with IV contrast should be performed in the condition of suspected intracranial mass or infection. Contrast administration will help in detection and evaluation of intracranial pathology.[8,130]

Several organizations such as the ACR,[8] the AHS,[131] the American College of Emergency Physicians (ACEP),[92] and the US Headache Consortium (USHC)[132] have all proposed guidelines on indications of headache imaging (**Table 5**). These guidelines provide a useful source of most available studies of the role of headache neuroimaging and are used at the beginning of clinical decision making, but they are not comprehensive. There are many indications that are not addressed by consensus or society standards, because the available literature has serious methodological limitations, or fails to address several important issues.[96,133] Different investigations and groups also consolidated imaging guidelines.[44,131,134] Finally, the clinician expertise and clinical judgment are crucial in choosing when to do imaging when available data are inadequate.

SUMMARY

Several variables must be considered when choosing whether to conduct imaging for headache, including headache features (typical or atypical), change of headache type or pattern, additional significant risk factors or red flags, sensitivities of imaging modalities, and impact of imaging on therapy.

Although most headaches are caused by a primary headache disease with a benign course, imaging is an essential component of the diagnostic assessment to exclude secondary causes of headache that may result in significant neurologic morbidity and death and require intervention. In headache patients without focal neurologic examination abnormalities, the yield of neuroimaging for significant intracranial findings is generally low. However, the incidence of clinically important intracranial abnormalities may be much greater in some subgroups of headache patients and headache presentations, necessitating neuroimaging.

CLINICS CARE POINTS

- The diagnostic work-up for headache begins with a complete history and physical examination including a comprehensive neurologic evaluation.
- Primary headache disorder (including migraine, cluster headache, and tension headaches) accounts for most headache presentations and can be diagnosed through detailed history and symptom pattern evaluation, without need for neuroimaging.
- Secondary headache disorder occurs as a consequence of pathologic process such as stroke, tumor, trauma, and vascular disease, and neuroimaging in these settings plays an important role.

- The decision to image by CT or MRI requires clinical expertise and judgment, but should take into account the headache pattern and clinical context.
- Numerous guidelines for neuroimaging in the headache setting exist, including the Appropriate Use Criteria put forth by the ACR, which provides evidence-based imaging recommendations for specific headache patterns in various clinical contexts.

DISCLOSURE

Dr S. Asadollahi has no financial disclosures. Dr D.M. Yousem receives compensation for medicolegal consultation, consultation fees, and honoraria from MRI Online, and royalties from Elsevier, Inc., for textbook publication but has no financial disclosures in the subject matter or materials discussed in the article or with any company making a competing product. Dr R. Nadgir receives royalties from Elsevier Inc., for textbook publication and Wolters Kluwer for article review but has no financial disclosures in the subject matter or materials discussed in the article or with any company making a competing product.

REFERENCES

1. Gaughran CG, Tubridy N. Headaches, neurologists and the emergency department. Ir Med J 2014;107:168–71.
2. Heetderks-Fong E. Appropriateness criteria for neuroimaging of adult headache patients in the emergency department: how are we doing? Adv Emerg Nurs J 2019;41:172–82.
3. Jordan JE, Flanders AE. Headache and neuroimaging: why we continue to do it. AJNR Am J Neuroradiol 2020;41:1149–55.
4. Saylor D, Steiner TJ. The global burden of headache. Semin Neurol 2018;38: 182–90.
5. Sandrini G, Friberg L, Coppola G, et al. European Federation of Neurological Sciences. Neurophysiological tests and neuroimaging procedures in non-acute headache (2nd edition). Eur J Neurol 2011;18:373–81.
6. Zhang Y, Kong Q, Chen J, et al. International classification of headache disorders 3rd edition beta-based field testing of vestibular migraine in China: demographic, clinical characteristics, audiometric findings and diagnosis statues. Cephalalgia 2016;36:240–8.
7. Olesen J. International classification of headache disorders. Lancet Neurol 2018;17:396–7.
8. Whitehead MT, Cardenas AM, Corey AS, et al. ACR appropriateness criteria headache. J Am Coll Radiol 2019;16:S364–77.
9. Schaefer PW, Miller JC, Singhal AB, et al. Headache: when is neurologic imaging indicated? J Am Coll Radiol 2007;4:566–9.
10. Ravishankar K. Which headache to investigate, when, and how? Headache 2016;56:1685–97.
11. Rosenkrantz AB, Hanna TN, Babb JS, et al. Changes in emergency department imaging: perspectives from national patient surveys over two decades. J Am Coll Radiol 2017;14(10):1282–90.
12. Jordan YJ, Lightfoote JB, Jordan JE. Computed tomography imaging in the management of headache in the emergency department: cost efficacy and policy implications. J Natl Med Assoc 2009;101:331–5.

13. Lepage R, Krebs L, Kirkland SW, et al. MP25: the role of advanced imaging in the management of benign headaches in the emergency department: a systematic review. CJEM 2017;19:S73.
14. Williams A, Friedman BW. 134 the yield of non-contrast cranial computed tomography for the detection of intracranial pathology in emergency department patients with headache: a systematic review. Ann Emerg Med 2014;64:S48.
15. Kuruvilla DE, Lipton RB. Appropriate use of neuroimaging in headache. Curr Pain Headache Rep 2015;19:1–7.
16. Rizzoli P, Iuliano S, Weizenbaum E, et al. Headache in patients with pituitary lesions: a longitudinal cohort study. Neurosurgery 2016;78:316–23.
17. Gooch CL, Pracht E, Borenstein AR. The burden of neurological disease in the United States: a summary report and call to action. Ann Neurol 2017;81:479–84.
18. Mafi JN, Edwards ST, Pedersen NP, et al. Trends in the ambulatory management of headache: analysis of NAMCS and NHAMCS data 1999–2010. J Gen Intern Med 2015;30:548–55.
19. Reports C. Many common medical tests and treatments are unnecessary: learn when to say 'whoa!' to your doctor. Consum Rep 2012;77:12–3.
20. Kahn CE Jr, Sanders GD, Lyons EA, et al. Computed tomography for nontraumatic headache: current utilization and cost-effectiveness. Can Assoc Radiol J 1993;44:189–93.
21. Centers for Medicare and Medicaid Services. Priority clinical areas. Available at: https://www.cms.gov/Medicare/Quality-Initiatives-Patient-Assessment-Instruments/Appropriate-Use-Criteria-Program/PCA.html. Accessed August 16, 2021.
22. Eller M, Goadsby PJ. MRI in headache. Expert Rev Neurother 2013;13:263–73.
23. Perry JJ, Stiell IG, Sivilotti ML, et al. Sensitivity of computed tomography performed within six hours of onset of headache for diagnosis of subarachnoid haemorrhage: prospective cohort study. BMJ 2011;343:d4277.
24. Blok KM, Rinkel GJ, Majoie CB, et al. CT within 6 hours of headache onset to rule out subarachnoid hemorrhage in nonacademic hospitals. Neurology 2015;84:1927–32.
25. Backes D, Rinkel GJ, Kemperman H, et al. Time-dependent test characteristics of head computed tomography in patients suspected of nontraumatic subarachnoid hemorrhage. Stroke 2012;43:2115–9.
26. Kocher KE, Meurer WJ, Fazel R, et al. National trends in use of computed tomography in the emergency department. Ann Emerg Med 2011;58:452–62.
27. Shinagare AB, Ip IK, Abbett SK, et al. Inpatient imaging utilization: trends of the past decade. AJR Am J Roentgenol 2014;202:W277–83.
28. Einstein AJ. Medical radiation exposure to the U.S. population: the turning tide. Radiology 2020;295:428–9.
29. Schultz CH, Fairley R, Murphy LS, et al. The risk of cancer from CT scans and other sources of low-dose radiation: a critical appraisal of methodologic quality. Prehosp Disaster Med 2020;35:3–16.
30. Edlow JA, Panagos PD, Godwin SA, et al. Clinical policy: critical issues in the evaluation and management of adult patients presenting to the emergency department with acute headache. J Emerg Nurs 2009;35:e43–71.
31. Mackenzie MJ, Hiranandani R, Wang D, et al. Determinants of computed tomography head scan ordering for patients with low-risk headache in the emergency department. Cureus 2017;9:e1760.
32. Lockhart ML, Bykowski J, Rybicki FJ. Introduction to the JACR appropriateness criteria November 2019 supplement. J Am Coll Radiol 2019;16:S315.

33. Guryildirim M, Kontzialis M, Ozen M, et al. Acute headache in the emergency setting. Radiographics 2019;39:1739–59.
34. Schwedt TJ. Thunderclap headache. Continuum (Minneap Minn) 2015;21: 1058–71.
35. Grasso G, Alafaci C, Macdonald RL. Management of aneurysmal subarachnoid hemorrhage: state of the art and future perspectives. Surg Neurol Int 2017;8:71.
36. Toth G, Cerejo R. Intracranial aneurysms: review of current science and management. Vasc Med 2018;23:276–88.
37. Mark DG, Kene MV, Vinson DR, et al. Outcomes following possible undiagnosed aneurysmal subarachnoid hemorrhage: a contemporary analysis. Acad Emerg Med 2017;24:1451–63.
38. Mills ML, Russo LS, Vines FS, et al. High-yield criteria for urgent cranial computed tomography scans. Ann Emerg Med 1986;15:1167–72.
39. Oh SY, Lim YC, Shim YS, et al. Initial misdiagnosis of aneurysmal subarachnoid hemorrhage: associating factors and its prognosis. Acta Neurochir (Wien) 2018; 160:1105–13.
40. Vannemreddy P, Nanda A, Kelley R, et al. Delayed diagnosis of intracranial aneurysms: confounding factors in clinical presentation and the influence of misdiagnosis on outcome. South Med J 2001;94:1108–11.
41. Connolly ES Jr, Rabinstein AA, Carhuapoma JR, et al. Guidelines for the management of aneurysmal subarachnoid hemorrhage: a guideline for healthcare professionals from the American Heart Association/American Stroke Association. Stroke 2012;43:1711–37.
42. Vermeulen MJ, Schull MJ. Missed diagnosis of subarachnoid hemorrhage in the emergency department. Stroke 2007;38:1216–21.
43. Detsky ME, McDonald DR, Baerlocher MO, et al. Does this patient with headache have a migraine or need neuroimaging? JAMA 2006;296:1274–83.
44. De Luca GC, Bartleson JD. When and how to investigate the patient with headache. Semin Neurol 2010;30:131–44.
45. Kowalski RG, Claassen J, Kreiter KT, et al. Initial misdiagnosis and outcome after subarachnoid hemorrhage. JAMA 2004;291:866–9.
46. Harling DW, Peatfield RC, Van Hille PT, et al. Thunderclap headache: is it migraine? Cephalalgia 1989;9:87–90.
47. Edlow JA, Caplan LR. Avoiding pitfalls in the diagnosis of subarachnoid hemorrhage. N Engl J Med 2000;342:29–36.
48. Policeni B, Corey AS, Burns J, et al. ACR Appropriateness criteria cranial neuropathy. J Am Coll Radiol 2017;14:S406–20.
49. Jayaraman MV, Mayo-Smith WW, Tung GA, et al. Detection of intracranial aneurysms: multi–detector row CT angiography compared with DSA. Radiology 2004;230:510–8.
50. Sahraian S, Beheshtian E, Haj-Mirzaian A, et al. Worst headache of life in a migraineur: marginal value of emergency department CT scanning. J Am Coll Radiol 2019;16:683–90.
51. Evans RW. Migraine mimics. Headache 2015;55:313–22.
52. Kassirer JP. Our stubborn quest for diagnostic certainty. A cause of excessive testing. N Engl J Med 1989;320:1489–91.
53. Evans RW. Negative online patient reviews in headache medicine. Headache 2018;58:1435–41.
54. Norman GR, Eva KW. Diagnostic error and clinical reasoning. Med Educ 2010; 44:94–100.

55. Evans RW, Johnston JC. Migraine and medical malpractice. Headache 2011;51: 434–40.
56. Liberman AL, Gialdini G, Bakradze E, et al. Misdiagnosis of cerebral vein thrombosis in the emergency department. Stroke 2018;49:1504–6.
57. Van Os HJ, Mulder IA, Broersen A, et al. Migraine and cerebrovascular atherosclerosis in patients with ischemic stroke. Stroke 2017;48:1973–5.
58. Milhaud D, Bogousslavsky J, van Melle G, et al. Ischemic stroke and active migraine. Neurology 2001;57:1805–11.
59. Kurth T, Diener HC. Migraine and stroke: perspectives for stroke physicians. Stroke 2012;43:3421–6.
60. Castillo M. Imaging of meningitis. Semin Roentgenol 2004;39:458–64.
61. Kastrup O, Wanke I, Maschke M. Neuroimaging of infections of the central nervous system. Semin Neurol 2008;28:511–22.
62. Tunkel AR, Hasbun R, Bhimraj A, et al. 2017 Infectious Diseases Society of America's clinical practice guidelines for healthcare-associated ventriculitis and meningitis. Clin Infect Dis 2017;64:e34–65.
63. Thompson N, Arulselvam K, Arulselvam K, et al. Technology and TBI: perspectives of persons with TBI and their family caregivers on technology solutions to address health, wellness, and safety concerns. Assist Technol 2019;33:1–12.
64. Taylor CA, Bell JM, Breiding MJ, et al. Traumatic brain injury-related emergency department visits, hospitalizations, and deaths - United States, 2007 and 2013. MMWR Surveill Summ 2017;66:1–16.
65. Lefevre-Dognin C, Cogné M, Perdrieau V, et al. Definition and epidemiology of mild traumatic brain injury. Neurochirurgie 2021;67:218–21.
66. Wintermark M, Sanelli PC, Anzai Y, et al. ACR head injury institute; ACR head injury institute. Imaging evidence and recommendations for traumatic brain injury: conventional neuroimaging techniques. J Am Coll Radiol 2015;12:e1–14.
67. Yamamoto S, Levin HS, Prough DS. Mild, moderate and severe: terminology implications for clinical and experimental traumatic brain injury. Curr Opin Neurol 2018;31:672–80.
68. Kontos AP, Elbin RJ, Lau B, et al. Posttraumatic migraine as a predictor of recovery and cognitive impairment after sport-related concussion. Am J Sports Med 2013;41:1497–504.
69. Holtkamp MD, Grimes J, Ling G. Concussion in the military: an evidence-base review of mTBI in US military personnel focused on posttraumatic headache. Curr Pain Headache Rep 2016;20:37.
70. Marcus DA. Disability and chronic posttraumatic headache. Headache 2003;43: 117–21.
71. Arnold M. Headache classification committee of the international headache society (IHS) the international classification of headache disorders. Cephalalgia 2018;38:1–211.
72. Shih RY, Burns J, Ajam AA, et al. ACR appropriateness criteria head trauma: 2021 update. J Am Coll Radiol 2021;18:S13–36.
73. Undén J, Ingebrigtsen T, Romner B. Scandinavian guidelines for initial management of minimal, mild and moderate head injuries in adults: an evidence and consensus-based update. BMC Med 2013;11:1–4.
74. Rau JC, Dumkrieger GM, Chong CD, et al. Imaging post-traumatic headache. Curr Pain Headache Rep 2018;22:1–9.
75. Jagoda AS, Bazarian JJ, Bruns JJ Jr, et al. Clinical policy: neuroimaging and decision making in adult mild traumatic brain injury in the acute setting. J Emerg Nurs 2009;35:e5–40.

76. George E, Khandelwal A, Potter C, et al. Blunt traumatic vascular injuries of the head and neck in the ED. Emerg Radiol 2019;26(1):75–85. https://doi.org/10.1007/s10140-018-1630-y. Epub 2018 Aug 10. PMID: 30097750.

77. Lenaerts ME. Post-traumatic headache: from classification challenges to biological underpinnings. Cephalalgia 2008;28:12–5.

78. Holle D, Obermann M. The role of neuroimaging in the diagnosis of headache disorders. Ther Adv Neurol Disord 2013;6:369–74.

79. Filler L, Akhter M, Nimlos P. Evaluation and management of the emergency department headache. Semin Neurol 2019;39:20–6.

80. Turner DP, Houle TT. Psychological evaluation of a primary headache patient. Pain Manag 2013;3:19–25.

81. Martin VT. The diagnostic evaluation of secondary headache disorders. Headache 2011;51:346–52.

82. Donohoe CD. The role of the physical examination in the evaluation of headache. Med Clin North Am 2013;97:197–216.

83. Dodick DW. Clinical clues and clinical rules: primary vs secondary headache. ASM 2003;3:S550–5.

84. Do TP, Remmers A, Schytz HW, et al. Red and orange flags for secondary headaches in clinical practice: SNNOOP10 list. Neurology 2019;92:134–44.

85. Suarez JI, Tarr RW, Selman WR. Aneurysmal subarachnoid hemorrhage. N Engl J Med 2006;354:387–96.

86. Friedman DI, Jacobson DM. Diagnostic criteria for idiopathic intracranial hypertension. Neurology 2002;59:1492–5.

87. Friedman DI, Liu GT, Digre KB. Revised diagnostic criteria for the pseudotumor cerebri syndrome in adults and children. Neurology 2013;81:1159–65.

88. Schoenen J, Sándor PS. Headache with focal neurological signs or symptoms: a complicated differential diagnosis. Lancet Neurol 2004;3:237–45.

89. Salmela MB, Mortazavi S, Jagadeesan BD, et al. ACR appropriateness criteria cerebrovascular disease. J Am Coll Radiol 2017;14:S34–61.

90. Vilela P, Rowley HA. Brain ischemia: CT and MRI techniques in acute ischemic stroke. Eur J Radiol 2017;96:162–72.

91. Munich SA, Shakir HJ, Snyder KV. Role of CT perfusion in acute stroke management. Cor et Vasa 2016;58:e215–24.

92. Leigh R, Knutsson L, Zhou J, et al. Imaging the physiological evolution of the ischemic penumbra in acute ischemic stroke. J Cereb Blood Flow Metab 2018;38:1500–16.

93. Jordan JE. Expert panel on neurologic imaging. Headache. AJNR Am J Neuroradiol 2007;28:1824–6.

94. Wolf SJ, Byyny R, Carpenter CR, et al. Clinical policy: critical issues in the evaluation and management of adult patients presenting to the emergency department with acute headache. Ann Emerg Med 2019;74:e41–74.

95. Jordan JE, Wippold FJ II, Cornelius RS, et al. Expert panel on neurologic imaging. ACR appropriateness criteria headache. Reston (VA): American College of Radiology (ACR); 2009.

96. Robbins MS, Farmakidis C, Dayal AK, et al. Acute headache diagnosis in pregnant women: a hospital-based study. Neurology 2015;85:1024–30.

97. Raffaelli B, Neeb L, Israel-Willner H, et al. Brain imaging in pregnant women with acute headache. J Neurol 2018;265:1836–43.

98. Lester MS, Liu BP. Imaging in the evaluation of headache. Med Clin North Am 2013;97:243–65.

99. American College of Radiology. ACR-SPR practice parameter for imaging pregnant or potentially pregnant adolescents and women with ionizing radiation. Available at: https://www.acr.org/-/media/ACR/Files/Practice-Parameters/pregnant-pts.pdf. Accessed August 16, 2021.

100. Kodzwa R. ACR manual on contrast media: 2018 updates. Radiol Technol 2019; 91:97–100.

101. American College of Obstetricians and Gynecologists, Committee on Obstetric Practice. Committee opinion no. 656: guidelines for diagnostic imaging during pregnancy and lactation. Obstet Gynecol 2016;127:e75–80.

102. Patel SJ, Reede DL, Katz DS, et al. Imaging the pregnant patient for nonobstetric conditions: algorithms and radiation dose considerations. Radiographics 2007;27:1705–22.

103. Saltybaeva N, Platon A, Poletti PA, et al. Radiation dose to the fetus from computed tomography of pregnant patients—development and validation of a Web-based tool. Invest Radiol 2020;55:762–8.

104. Tirada N, Dreizin D, Khati NJ, et al. Imaging pregnant and lactating patients. Radiographics 2015;35:1751–65.

105. Tremblay E, Thérasse E, Thomassin-Naggara I, et al. Quality initiatives: guidelines for use of medical imaging during pregnancy and lactation. Radiographics 2012;32:897–911.

106. van Welie N, Portela M, Dreyer K, et al. Iodine contrast prior to or during pregnancy and neonatal thyroid function: a systematic review. Eur J Endocrinol 2021; 184:189–98.

107. Gronseth G, Cruccu G, Alksne J, et al. Practice parameter: the diagnostic evaluation and treatment of trigeminal neuralgia (an evidence-based review): report of the Quality Standards Subcommittee of the American Academy of Neurology and the European Federation of Neurological Societies. Neurology 2008;71: 1183–90.

108. Prakash C, Tanwar N. Trigeminal neuralgia secondary to cerebellopontine angle tumor: a case report and brief overview. Natl J Maxillofac Surg 2019;10:249.

109. Subha M, Arvind M. Role of magnetic resonance imaging in evaluation of trigeminal neuralgia with its anatomical correlation. Biomed Pharmacol J 2019; 12:289–96.

110. Darrow DP, Quinn C, McKinney A, et al. The role of magnetic resonance imaging in diagnosing trigeminal neuralgia. Neurosurgery 2020;67. nyaa447_563.

111. Tai AX, Nayar VV. Update on trigeminal neuralgia. Curr Treat Options Neurol 2019;21:42.

112. Sampaio PG, Maracajá HD, Figueiredo SR, et al. Sociodemographic characteristics of patients with chronic headache. Headache Med 2020;22–4.

113. Yancey JR, Sheridan R, Koren KG. Chronic daily headache: diagnosis and management. Am Fam Physician 2014;89:642–8.

114. Young NP, Elrashidi MY, McKie PM, et al. Neuroimaging utilization and findings in headache outpatients: significance of red and yellow flags. Cephalalgia 2018; 38:1841–8.

115. Forde G, Duarte RA, Rosen N. Managing chronic headache disorders. Med Clin North Am 2016;100:117–41.

116. Choosing wisely. An initiative of the ABIM foundation. Clinician lists. Available at: http://www.choosingwisely.org/clinician-lists/. Accessed August 18, 2021.

117. American College of Radiology. ACR appropriateness criteria Ò radiation dose assessment introduction. Available at: https://www.acr.org/-/media/ACR/Files/

Appropriateness-Criteria/RadiationDoseAssessmentIntro.pdf. Accessed August 18, 2021.

118. Thukral BB. Problems and preferences in pediatric imaging. Indian J Radiol Imaging 2015;25:359.

119. Wrixon AD. New recommendations from the International Commission on Radiological Protection—a review. Phys Med Biol 2008;53:R41.

120. Cohen MD. ALARA, image gently and CT-induced cancer. Pediatr Radiol 2015; 45:465–70.

121. Slovis TL. The ALARA concept in pediatric CT: myth or reality? Radiology 2002; 223:5–6.

122. Jordan DW, Becker MD, Brady S, et al. Validation of adult relative radiation levels using the ACR dose index registry: report of the ACR appropriateness criteria radiation exposure subcommittee. J Am Coll Radiol 2019;16:236–9.

123. Martin CJ. Effective dose: how should it be applied to medical exposures? Br J Radiol 2007;80:639–47.

124. National Cancer Institute. Radiation risks and pediatric computed tomography (CT): a guide for health care providers. Available at: http://www.cancer.gov/cancertopics/causes/radiation-risks-pediatric-CT. Accessed August 18, 2021.

125. Image Gently. The alliance for radiation safety in pediatric imaging. Available at: http://www.imagegently.org/. Accessed August 18, 2021.

126. Slovis TL. Sedation and anesthesia issues in pediatric imaging. Pediatr Radiol 2011;41:514–6.

127. Wilder RT, Flick RP, Sprung J, et al. Early exposure to anesthesia and learning disabilities in a population-based birth cohort. Anesthesiology 2009;110: 796–804.

128. Jaimes C, Murcia DJ, Miguel K, et al. Identification of quality improvement areas in pediatric MRI from analysis of patient safety reports. Pediatr Radiol 2018;48: 66–73.

129. Burstein B, Saint-Martin C. The feasibility of fast MRI to reduce CT radiation exposure with acute traumatic head injuries. Pediatrics 2019;144:e20192387.

130. Loder E, Weizenbaum E, Frishberg B, et al, American Headache Society Choosing Wisely Task Force. Choosing wisely in headache medicine: the American Headache Society's list of five things physicians and patients should question. Headache 2013;53:1651–9.

131. Evans RW, Burch RC, Frishberg BM, et al. Neuroimaging for migraine: the American Headache Society systematic review and evidence-based guideline. Headache 2020;60:318–36.

132. Frishberg BM, Rosenberg JH, Matchar DB, et al. Evidence-based guidelines in the primary care setting: neuroimaging in patients with nonacute headache. St Paul, MN: US Headache Consortium;; 2000. p. 1–25.

133. Sudlow C. US guidelines on neuroimaging in patients with non-acute headache: a commentary. J Neurol Neurosurg Psychiatr 2002;72:ii16–8.

134. Jang YE, Cho EY, Choi HY, et al. Diagnostic neuroimaging in headache patients: a systematic review and meta-analysis. Psychiatry Investig 2019;16:407–17.

Imaging Appearance of Migraine and Tension Type Headache

Abdelkader Mahammedi, MD*, Lily L. Wang, MBBS, MPH,
Achala S. Vagal, MD, MS

KEYWORDS

- Computed tomography • Magnetic resonance imaging • Migraine-type headache
- Neuroimaging • Tension-type headache

KEY POINTS

- Primary headaches, such as migraine-type headache (MTH) and tension-type headache (TTH), are the most prevalent type of headache disorders.
- Neuroimaging is warranted to distinguish primary headaches from secondary causes.
- Neuroimaging is not warranted in patients with migraine and normal findings on neurologic examination.
- However, the recommendations for TTH are still not well-defined.
- Magnetic resonance imaging (MRI) is unrewarding in the evaluation of patients with chronic or recurrent headache and normal neurologic findings, and that neither contrast administration nor repeated MR examinations contributed to diagnosis.

DEFINITION AND EPIDEMIOLOGY

Headache disorders rank third among the worldwide causes of disability, measured in years of life lost to disability.[1] Primary headaches, such as migraine-type headache (MTH) and tension-type headache (TTH), are the most prevalent type of headache disorders. According to the Global Burden of Disease Study 2010 (GBD2010), TTH and migraine were reported as the second (20.1%) and third (14.7%) most prevalent disorders in the world, respectively, (after dental caries first).[2] The global prevalence of TTH is 40% and migraine 10%.[3]

MTH is a common and chronic condition with multifactorial neurovascular etiologies characterized by recurrent paroxysmal attacks of throbbing headache with or without autonomic nervous system dysfunction. According to the International Classification of Headache Disorders, 3rd Edition (ICHD-III beta) criteria,[4] the characteristics of MTH and TTH are well distinct (**Table 1**). In clinical practice, however, MTH and

Department of Radiology, University of Cincinnati Medical Center, 234 Goodman Street, Cincinnati, OH 45219, USA
* Corresponding author.
E-mail address: abdelkm2@gmail.com

Neurol Clin 40 (2022) 491–505
https://doi.org/10.1016/j.ncl.2022.02.002
0733-8619/22/Published by Elsevier Inc.
neurologic.theclinics.com

Abbreviations	
ASL	Arterial Spin Labeling
CSD	cortical spreading depression
DCE	dynamic contrast-enhanced
DSC	dynamic susceptibility-weighted
FLAIR	fluid-attenuated inversion recovery
fMRI	Functional MRI
GM	gray matter
MRS	magnetic resonance spectroscopy
MTH	migraine-type headache
NAA	N-acetylaspartate
rCBF	relative cerebral blood flow
rCBV	relative cerebral blood volume
rMTT	delayed relative mean transit time
rs-fMRI	Resting-state fMRI
SWI	susceptibility weighted images
TOF	time of flight
TTH	tension-type headache
TTP	time-to-peak
WM	white matter
WMH	white matter hyperintensities

TTH can exhibit similar clinical features, respond to similar medications, share identical demographics, have common triggers and psychiatric comorbidities, and even may coexist in the same patient.[5]

PATHOPHYSIOLOGY

The pathophysiological mechanisms of MTH and TTH have been widely debated over the decades. Both types of headaches have been characterized by central sensitization, as revealed in many neurophysiological studies.[6,7] While there is solid evidence supporting the involvement of the trigeminovascular system in the pain phase of MTH, there is no evidence that vascular changes can solely explain the many nonnociceptive symptoms typically experienced during the different stages of MTH.[8,9] However, functional neuroimaging has shed light on the pathophysiology of migraine, from

Table 1
Diagnostic criteria for MTH and TTH according to the International Classification of Headache Disorders, 3rd Edition (ICHD-III beta)

MTH	TTH

• Should last between 4 and 72 h
• At least 2 of the following:
  1 .Unilateral location
  2 .Pulsating pain
  3 .Moderate to severe intensity
  4 .Aggravated by routine physical activity
	Bilateral pain
	Nonpulsatile pain
	Mild-to-moderate in intensity
	Not aggravated by daily activities

At least 1 of the following: 1 .Nausea or vomiting 2 .Photophobia and phonophobia	No Nausea/vomiting Photophobia or phonophobia but not both

Data from Headache Classification Committee of the International Headache Society (IHS). The International Classification of Headache Disorders, 3rd edition (beta version). Cephalalgia. 2013;33(9):629-808. https://doi.org/10.1177/0333102413485658

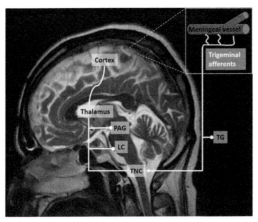

Fig. 1. Migraine headache is caused by the activation of the trigeminovascular system. The trigeminovascular system consists of nociceptive trigeminal sensory afferents surrounding cranial blood vessels. On activation of these perivascular trigeminal afferents, the signal travels through the trigeminal ganglion to neurons in the trigeminocervical complex, using CGRP as the main neurotransmitter. The signals are then relayed to the thalamus; because all nociceptive inputs are integrated through this structure, it has been named the pain matrix of the brain. Modulation of the signal occurs through extensive connections with brainstem regions such as the periaqueductal gray and the locus coeruleus. Symptoms accompanying the headache, such as allodynia, photophobia, and phonophobia, are generated by the sensitization of neurons along the pain pathway, mainly in the trigeminocervical complex and the thalamus. LC, locus coeruleus; PAG, periaqueductal gray; TG, trigeminal ganglion; TNC, trigeminal nucleus caudalis. *From* Ferrari MD, Klever RR, Terwindt GM, Ayata C, van den Maagdenberg AM. Migraine pathophysiology: lessons from mouse models and human genetics. Lancet Neurol. 2015;14(1):65-80. doi:10.1016/S1474-4422(14)70220-0; Reprinted with permission from Elsevier.)

demonstrating that hypoperfusion and cortical spreading depression (CSD) are the underlying mechanisms of visual aura[10] to elucidating the role of the brainstem as a potential "migraine generator."[6] Dodick and colleagues[11] showed that migraine is characterized by multiple phases: premonitory, aura, headache, postdrome, and interictal. The premonitory phase starts as early as 3 days before the headache phase and involves a complex interplay between various cortical and subcortical brain regions, including the hypothalamus and brainstem nuclei that modulate nociceptive signaling. The headache phase involves the activation of the trigeminovascular system that enervates pain-sensitive intracranial structures, a pathway that is well characterized and whereby calcitonin gene-related peptide (CGRP) is the main neurotransmitter involved[12] (**Fig. 1**). Approximately one-third of patients may have an aura phase which is associated with CSD; a slowly propagating wave of extreme depolarization and hyperpolarization of glial and neuronal cell membranes that disrupts ionic gradients leading to glutamate release, which affects cerebral blood flow.[11,12] These regional cerebral blood flow changes usually begin in the occipital cortex and slowly spread in the frontal direction (**Fig. 2**).[12]

Furthermore, neuroimaging findings demonstrated widespread brain structural[13,14] and functional[15,16] alterations in MTH and TTH, suggesting that these 2 entities seem more interrelated than would be indicated by their diagnostic criteria (**Table 2**). On the

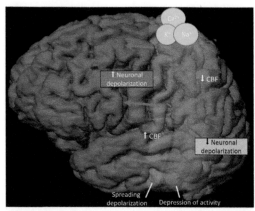

Fig. 2. Migraine aura is caused by cortical spreading depression Cortical spreading depression is regarded as the electrophysiological substrate of migraine aura. In animal models, cortical spreading depression is characterized by a short-lasting, intense wave of neuronal and glial depolarization that spreads slowly over the cortex at a rate of approximately mm/min. The depolarization wave is accompanied by massive transmembrane ion fluxes (eg, Ca^{2+}, Na^+, and K^+) along their concentration gradients, followed by a long-lasting inhibition of spontaneous and evoked neuronal activity. The biphasic electrophysiological changes are associated with an apparent initial increase and longer-lasting decrease in regional cerebral blood flow. Direct evidence that cortical spreading depression underlies migraine aura stems from functional neuroimaging studies in patients displaying similar regional cerebral blood flow changes during aura as those seen in cortical spreading depression in animal experiments. These regional cerebral blood flow changes usually start in the occipital cortex and slowly spread in the frontal direction. CBF, cerebral blood flow. (*From* Ferrari MD, Klever RR, Terwindt GM, Ayata C, van den Maagdenberg AM. Migraine pathophysiology: lessons from mouse models and human genetics. Lancet Neurol. 2015;14(1):65-80. doi:10.1016/S1474-4422(14)70220-0; Reprinted with permission from Elsevier.)

contrary, few recent studies revealed distinct gray matter (GM) volume patterns that distinguish between patients with MTH and TTH,[17] reflecting the differences in the pathophysiologic mechanisms underlying each entity.

ROLE OF NEUROIMAGING IN PRIMARY HEADACHES

Most primary headaches can be evaluated via history and physical examination alone. Neuroimaging is warranted to distinguish primary headaches from secondary causes. Current guidelines such as the ACR Appropriateness Criteria,[18] the American Headache Society (AHS),[19] multispecialty consensus on diagnosis and treatment of headache,[20] and the Headache Consortium guidelines in migraine work-up,[21] provide a precise consensus that neuroimaging is not warranted in patients with migraine and normal findings on neurologic examination.[22] However, the recommendations for TTH are still not well-defined. The prevalence of significant intracranial abnormalities on neuroimaging among patients with migraine and a normal neurologic examination ranges from 0% to 3.1%, and combining this data in a meta-analysis resulted in a prevalence of 0.18%.[23] Although MR imaging is more sensitive than CT in detecting intracranial abnormality, multiple clinical studies showed that even magnetic resonance imaging (MRI) is unrewarding in the evaluation of patients with chronic or

Table 2		
Modality-based neuroimaging findings of migraine and tension-type headache		
		Imaging Characteristics
Structural Neuroimaging	White Matter	• Nonspecific subcortical and deep white matter, scattered small foci of FLAIR hyperintensities • Changes of white matter microstructures in areas such as corpus callosum and cingulate gyrus on DTI
	Gray Matter	• Atrophy of GM in multiple brain areas, with predilection sites for frontal lobe, limbic system, parietal lobe, basal ganglia, brainstem, and cerebellum • Reduced cortical thickness and surface area in regions subserving pain processing and increased cortical thickness and surface area in regions involved in migraine • Both attack frequency and duration are indicators for GM atrophy • High attack frequency associated with reduced GM density in fronto-limbic and parietal regions; and decreased WM density in the frontal lobe • Dynamic alteration of fractional anisotropy noted at thalami, in relation with peri-ictal/ictal status • Long attack duration have reduced frontal anisotropy, and increased WM density in the cerebellum, bilaterally, and reduced GM density of the brainstem and lentiform nucleus
	DWI	• Early increased ADC in the hippocampus, brain stem, thalamus, and amygdala in MTH. • Early increased ADC in the hippocampus and brain stem in TTH
MR Perfusion	DCE-MRI	• Increased BBB permeability in some migraine-associated brain regions • A lower fractional plasma volume (V_p) in the left amygdala
	DSC-MRI and ASL	• Hypoperfusion in 70% of acute migraine aura with delayed rMTT and TTP, decreased rCBF, and minimal decrease in rCBV, >1 vascular territory • Hypoperfusion during the aural phase and hyperperfusion during the headache phase • SWI can detect dilated cortical veins draining regions associated with increased oxygen extraction in the hypoperfused parenchyma
Functional Neuroimaging		• Altered functional connectivity between the pain modulatory system and the limbic system • Greater response to visual stimulation in visual cortex and lateral geniculate nuclei in migraine with aura as compared to healthy controls and migraine without aura • Suggests connection between cortical hyperresponsiveness and migraine aura • Resting-state fMRI has detected altered connectivity during ictal and interictal migraineurs

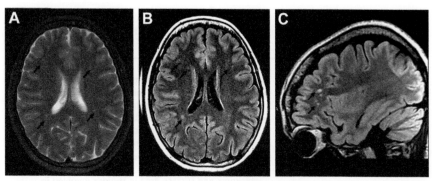

Fig. 3. A 30-year-old female with chronic migraine headache. Few scattered T2 (*arrows* in *A*) and FLAIR (*arrows* in *B* and *C*) hyperintense foci within the subcortical white matter of the bilateral frontal lobes, right greater than left. No abnormal signal on DWI, SWI, and post-contrast images.

recurrent headache and normal neurologic findings, and that neither contrast administration nor repeated MR examinations contributed to diagnosis.[24]

MAGNETIC RESONANCE IMAGING IMAGING
Structural Neuroimaging

White matter
No single imaging examination has yet been able to define or differentiate between primary headache disorders. Multiple studies reported that migraineurs are at increased risk of more diffuse subclinical lesions in the deep white matter or periventricular areas, which demonstrate increased signal on fluid-attenuated inversion recovery (FLAIR) images (**Fig. 3**).[25–29] It was reported that subcortical and periventricular white matter lesions are present in 12% to 48% of migraineurs compared with 2% to 11% of control subjects.[29] However, these lesions remain nonspecific as they can also be associated with cardiovascular risk factors, use of vasoconstrictor (migraine) agents, inflammatory or infectious etiologies. Clinical studies suggested that migraine may be a risk factor for the development of infarct-like lesions, particularly in the territory of the posterior circulation,[28,30] although whether the white matter changes in MTH and/or TTH are true or marker of future vascular infarcts remains debated.[31,32] White matter hyperintensities (WMH) and silent infarct-like abnormalities in migraineurs, have been demonstrated in women with migraine with aura;[33] however, a more recent study has disputed this finding with no association between silent brain infarcts, WMH, and migraine with aura.[34]

Gray matter
Multiple morphologic studies show that patients with migraine have atrophy of GM in brain areas that broadly overlap with the "pain-matrix" which are part of the network subserving supraspinal nociceptive processing.[13,35–38] The concept that long-term exposure to pain might cause a loss of GM volume is supported by the results obtained in a wide variety of other chronic pain conditions, including facial and chronic back pain,[39,40] fibromyalgia,[41] and rheumatoid arthritis.[42] The GM volume changes can correlate with the frequency and duration of the attacks[38] and between ictal and interictal periods.[43]

Studies demonstrate conflicting results in assessing GM cortical thickness in patients with migraine.[44–48] While studies that examined only a few cortical areas[44,45]

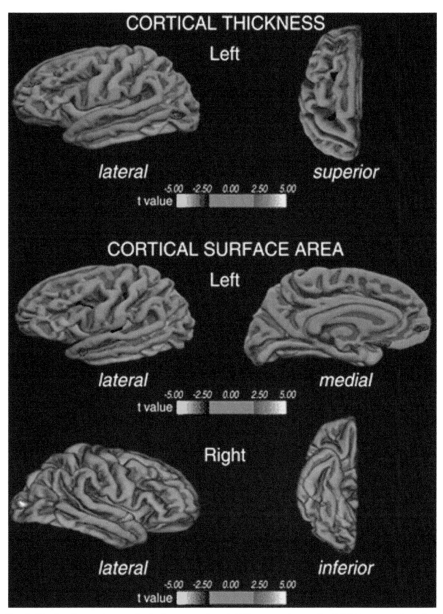

Fig. 4. Vertex-by-vertex analysis shows regional differences in cortical thickness and cortical surface area in patients with migraine compared with healthy control subjects (*P* < .01) represented on an averaged brain map. Regions of increased cortical thickness or surface area are shown in red (color coded according to *t* value), and regions of decreased cortical thickness or surface area are shown in blue (color-coded according to *t* value). Only the most representative views are shown. (*From* Messina R, Rocca MA, Colombo B, et al. Cortical abnormalities in patients with migraine: a surface-based analysis. Radiology. 2013;268(1):170-180. https://doi.org/10.1148/radiol.13122004; with permission)

showed an increased cortical thickness of the primary sensorimotor cortex, another study did not.[48] Another study[46] found concomitant cortical thickness and functional MR imaging differences between patients with migraine and control subjects. Furthermore, a most recent comprehensive study[13] that explored the patterns of both cortical thickness and cortical surface area abnormalities found that compared with control subjects, patients with migraine had a reduced cortical thickness and surface area in regions subserving pain processing and increased cortical thickness and surface area in regions involved in migraine pathogenesis (**Fig. 4**). However, these 2 metrics were related to aura and WMHs ($P < .01$) but not to disease duration and attack frequency.[13] Finally, it is still not clear whether these GM abnormalities are the trigger or the result of migraine attacks.

A decrease in GM volume was also reported in patients with chronic TTH, which involves the anterior cingulate cortex, insula, orbitofrontal cortex, parahippocampal gyrus, and dorsal rostral pons,[49] which were positively correlated with headache duration, and might be the consequence of central sensitization.

MR Perfusion

There are two general methods by which MR perfusion can be performed: bolus techniques and arterial spin labeling (ASL). Bolus perfusion techniques include either dynamic susceptibility-weighted (DSC) or dynamic contrast-enhanced (DCE) MRI. Both bolus techniques derive physiologic information from the assessment of the concentration of gadolinium passing through the tissue microcirculation over time.

ASL is used to assess cerebral blood flow noninvasively without an exogenous contrast agent, but instead uses a radiofrequency pulse to invert the spins of protons in flowing blood prior to their entry into the tissue of interest (eg, while blood is in the neck prior to cerebral perfusion imaging). The inflow of these protons into a given voxel, therefore, results in a reduction in its signal intensity. The labeled image volume can then be subtracted from the dataset obtained using an identical MR sequence performed without the labeling pulse. The result is an image with contrast that is based primarily on tissue perfusion.[50]

a. dynamic susceptibility-weightedmagnetic resonance imaging

Although patients with acute-onset migraine aura can have unremarkable standard MRI examination including DWI, T1-WI, T2-WI, and FLAIR, approximately 70% of these patients will demonstrate hypoperfusion on perfusion-weighted imaging (PWI)

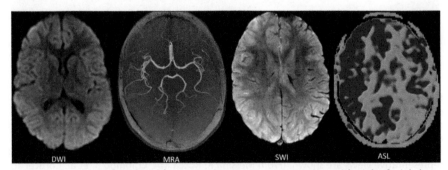

Fig. 5. A 12-year-old female with acute migraine aura presenting with right facial droop and garbled speech. FLAIR (not shown) and DWI images are unremarkable. "Pruning" in the left MCA branches on TOF-MRA without significant stenosis. Asymmetric vascular susceptibility effect in left MCA territory on SWI; indicating slow flow; with associated hypoperfusion on ASL. All findings resolved on follow-up exam (not shown).

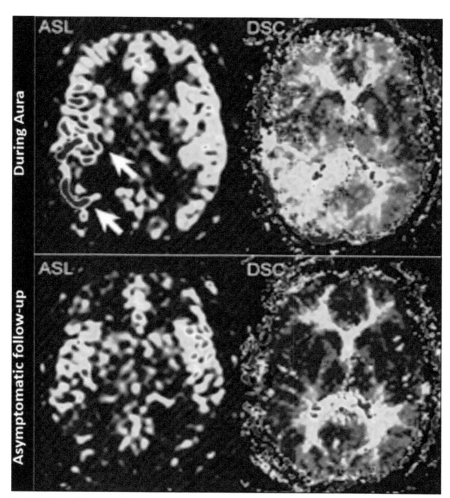

Fig. 6. ASL and DSC perfusion imaging in a 32-year-old woman during migraine aura illustrates a right temporal hyperperfusion and right parietooccipital hypoperfusion (upper row) that normalized on follow-up (bottom row). On the initial ASL imaging, an arterial transit artifact could be identified (*arrows*). (*From* Wolf ME, Okazaki S, Eisele P, et al. Arterial Spin Labeling Cerebral Perfusion Magnetic Resonance Imaging in Migraine Aura: An Observational Study. J Stroke Cerebrovasc Dis. 2018;27(5):1262-1266. https://doi.org/10.1016/j.jstrokecerebrovasdis.2017.12.002; with permission)

with delayed relative mean transit time (rMTT) and time-to-peak (TTP), decreased relative cerebral blood flow (rCBF) and minimal decreased relative cerebral blood volume (rCBV).[51] Unlike ischemic stroke, this hypoperfusion affects more than one arterial territory in a migraine aura, can be bilateral in 20% of cases, have a propensity for the posterior regions, and have negative clinical and imaging follow-up findings.[51] TOF-MRA may reveal regional and distal areas of arterial narrowing in relation to the hypoperfused areas.[52] Furthermore, T2-GRE or SWI may show dilated cortical veins draining these areas of hypoperfusion due to the increased oxygen extraction and relative increase of deoxyhemoglobin in these regions[52,53] (**Fig. 5**). On the other

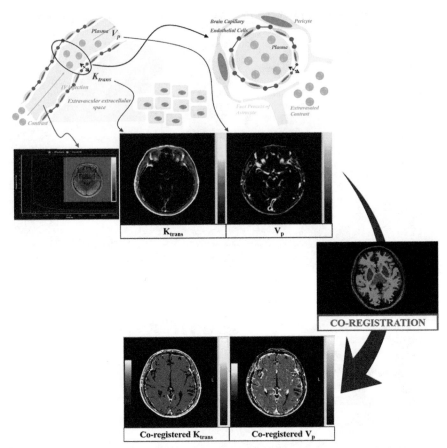

Fig. 7. Flow diagram of the perfusion analysis and co-registration between perfusion maps and region-of-interest masks. A schematic illustrates the measurement of blood–brain barrier (BBB) disruption using dynamic contrast-enhanced (DCE) MRI. The BBB is formed by brain capillary endothelial cells (*pink ovals*) sealed by tight junctions (*red dumbbells*), pericytes (*light blue ovals*), and foot processes of astrocytes (*yellow*). After the administration of low-molecular-weight MRI contrast agent (*green circles*), BBB disruption (*dotted black arrow*) can enable the contrast agent extravasation and its accumulation in the extravascular extracellular space. The volume transfer constant (K^{trans}) represents the rate at which the contrast agent is delivered to the extravascular extracellular space per volume of tissue, and the fractional plasma volume (V_p) represents blood plasma volume per unit volume of tissue. The arterial input function (AIF) graph (*red graph*) and DCE-derived pharmacokinetic parameters (K^{trans} and V_p maps) are automatically extracted; the yellow box in the AIF graph represents a searching box at the level of the middle cerebral artery horizontal segment. After coregistration between K^{trans} and V_p maps, the total volumes of interest of automatically segmented brain region masks were determined. (*From* Kim YS, Kim M, Choi SH, et al. Altered Vascular Permeability in Migraine-associated Brain Regions: Evaluation with Dynamic Contrast-enhanced MRI. Radiology. 2019;292(3):713-720. https://doi.org/10.1148/radiol.2019182566; with permission)

hand, multiple studies reported hyperfusion changes on PWI and ASL in the headache phase of migraine distance to the aural phase[54,55]

b. Arterial spin labeling perfusion
ASL demonstrates similar perfusion changes to DSC MRI, which might reveal insights into the pathophysiology of migraine.[50,55] In a recent study,[55] ASL showed biphasic perfusion changes with areas of hypoperfusion or hyperperfusion during the acute phase and normalized perfusion at follow-up (**Fig. 6**). A case series[54] demonstrated regional cerebral hyperperfusion in 3 of 11 patients during a headache episode that corresponded to previous aura symptoms. Although these pilot studies show intriguing preliminary findings, future larger-scale ASL studies will be interesting for two main reasons. First, ASL is a noninvasive technique, which allows repetitive perfusion imaging during different phases of migraine attacks which enables a better understanding of its spatiotemporal dynamics. Second, ASL can characterize cortical blood flow dynamic in migraine, which allows a better understating of its cortical phenomenon of spreading depression pathophysiology.

c. Dynamic contrast material-enhanced magnetic resonance imaging
DCE MRI can determine the microcirculation permeability and perfusion properties of tissue by using the T1-shortening effect to measure the degree of signal enhancement.[56,57] However, due to the lack of fast imaging techniques[58] and imaging parameter modeling, the measurement of BBB remains challenging, particularly in migraine.[59] Despite these challenges, multiple studies showed that some migraine-associated brain regions might have greater BBB permeability by using DCE MRI, which can suggest the pathophysiologic loci of brain in migraine.[56] Interestingly, in a recent study,[56] migraine suffers were found to have a lower fractional plasma volume (V_p) in the left amygdala compared to healthy participants, in association with increased permeability in the BBB, as depicted on DCE MRI (**Fig. 7**).

Functional Neuroimaging

Functional MRI (fMRI) recordings of the brain as an indirect measure of neuronal activity that reflects changes in regional cerebral blood flow, volume, and oxygenation. There are two types of fMRI studies that can be performed: resting-state and task-based. Resting-state fMRI (rs-fMRI) examines the synchronicity of spontaneous fluctuations in the BOLD signal as a measure of neuronal connectivity without a specific task or stimulus. In task-based fMRI, the subject performs a task while being scanned.[33]

fMRI studies have provided several insights into the pathophysiological mechanisms of migraines. For instance, the pivotal role of both the brainstem and the hippocampus in the first phase of a migraine attack, the involvement of limbic pathway in the constitution of a migrainous pain network, the disrupted functional connectivity in cognitive brain networks, as well as the abnormal function of the visual network in patients with migraine with aura are the main milestones in migraine imaging achieved through advances in fMRI.[16] Interestingly, Martin and colleagues[60] reported that fMRI could show a greater response to visual stimulation within primary visual cortex and lateral geniculate nuclei in migraine aura compared to healthy controls, which suggested a direct connection between cortical hyperresponsiveness and migraine aura.

Furthermore, multiple rs-fMRI studies demonstrated functional changes in some regions of the brain during the interictal and headache phases and have also noted an association between the degree of connectivity and clinical variables, such as headache frequency and duration.[33,61] For example, during the interictal phase, there is increased activation of the visual cortex, primary sensorimotor cortex, superior-anterior middle temporal complex, and perigenual anterior cingulate cortex, with an increased connection between nociceptive areas and the periaqueductal gray.[33] During the headache phase, there is altered connectivity involving the salience network, the somatosensory network, the default mode network, the pons, and the thalamus.[62]

CONCLUSIONS AND FUTURE DIRECTIONS

Despite several guidelines and studies demonstrating a lack of cost-effectiveness, neuroimaging of primary headaches remains a challenging decision for clinicians who continue to image patients with nonfocal migraine. Although the reasons are complex and mainly include the fear of missing a significant lesion and consequent litigation, radiologists and clinicians should remain conversant regarding the value of imaging tests with negative findings because they appear to provide reassurance to patients. While routine neuroimaging in MTH and TTH is frequently low yield for clinically relevant findings, functional imaging and perfusion MR have shown widespread brain structural abnormalities in patients with primary headache.

DISCLOSURE

A. Mahammedi None. L.L. Wang. None. A. Vagal. NIH/NINDS NS103824, NINDS/NIA NS117643, NIH/NINDS NS100417, NIH/NINDS 1U01NS100699, NIH/NINDS U01NS110772, PI, Imaging Core Lab, ENDOLOW Trial, Cerenovus

REFERENCES

1. Steiner TJ, Birbxeck GL, Jensen RH, et al. Headache disorders are third cause of disability worldwide. J Headache Pain 2015;16(1):58.
2. Vos T, Flaxman AD, Naghavi M, et al. Years lived with disability (YLDs) for 1160 sequelae of 289 diseases and injuries 1990–2010: a systematic analysis for the Global Burden of Disease Study 2010. Lancet 2012;380(9859):2163–96.
3. Jordan JE, Flanders AE. Headache and neuroimaging: why we continue to do it. Am J Neuroradiol 2020;41(7):1149–55.
4. The International Classification of Headache Disorders, 3rd edition (beta version). Cephalalgia 2013;33(9):629–808.
5. Vargas BB. Tension-type headache and migraine: two points on a continuum? Curr Pain Headache Rep 2008;12(6):433–6.
6. Lai T-H, Protsenko E, Cheng Y-C, et al. Neural Plasticity in Common Forms of Chronic Headaches. Neural Plast 2015;2015:205985.
7. de Tommaso M, Ambrosini A, Brighina F, et al. Altered processing of sensory stimuli in patients with migraine. Nat Rev Neurol 2014;10(3):144–55.
8. Goadsby PJ, Holland PR, Martins-Oliveira M, et al. Pathophysiology of migraine: a disorder of sensory processing. Physiol Rev 2017;97(2):553–622.
9. Messina R, Filippi M, Goadsby PJ. Recent advances in headache neuroimaging. Curr Opin Neurol 2018;31(4):379–85.
10. Hadjikhani N, Rio MS del, Wu O, et al. Mechanisms of migraine aura revealed by functional MRI in human visual cortex. Proc Natl Acad Sci 2001;98(8):4687–92.
11. Dodick DW. A Phase-by-Phase Review of Migraine Pathophysiology. Headache J Head Face Pain 2018;58(S1):4–16.
12. Ferrari MD, Klever RR, Terwindt GM, et al. Migraine pathophysiology: lessons from mouse models and human genetics. Lancet Neurol 2015;14(1):65–80.

13. Messina R, Rocca MA, Colombo B, et al. Cortical abnormalities in patients with migraine: a surface-based analysis. Radiology 2013;268(1):170–80.
14. Jia Z, Yu S. Grey matter alterations in migraine: a systematic review and meta-analysis. Neuroimage Clin 2017;14:130–40.
15. Chong CD, Schwedt TJ, Hougaard A. Brain functional connectivity in headache disorders: a narrative review of MRI investigations. J Cereb Blood Flow Metab Off J Int Soc Cereb Blood Flow Metab 2019;39(4):650–69.
16. Russo A, Silvestro M, Tedeschi G, et al. Physiopathology of migraine: what have we learned from functional imaging? Curr Neurol Neurosci Rep 2017;17(12):95.
17. Chen W-T, Chou K-H, Lee P-L, et al. Comparison of gray matter volume between migraine and "strict-criteria" tension-type headache. J Headache Pain 2018; 19(1):4.
18. Douglas AC, Wippold FJ, Broderick DF, et al. ACR appropriateness criteria headache. J Am Coll Radiol 2014;11(7):657–67.
19. Evans RW, Burch RC, Frishberg BM, et al. Neuroimaging for Migraine: The American Headache Society Systematic Review and Evidence-Based Guideline. Headache J Head Face Pain 2020;60(2):318–36.
20. Silberstein SD. Practice parameter: Evidence-based guidelines for migraine headache (an evidence-based review): Report of the Quality Standards Subcommittee of the American Academy of Neurology. Neurology 2000;55(6):754–62.
21. Morey SS. Headache Consortium releases guidelines for use of CT or MRI in migraine work-up. Am Fam Physician 2000;62(7):1699–701.
22. Buethe J, Nazarian J, Kalisz K, et al. Neuroimaging wisely. Am J Neuroradiol 2016;37(12):2182–8.
23. Micieli A, Kingston W. An approach to identifying headache patients that require neuroimaging. Front Public Health 2019;7:52.
24. Tsushima Y, Endo K. MR imaging in the evaluation of chronic or recurrent Headache1. Radiology 2005. Available at: https://pubs.rsna.org/doi/abs/10.1148/radiol.2352032121.
25. The Prevalence of cerebral damage varies with migraine type: A MRI Study - Fazekas - 1992 - Headache: The Journal of Head and Face Pain. Available at: https://headachejournal.onlinelibrary.wiley.com/doi/abs/10.1111/j.1526-4610. 1992.hed3206287.x. Accessed June 1992.
26. Pavese N, Canapicchi R, Nuti A, et al. White matter MRI hyperintensities in a hundred and twenty-nine consecutive migraine patients. Cephalalgia 1994;14(5): 342–5.
27. Benedittis GD, Lorenzetti A, Sina C, et al. Magnetic Resonance Imaging in Migraine and Tension-Type Headache. Headache J Head Face Pain 1995; 35(5):264–8.
28. Kruit MC, van Buchem MA, Hofman PAM, et al. Migraine as a risk factor for subclinical brain lesions. JAMA 2004;291(4):427–34.
29. Silberstein SD, Lipton RB, Dalessio DJ. Wolff's headache and other head pain. Oxford University Press; 2001. p. 647.
30. Kruit MC, Launer LJ, Ferrari MD, et al. Infarcts in the posterior circulation territory in migraine. The population-based MRI CAMERA study. Brain 2005;128(9): 2068–77.
31. May A. New insights into headache: an update on functional and structural imaging findings. Nat Rev Neurol 2009;5(4):199–209.
32. Tietjen GE. Stroke and migraine linked by silent lesions. Lancet Neurol 2004; 3(5):267.

33. Ashina S, Bentivegna E, Martelletti P, et al. Structural and functional brain changes in migraine. Pain Ther 2021;10(1):211–23.
34. Gaist D, Garde E, Blaabjerg M, et al. Migraine with aura and risk of silent brain infarcts and white matter hyperintensities: an MRI study. Brain 2016;139(7): 2015–23.
35. Rocca MA, Ceccarelli A, Falini A, et al. Brain gray matter changes in migraine patients with T2-visible lesions. Stroke 2006;37(7):1765–70.
36. Schmidt-Wilcke T, Gänßbauer S, Neuner T, et al. Subtle Grey matter changes between migraine patients and healthy controls. Cephalalgia 2008;28(1):1–4.
37. Schmitz N, Arkink EB, Mulder M, et al. Frontal lobe structure and executive function in migraine patients. Neurosci Lett 2008;440(2):92–6.
38. Schmitz N, Admiraal-Behloul F, Arkink EB, et al. Attack frequency and disease duration as indicators for brain damage in migraine. Headache J Head Face Pain 2008;48(7):1044–55.
39. Schmidt-Wilcke T, Hierlmeier S, Leinisch E. Altered Regional Brain Morphology in Patients With Chronic Facial Pain. Headache J Head Face Pain 2010;50(8): 1278–85.
40. Apkarian AV, Sosa Y, Sonty S, et al. Chronic back pain is associated with decreased prefrontal and thalamic gray matter density. J Neurosci 2004;24(46): 10410–5.
41. Decreased gray matter volumes in the cingulo-frontal cortex... : Psychosomatic Medicine. Available at: https://journals.lww.com/psychosomaticmedicine/Fulltext/2009/06000/Decreased_Gray_Matter_Volumes_in_the.12.aspx.
42. Structural changes of the brain in rheumatoid arthritis - Wartolowska - 2012 - Arthritis & Rheumatism. Available at: https://onlinelibrary.wiley.com/doi/full/10.1002/art.33326. Accessed February 2, 2012.
43. Coppola G, Di Renzo A, Tinelli E, et al. Evidence for brain morphometric changes during the migraine cycle: a magnetic resonance-based morphometry study. Cephalalgia 2015;35(9):783–91.
44. DaSilva AFM, Granziera C, Snyder J, et al. Thickening in the somatosensory cortex of patients with migraine. Neurology 2007;69(21):1990–5.
45. Granziera C, DaSilva AFM, Snyder J, et al. Anatomical alterations of the visual motion processing network in migraine with and without aura. PLoS Med 2006; 3(10):e402.
46. Maleki N, Becerra L, Brawn J, et al. Concurrent functional and structural cortical alterations in migraine. Cephalalgia 2012;32(8):607–20.
47. Jouvent E, Mangin J-F, Hervé D, et al. Cortical folding influences migraine aura symptoms in CADASIL. J Neurol Neurosurg Psychiatry 2012;83(2):213–6.
48. Datta R, Detre JA, Aguirre GK, et al. Absence of changes in cortical thickness in patients with migraine. Cephalalgia 2011;31(14):1452–8. Available at: https://journals.sagepub.com/doi/full/10.1177/0333102411421025.
49. Schmidt-Wilcke T, Leinisch E, Straube A, et al. Gray matter decrease in patients with chronic tension type headache. Neurology 2005;65(9):1483–6.
50. Haller S, Zaharchuk G, Thomas DL, et al. Arterial spin labeling perfusion of the brain: emerging clinical applications. Radiology 2016;281(2):337–56.
51. Floery D, Vosko MR, Fellner FA, et al. Acute-onset migrainous aura mimicking acute stroke: mr perfusion imaging features. Am J Neuroradiol 2012;33(8): 1546–52.
52. Adam G, Ferrier M, Patsoura S, et al. Magnetic resonance imaging of arterial stroke mimics: a pictorial review. Insights Imaging 2018;9(5):815–31.

53. Karaarslan E, Ulus S, Kürtüncü M. Susceptibility-weighted imaging in migraine with aura. Am J Neuroradiol 2011;32(1):E5–7.
54. Pollock JM, Deibler AR, Burdette JH, et al. Migraine associated cerebral hyperperfusion with arterial spin-labeled MR Imaging. Am J Neuroradiol 2008;29(8): 1494–7.
55. Wolf ME, Okazaki S, Eisele P, et al. Arterial spin labeling cerebral perfusion magnetic resonance imaging in migraine aura: an observational study. J Stroke Cerebrovasc Dis 2018;27(5):1262–6.
56. Kim YS, Kim M, Choi SH, et al. Altered vascular permeability in migraine-associated brain regions: evaluation with dynamic contrast-enhanced MRI. Radiology 2019;292(3):713–20.
57. Larsson HBW, Courivaud F, Rostrup E, et al. Measurement of brain perfusion, blood volume, and blood-brain barrier permeability, using dynamic contrast-enhanced T1-weighted MRI at 3 tesla. Magn Reson Med 2009;62(5):1270–81.
58. Quantitative measurement of blood-brain barrier permeability in human using dynamic contrast-enhanced MRI with fast T1 mapping - Taheri - 2011 - Magnetic Resonance in Medicine - Wiley Online Library [Internet]. Available at: https://onlinelibrary.wiley.com/doi/full/10.1002/mrm.22686. Accessed December 13, 2010.
59. Ewing JR, Brown SL, Lu M, et al. Model selection in magnetic resonance imaging measurements of vascular permeability: Gadomer in a 9L Model of Rat Cerebral Tumor. J Cereb Blood Flow Metab 2006;26(3):310–20.
60. Martín H, Río MS del, Silanes CL de, et al. Photoreactivity of the occipital cortex measured by functional magnetic resonance imaging–blood oxygenation level dependent in migraine patients and healthy volunteers: pathophysiological implications. Headache J Head Face Pain 2011;51(10):1520–8.
61. Schwedt TJ, Chiang C-C, Chong CD, et al. Functional MRI of migraine. Lancet Neurol 2015;14(1):81–91.
62. Skorobogatykh K, van Hoogstraten WS, Degan D, et al. Functional connectivity studies in migraine: what have we learned? J Headache Pain 2019;20(1):108.

Imaging of Headache Attributed to Vascular Disorders

Lily L. Wang, MBBS, MPH*, Abdelkader Mahammedi, MD,
Achala S. Vagal, MD, MS

KEYWORDS

- Neuroimaging • Computed tomography • Magnetic resonance imaging
- Digital subtracted angiography • Cerebral angiography • Vascular disease

KEY POINTS

- A myriad of vascular causes of headaches with overlapping clinical and imaging features can confound the diagnosis.
- Careful selection, utilization, and interpretation of imaging findings are crucial in the management of vascular causes of headaches.
- A multidisciplinary team of neurologists, neurosurgeons, and diagnostic and interventional neuroradiologists is critical for the diagnosis and management of patients with cerebral vascular disorders.

INTRODUCTION

This article will focus on imaging pearls and pitfalls of vascular causes of headaches. These include aneurysms, vascular malformations, vasculitides, and cerebral venous thrombosis.

ANEURYSMS AND SUBARACHNOID HEMORRHAGE

The classic ruptured aneurysm presents with sudden onset of "the worst headache of life" and is often associated with photophobia and meningism. Sentinel headaches can occur in patients with unruptured aneurysms due to leaks or fissuring.[1] The majority (90%–85%) of spontaneous SAH are due to ruptured cerebral aneurysms.[2]

For suspected SAH, a noncontrast CT head is the first study of choice, typically accompanied by CTA of the head. CT findings of SAH show hyperdense blood, typically in the basal cisterns, around the circle of Willis (**Fig. 1**). Aneurysms can seem

Department of Radiology, University of Cincinnati, University of Cincinnati Medical Center, 234 Goodman Street, Cincinnati, OH 45219, USA
* Corresponding author.
E-mail address: Lily.wang@uc.edu

Neurol Clin 40 (2022) 507–530
https://doi.org/10.1016/j.ncl.2022.02.004
0733-8619/22/© 2022 Elsevier Inc. All rights reserved.

Abbreviations	
ADC	apparent diffusion coefficient
AVF	arteriovenous fistula
AVM	arteriovenous malformation
CSF	cerebral spinal fluid
CT	computed tomography
CTA	computed tomography angiogram
CTV	computed tomography venography
CVT	cerebral venous thrombosis
DAVFs	dural arteriovenous fistulas
DSA	digital subtracted angiography
DVA	developmental venous anomaly
DWI	diffusion weighted imaging
FLAIR	fluid attenuated inversion recovery
MR	magnetic resonance
MRA	magnetic resonance angiography
MRV	magnetic resonance venography
PACNS	primary angiitis of the central nervous system
PRES	posterior reversible encephalopathy syndrome
RCVS	reversible cerebral vasoconstriction syndrome
SAH	subarachnoid hemorrhage
SWI	susceptibility weighted images
TOF	time-of-flight
WI	weighted image

hyperdense on noncontrast CT (**Fig. 2**). A perimesencephalic pattern, when there is only localized SAH in the interpeduncular fossa, may be due to a nonaneurysmal cause (**Fig. 3**). Susceptibility weighted imaging (SW) on MRI is sensitive to SAH[3] (**Fig. 4**).

Most patients receive a CTA or MRA before a DSA. The advantages and disadvantages of each modality are summarized in **Table 1**. 3D volume-rendered images can be helpful for visualization (see **Figs. 1** and **2**). For smaller aneurysms (<3 mm), studies have shown that DSA has greater sensitivity.[10] In SAH patients with a negative CTA, a DSA can be performed to detect additional pathologic conditions such as vasculitis, aneurysm, AVM, and AVF.[11] A repeat DSA can detect additional small aneurysms if the first DSA is negative.[12] DSA 3D rotational angiography provides more details about the aneurysm with the ability to select the vessel and image at different phases. The

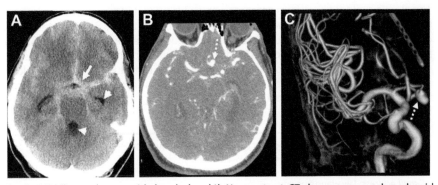

Fig. 1. Middle-aged man with headache. (*A*) Noncontrast CT shows severe subarachnoid hemorrhage in the basilar cisterns (*white arrow*) with moderate hydrocephalus (*arrowheads*). (*B*, *C*) CTA and volume rendered image show a large anterior communicating artery aneurysm (dashed *arrows*).

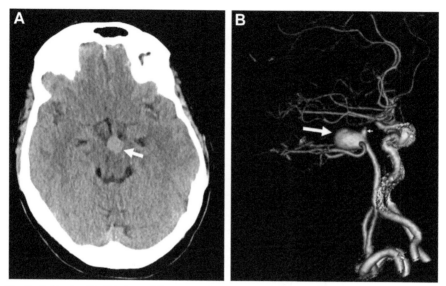

Fig. 2. Patient with third cranial nerve palsy presented with a large basilar aneurysm (*arrows*) which is hyperdense on noncontrast CT (*A*). CTA confirms the aneurysm. 3D volume rendered image shows that it is posterosuperiorly directed with a second outpouching (small *arrow*) (*B*).

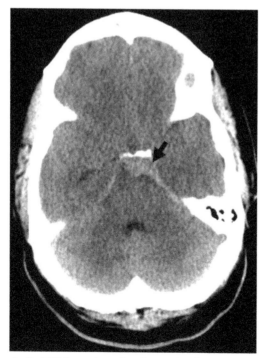

Fig. 3. Perimesencephalic SAH (*arrow*) can be the result of venous (nonaneurysmal) cause. The CTA on this patient was negative for aneurysms.

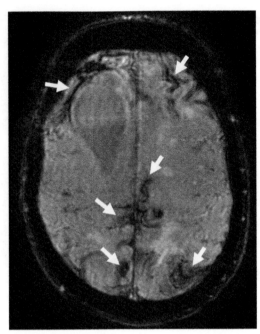

Fig. 4. Superficial siderosis with Indian ink appearance on SWI of the subarachnoid spaces in this patient with cerebral amyloid angiopathy (*arrows*).

arterial side branches arising from the aneurysm sac, neck, and the dimensions are better assessed on DSA, and treatment can be performed concurrently (**Fig. 5**).

The risk factors include autosomal dominant polycystic renal disease, hereditary connect tissue disorders, coarctation of the aorta, systemic lupus erythematosus, or positive family history[13] (**Fig. 6**). However, only a small proportion of unruptured aneurysms are associated with these disorders.[14] MRA is an excellent study of choice in screening patients with suspected aneurysms without rupture (**Fig. 7**). Depending on the type of treatment and preference, a combination of MRA, CTA, and DSA can be used for follow-up postcoiling or clipping.[15]

Anterior circle of Willis accounts for 85% of the intracranial aneurysms.[16] About 20% of patients have multiple aneurysms.[17] Risk factors and predictors of rupture include size, location, history of SAH, and morphologic characteristics. Unruptured aneurysms are more common in women and the elderly.[18,19] Aneurysms can also cause symptoms by compression of cranial nerves in the cavernous sinus or oculomotor nerve compression from a large posterior communicating artery or basilar artery aneurysms (see **Fig. 2**).

Complications of SAH such as hydrocephalus and vasospasm are imaged on CT and CTA. Vasospasm peaks 4–12 days after rupture and cause ischemia and occurs in about one-third of SAH patients. CT may show multiple areas of infarction (**Fig. 8**). CTA may show multiple vessels with irregularity and narrowing (**Fig. 9**). DSA is the gold standard. Early intra-arterial treatment of vasospasm can improve the outcome.[20]

VASCULIDES
Reversible Cerebral Vasoconstriction Syndrome

Reversible cerebral vasoconstriction syndrome (RCVS) is an excellent mimic of aneurysmal SAH in presentation (thunderclap headache). About 70% of RCVS patients

Table 1	
Vascular imaging in SAH and aneurysm	
CTA	
Advantages	Disadvantages
• Fast	• Radiation
• Readily available	• Iodinated contrast required
• Well tolerated	• Metallic artifact from coils/clips can
• Noninvasive	obscure recurrence
• Excellent sensitivity and specificity.	• Decreased sensitivity around bone
About 90%–100% sensitivity for	• Less sensitive for small (<3 mm) aneurysms
detecting aneurysms >4 m.[4–6,11]	
• Study of choice for initial acute	
diagnosis, follow up of known	
untreated aneurysms	
MRA	
Advantages	Disadvantages
• No radiation	• Lower availability than CT, especially in
• No contrast agent required, except	the acute setting
when there is prior coiling,	• Length of study (typical study ~30 min)
gadolinium may increase the sensitivity[7]	• Prone to artifacts such as motion, flow,
• Noninvasive	metal and blood
• Provides best details of the brain	• Contraindications to MRI (pacemaker,
and can help rule out other causes	implants, claustrophobia, and so forth)
of headaches	• False positives are more common than CTA[9]
• The pooled sensitivity of MRA was	
95% and specificity was 89% in a	
meta-analysis[8]	
• Study of choice for screening, follow	
of a known unruptured aneurysm	
and post-treatment follow up	
DSA	
Advantages	Disadvantages
• Best spatial resolution	• Radiation
• Best temporal resolution	• (Minimally) invasive
• Best sensitivity for small aneurysms	• Risk of stroke
• Able to select vessel individually	• Iodinated contrast required
• Treatment planning	• Needs technical expertise

have a precipitating factor such as cannabis, antidepressants, nasal decongestants, postpartum, alcohol, steroids, epinephrine, strenuous sexual activity, and direct vessel injury.[21]

On CT, a small volume of SAH is typically identified at the convexity, with no evidence of aneurysm (**Fig. 10**). Lobar hemorrhage, watershed infarcts, and vasogenic edema can be seen on CT and MRI.[22] The imaging spectrum of RCVS is summarized in **Table 2**.[22] It is important to note that cerebral vasoconstriction may not be visualized in up to one-third of patients with RCVS during the first week following symptom onset, making the diagnosis challenging.[23] Longitudinal monitoring of RCVS can be performed with MRA, CTA, and DSA, in the order of increasing sensitivity.[24] RCVS is usually self-limiting. The resolution of symptoms and imaging abnormalities usually occur by 3 months.

Reversible Cerebral Vasoconstriction Syndrome and Aneurysmal SAH Imaging

In the presence of SAH and vasoconstriction, it can be difficult to distinguish RCVS and aneurysmal SAH. The most obvious difference is if an aneurysm can be identified

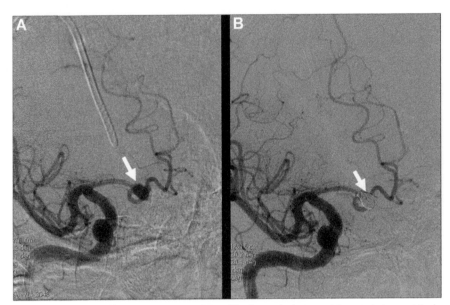

Fig. 5. DSA in a patient with SAH complicated hydrocephalus requiring an intraventricular shunt catheter due to ruptured anterior communicating artery aneurysm before (*A*) and after coiling (*B*) (*arrows*).

on angiogram. SAH from aneurysm is more common in the basal cisterns, whereas RCVS tends to cause focal superficial sulcal SAH.[22] The presence of increased intracranial pressure and hydrocephalus is more common in aneurysmal SAH. In RCVS, the vasoconstriction involves distal second and third order branches and tends to develop in the first week of symptom onset, whereas in aneurysmal SAH, the narrowing is smooth and long segment of proximal arteries and peaks between day 4 and

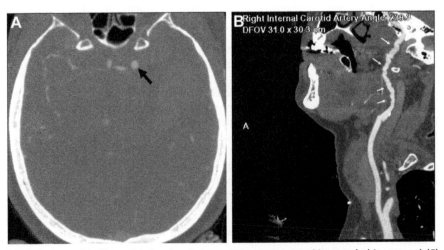

Fig. 6. Patient with fibromuscular dysplasia on CTA reconstructed images (*white arrows*) (*B*) and a ruptured internal carotid artery aneurysm (*black arrow*) on CTA (*A*).

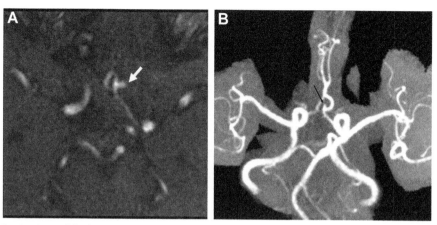

Fig. 7. Time-of-flight MRA (*A*) and maximum intensity projection (*B*) in an asymptomatic patient shows a 3 mm anterior communicating artery aneurysm involving the origin of left A2 segment.

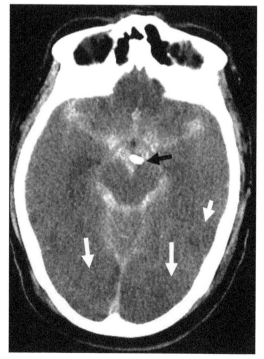

Fig. 8. Middle-aged woman with ruptured aneurysm, SAH, complicated by hydrocephalus, which was shunted (*black arrow*), and multiple infarctions in different vascular territories (*white arrows*) from vasospasm.

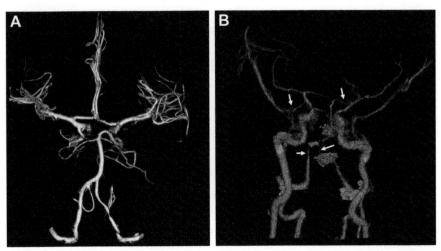

Fig. 9. Young man with vasospasm due to head trauma with subdural and subarachnoid hemorrhage on presentation. The CTA was normal 1 week prior (A). (B) Multiple vessels are attenuated and irregular one week later. The vertebral arteries, MCA, ACA, and PCA branches are all involved (*arrows*).

14.[22] Vasospasm due to aneurysmal SAH typically involves longer segments of proximal vessels and RCVS is more peripheral.[22]

Vasculitis

Vasculitis is an inflammatory disease of the blood vessel walls and can affect vessels of different sizes. The clinical presentation, such as headache, confusion, paresis,

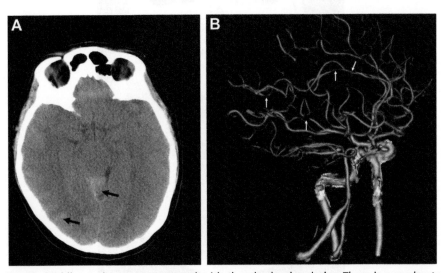

Fig. 10. Middle-aged woman presented with thunderclap headache. There is a moderate subarachnoid hemorrhage in the quadrigeminal cistern and cerebral convexity (*black arrows*) (A). The CTA 3D volume rendered image (B) shows multifocal narrowing of anterior and middle cerebral artery branches (*white arrows*). The vascular findings resolved on follow up cerebral angiogram in a few weeks.

Table 2
Imaging findings of reversible cerebral vasoconstriction syndrome and roles of imaging

CT	SAH in the cerebral convexity (nonaneurysmal pattern) Watershed infarcts Lobar hemorrhage
MR	SWI: SAH. Lobar hemorrhage T2/FLAIR: SAH, cerebral edema, hyperintense vessels along cerebral sulci DWI: watershed infarcts Vessel wall imaging: vessel wall rarely enhance Help to exclude other causes such as PRES, vasculitis, and CVT
CTA, MRA	Vasoconstriction involving multiple vascular territories with multifocal areas of beaded narrowing interspersed with normal-caliber segments Distal second and third order branches Disproportionate degree and extent of vasoconstriction relative to the amount of SAH Help to exclude atherosclerotic disease, aneurysm, and dissection
DSA	Vasoconstriction Deliver treatment with vasodilator or balloon angioplasty Reversibility following intra-arterial vasodilator Vasospasm due to SAH typically involves longer segments of proximal vessels and RCVS is more peripheral
MR and CT perfusion imaging	Multifocal areas of hypoperfusion, often include cerebral watershed zones[22] Monitor and follow treatment response
Transcranial Doppler sonography	Vasoconstriction

cranial nerve involvement, or loss of consciousness, may be nonspecific. The patients typically have a slower progressive insidious headache presentation compared with RCVS. CSF markers typically demonstrated increased CSF protein levels and white cells, not typically seen with RCVS.

CNS vasculitis may be secondary to a systemic vasculitis or primary cause. Primary angiitis of the central nervous system (PACNS) can have similar clinical and imaging findings as RCVS. Secondary vasculitis includes giant cell arteritis, polyarteritis nodosa, Kawasaki disease, IgA arteritis, microscopic polyangiitis, Behcet disease, systemic lupus erythematosus, rheumatoid arthritis, Sjogren syndrome, scleroderma, and drug-induced, radiation-induced, or infectious etiologies. Infectious vasculitis can result from tuberculosis, syphilis, Varicella-Zoster, HIV, and fungal infections.

CT and MR may show multifocal bilateral infarcts of varying ages, microhemorrhages, parenchyma hemorrhagic, and SAH. Postcontrast MRI may show leptomeningeal enhancement, enhancing infarcts, and vessel wall imaging may show thickening and enhancement of the vessel wall affecting large brain arteries[25] (**Fig. 11**). Vascular imaging can show multifocal narrowing and irregularity of mid-to-distal arteries and occlusion of vessels (see **Fig. 11**). Some features such as eccentric narrowing, abrupt vessel occlusion, and no response to intra-arterial vasodilator therapy are more suggestive of PACNS.[24,26] This is a challenging diagnosis. For small vessel vasculitis, MRA has a limited resolution, and CTA does not visualize small

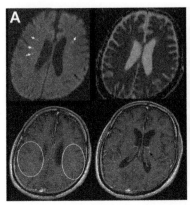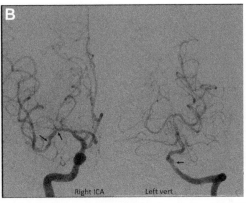

Fig. 11. Middle-aged man presented with headache and dizziness for 3 months. (*A*) MRI shows multiple subacute infarcts in the corona radiata on DWI and ACD map (*white arrows*), multiple enhancing medullary vessels (*circles*), and an enhancing subacute infarct in the left thalamus. (*B*) DSA shows multifocal eccentric stenosis in the right MCA and left vertebral artery (*arrows*). He had no systemic findings of vasculitis. Biopsy showed PACNS.

vessels well. DSA, despite being the most sensitive technique for detecting vasculitis vessel narrowing, has a sensitivity of only 20%–64%.[26] Biopsy of the vessel or brain may be necessary for diagnosis, although biopsy also may be negative. Immunosuppressive therapy is the mainstay of treatment.

Reversible cerebral vasoconstriction syndrome and vasculitis on imaging

Distinguishing RCVS and PACNS clinically and radiographically is challenging. Brain CT/MRI is abnormal in vasculitis patients, whereas only one-third of RCVS patients have imaging abnormalities on presentation. Acute ischemic stroke and infarcts of varying ages are more common with vasculitis than RCVS.[21,22] SAH and vasogenic edema is more common in RCVS. Multiple small deep infarcts, extensive deep white matter lesions, and contrast enhancement are only present in vasculitis. Vasospasm in vasculitis is more likely to be eccentric and abrupt.[22] Reversibility of vasospasm following vasodilator on DSA is seen with RCVS, which is a useful distinguishing feature.[22] Cervical artery dissection can be seen with RCVS but not vasculitis. Both entities can have arterial wall thickening on MR vessel wall imaging, and wall enhancement was present only in cases of CNS vasculitis in one study, but the utility is debated.[27,28]

Posterior Reversible Encephalopathy Syndrome

PRES manifests with headache, seizures, altered mental status, encephalopathy, vomiting, and visual disturbance.[29,30] There are many associations such as hypertension, eclampsia, organ transplantation, autoimmune disease, renal disease, immunosuppressive drugs, and viral infections (eg, HIV and COVID-19). The postulated etiologies include disturbance of cerebral vasculature autoregulation and systemic inflammatory state causing endothelial dysfunction.[31]

CT shows symmetric vasogenic edema in the parietal and occipital lobes (98%), followed by the frontal lobes and the cerebellum[32] (**Fig. 12**). MRI shows a pattern involving the watershed zones (see **Fig. 12**). Restricted diffusion and hemorrhage may be present in these areas, raising the differential diagnosis of posterior circulation ischemia.[32] There are also less common patterns associated with parenchymal

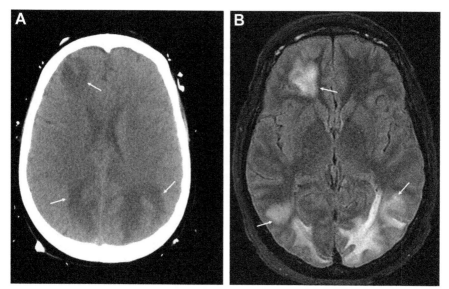

Fig. 12. Young woman presents with headache posthepatectomy and chemotherapy for metastatic adenocarcinoma of the liver on non-contrast CT (*A*) and FLAIR MRI (*B*).

hemorrhage, SAH, and hematomas, best seen on the SWI sequence on MRI.[31–33] In a large series, three major patterns of PRES were observed: the holohemispheric watershed (23%), superior frontal sulcal (27%), and dominant parietal-occipital (22%), with additional common partial or asymmetric expression of these primary PRES patterns (28%).[32] Brainstem involvement, hemorrhage, and a large amount of edema confer a poor prognosis.[28] PRES is usually self-limiting following treatment or removal of the potential causes.

Reversible cerebral vasoconstriction syndrome and PRES on imaging

RCVS and PRES have overlapping clinical and imaging features such as white matter signal abnormality, hemorrhage, and vasoconstriction, suggestive of a shared pathophysiologic pathway. As discussed above, it is common for PRES to be symmetric, involving parietal-occipital and watershed regions.[32] However, about 10% of RCVS patients is observed with symmetric signal abnormality at the cerebral convexity.[34] Ischemia, SAH, intracranial hemorrhage, and vasoconstriction are much more common in RCVS.[35] Hemorrhage in PRES is more likely to be punctate. Enhancement in PRES can be leptomeningeal and gyriform. PRES can show rapid reversibility on imaging.

VASCULAR MALFORMATIONS

Cerebral vascular malformations encompass many different pathologic entities. Distinguishing different types of cerebral vascular malformations is vital because their treatment and prognosis differ.

Arteriovenous Malformations

Brain AVMs are congenital abnormal high-flow connections between arteries (pial vessels) and normal veins that drain the brain. Although congenital, the presentation is typically in young adulthood due to hemorrhage.[36] Supratentorial location accounts for 85% of AVMs. When ruptured, SAH and parenchymal hemorrhage can result. CT and CTA are the examinations of choice for the first acute presentation suspected AVM. An uncomplicated AVM may be occult on noncontrast CT as the nidus has the same density as the brain parenchyma (**Fig. 13**). The nidus refers to the tangle of vessels, consisting of shunting arterioles and interconnected venous loops in the brain parenchyma (see **Fig. 13**). Early venous drainage is a diagnostic criterion. Other imaging characteristics pertinent to the diagnosis and treatment include feeding arteries and draining veins, which are usually enlarged (see **Fig. 13**). Venous aneurysms and dystrophic calcification may be present. DSA provides more spatial and temporal information, although dynamic MRA and dynamic CTA are being used increasingly. When multiple AVMs are present (2% of all AVMs), hereditary hemorrhagic telangiectasia and craniofacial AV metameric syndrome should be considered. The

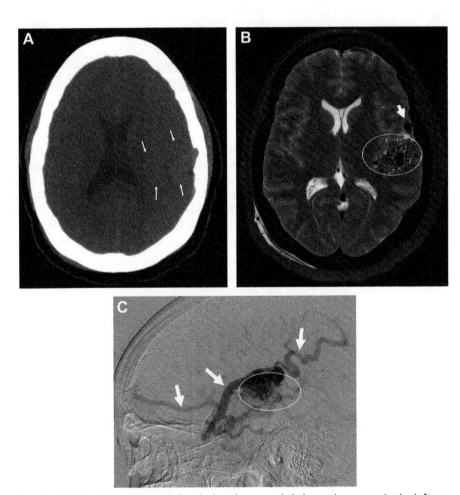

Fig. 13. (A) CT in this patient with headaches shows a subtle hyperdense area in the left posterior frontal lobe (small *arrows*). (B) MRI shows flow voids in the nidus in this location (*circle*) and a large draining vein (*arrow*), consistent with an AVM. (C) There are multiple enlarged draining veins (*arrows*) on the DSA. The nidus (*circle*) fills in early in the arterial phase and remains enhancing in the early venous phase.

Spetzler-Martin AVM grading system commonly used to assess risk–higher points confers a higher risk of hemorrhage and surgery.[37] Large lesions can recruit transdural arteries, which can supply the normal brain, resulting in an arterial steal phenomenon.

Arteriovenous Fistula

An AVF consists of a feeding artery directly connected to draining meningeal or cortical veins or dural venous sinuses, without an intervening nidus. Migraine-like headache was the major onset symptom of dural arteriovenous fistulas, whereas ocular symptoms and nonmigraine-like headaches were a typical characteristic of carotid-cavernous fistulas[38] (**Fig. 14**). The most common locations are transverse, sigmoid, and cavernous sinuses. DAVFs are associated with dural sinus thrombosis, venous hypertension, previous craniotomy, and trauma.[39] A noncontrast CT is typically unremarkable. MRI features include dilated vessels, venous pouches, enhancement, and signs of venous hypertension[39] (**Figs. 15** and **16**). Low-flow lesions may have only subtle findings. If there are suspicious findings on MR, a CTA or MRA could be performed. DSA remains the gold standard, and it can give the best details about vascular supply and drainage and is essential for endovascular treatment planning. Other treatment options include radiation and surgery. Borden[40] and Cognard[41] classification systems are used to determine the risk of hemorrhage. The presence of cortical venous drainage confers a higher risk of hemorrhage.[39]

Cavernous Malformations

Cavernous malformations, the most common cerebral vascular malformations in adults are low-flow vascular malformations with hyalinized dilated thin-walled capillary. These bleed chronically, usually a small amount each episode, which can cause headaches. The incidence of hemorrhage is 1%–3%, with rebleeding risk of 4%–23% per year.[42] Seizures are common due to irritation of the hemosiderin. Cavernous

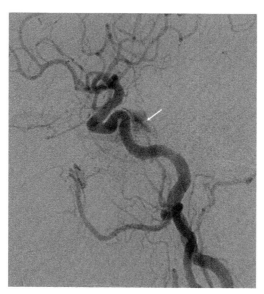

Fig. 14. In this arterial phase injection of the common carotid artery in a patient with headache and eye pain, there is early venous filling of the cavernous sinus (*arrow*), consistent with a carotid-cavernous fistula.

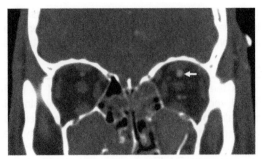

Fig. 15. Dilated superior ophthalmic vein (*arrow*) in a patient with carotid-cavernous fistula.

malformations may be invisible on noncontrast CT, especially when small. Hemorrhage and edema can be seen when acutely bled. Chronic cavernous malformations may seem as a calcified mass (**Fig. 17**). MRI SWI is the most sensitive sequence with blooming of the lesions. They seem as T1 and T2 heterogeneous (popcorn) due to various ages of blood products from insidious bleeding. A T2 hypointense rim is often seen. Multiple cavernous malformations can be familial (see **Fig. 17**). They do not typically enhance, but contrast injection can help to diagnose DVAs, which supports the diagnosis (see **Fig. 17**). Symptomatic lesions causing hemorrhage, mass effect, or seizures can be surgically resected.

Developmental Venous Anomaly

Developmental venous anomalies are common asymptomatic incidental findings on neuroimaging, particularly MRIs, with an incidence 2%–6%.[43,44] About 5% of DVAs are associated with cavernous malformations, and ~10% of cavernous malformations are associated with DVAs.[44,45] DVAs consist of radial clusters of dilated

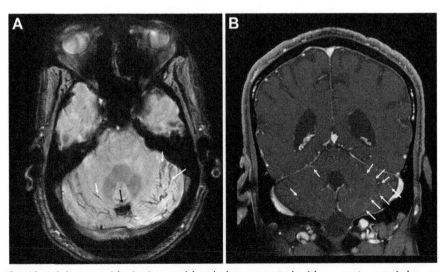

Fig. 16. Adult man with tinnitus and headaches presented with an acute vermis hemorrhage (*black arrow*) on SWI (*A*). Multiple prominent tentorial veins (*white arrrows*) which enhance post contrast (*B*) consistent with an ateriovenous fistula.

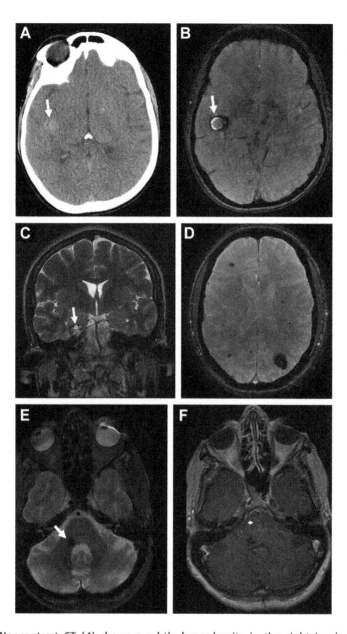

Fig. 17. 'Noncontrast CT (*A*) shows a subtle hyperdensity in the right insula and MRI SWI (*B*) shows susceptibility artifact and blooming, consistent with a cavernous malformation. Different patient with refractory seizures show typical popcorn appearance on T2-weight sequence (*C*). Multiple susceptibility artifacts on SWI in a patient with familial cavernous malformations (*D*). Cavernous malformation (big *arrow*) on T2-weight sequence (*E*) with a small developmental venous anomaly (small *arrow*) in the pons (*F*).

centripetally draining medullary veins that drain into a central vein ("caput medusa," "tree root"). It drains normal brain parenchyma. Rare complications such as hemorrhage and venous infarction can occur with the obstruction of the venous outflow[46,47] (**Fig. 25**). The presenting symptoms include headaches, neurologic deficits, and seizures.[48] MRI is sensitive for small DVAs. Thrombosed veins may show more blooming than normal veins. The filling defects are best seen on CTV and postcontrast MRI T1 sequence (see **Fig. 25**). MRV is not generally as helpful.

CEREBRAL VENOUS THROMBOSIS

Cerebral venous thrombosis is an uncommon but potentially treatable condition in which prompt diagnosis is crucial. It is more common in women, given the associated risk factors (**Box 1**).[49,50] Presenting symptoms are nonspecific, including headache, seizures, change in level of consciousness, and focal neurologic deficits.[50]

Dural Venous Sinus Thrombosis

Diagnosis of dural venous sinus thrombosis on noncontrast CT can be subtle. An acute thrombus may seem hyperdense but only present in 20% of cases[50] (**Fig. 18**). A venous infarct or hemorrhage can occur in one-third of cases of CVT[50] (**Fig. 19**). The location of the hemorrhage in suspicious locations (parasagittal superior frontal/parietal lobe, and posterior temporal/temporal lobe) warrant further investigation with venography in nonhypertensive young patients.

CT venogram (CTV) and MR venogram (MRV) are the imaging modalities of choice. CTV is fast, readily available, and well tolerated. It has excellent spatial resolution and, at least, equivalent accuracy for the detection.[51] The classic "empty delta" sign, seen in about one-third of cases, is due to enhancing dural collateral venous channels and cavernous spaces within the dural envelope44 (see **Fig. 18**). Contrast MRV is superior and complementary to TOF MRV for cerebral and venous sinus thrombosis[52] (**Fig. 20**). In pregnancy and renal failure, TOF MRA without contrast is the preferred modality. TOF MRV, similar to TOF MRA, is prone to artifacts. On TOF, the signal is best when perpendicular to the flow in the sinus. It is typically performed in at least two planes due to the anatomy of the dural venous sinuses. Flow gaps, turbulence, and slow flow are imaging pitfalls as they can cause loss of flow signal.[53] Additionally, it is important to recognize anatomic variations. For example, 60% of people have a larger right transverse sinus.[54]

The thrombus can manifest on MRI as loss of flow void in the sinus, best seen on T2-WI (see **Figs. 19, 20** and **21**). T1 hyper CTV and contrast MRV show filling defects in the sinuses.[55] The signal in the thrombus on T1 and T2 depends on the age of the thrombus.[50] If the thrombus is acute and has T1 hyperintense signal, it can be mistaken as normal sinus enhancement on postcontrast T1 (**Fig. 21**). On TOF MRV, the T1 hyperintense signal can also mimic the bright flow signal. Therefore, it is important to correlate with the postcontrast MRV, where the thrombus will seem as a filling defect.[53] With anticoagulation and time, the thrombus can resolve with recanalization and collateral vessels formation. In extensive thrombosis, chronic thrombosis can result in narrowed or obliterated sinus,[50] and chronic thrombi can have varying signals.

Cavernous Sinus Thrombosis

Although considered a subtype of dural venous sinus thrombosis, the cause of cavernous sinus thrombosis is associated with paranasal sinus infection (**Fig. 22**).

Box 1
Risk factors for cerebral venous thrombosis

Local factors
- Trauma
- CNS neoplasm
- Infections
- Intracranial hypertension

Systemic factors
- Pregnancy and peripartum state
- Hypercoagulable state
  ○ Anemia
  ○ Malignancy
  ○ Oral contraceptive use
  ○ Dehydration

The diagnosis may be challenging on CT and MRI as the cavernous sinus typically enhances heterogeneous ("the caverns" fill at different time points). There is a positive mass effect with a convex margin, and the thrombus may involve the superior ophthalmic vein (see **Fig. 22**).

Deep Venous Thrombosis

Internal cerebral vein, straight sinus, and vein of Galen thrombosis is present in 16% of CVT cases[50] (**Fig. 23**). Symmetric thalamic edema with or without hemorrhage can be seen on both CT and MRI. The mortality is high, but about half of the patients have no neurologic sequelae.[56]

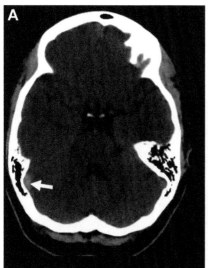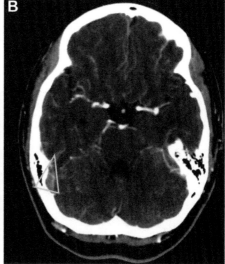

Fig. 18. Young woman with headache. (*A*) CT shows a hyperdense thrombus in the right transverse sinus (*arrow*). (*B*) CTV shows an empty delta sign, with the central nonenhancing thrombus surrounded by the enhancing venous collaterals.

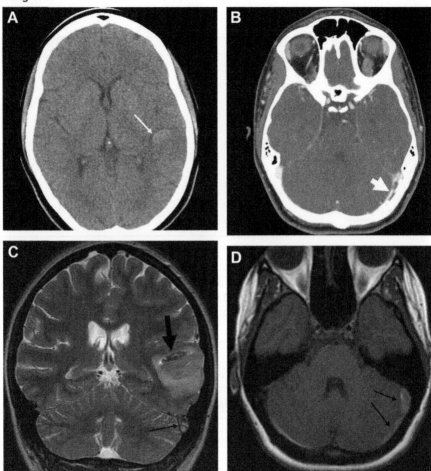

Fig. 19. Young woman presented with headache and altered mental status. (*A*) Noncontrast CT shows hyperdense hemorrhage in the left posterior temporal lobe (thin *white arrow*). (*B*) CTV shows filling defects in the left transverse sinus (big *white arrow*). (*C, D*) MRI shows hemorrhage surrounded by edema (large *black arrow*) loss of flow void on T2WI and T1 hyperintense thrombus in the left transverse sinus (thin *black arrows*).

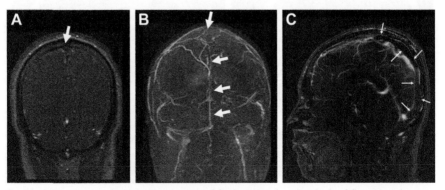

Fig. 20. Sagittal sinus thrombosis on time-of-flight MRV showing lack of flow signal on coronal TOF MRV (*A*) and 3D rotation (*B*) (*arrows*). On the postcontrast 3D MRV (*C*), there is large filling defect (*thin arrows*) throughout the superior sagittal sinus.

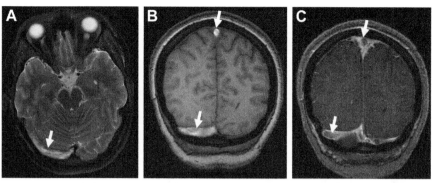

Fig. 21. Young woman with headache. The thrombus in the right transverse sinus is T2 hyperintense, with loss of flow void (*A*); T1 hyperintense (*B*) and seems heterogeneous on postcontrast T1 (*C*). The T1 hyperintensity of the thrombus can mimic enhancement.

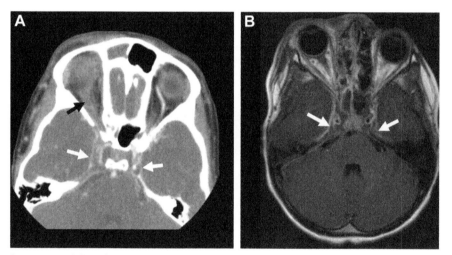

Fig. 22. CTV (*A*) and postcontrast MR (*B*) showing cavernous sinus thrombosis (*white arrows*) in a teenager with sinusitis. There is enlargement and no opacification of the right superior ophthalmic vein (*black arrow*) and the cavernous sinuses (*black arrows*) on CT and MRI.

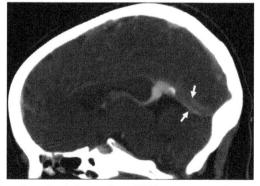

Fig. 23. Straight sinus thrombosis (*arrows*) on CTV in a young patient on oral contraceptive pill.

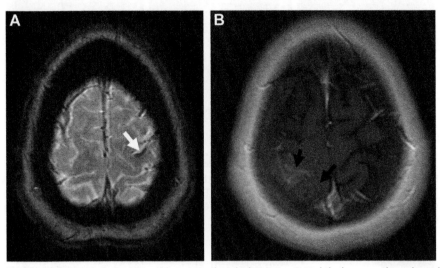

Fig. 24. Middle-aged woman with a new headache type. SWI (*A*) shows a thrombosed cortical vein with susceptibility artifact (*white arrow*). Postcontrast T1-weighted imaging (*B*) on a different patient shows a filling defect thrombus in cortical vein (*black arrow*) and pial enhancement.

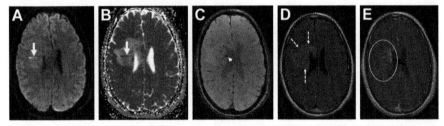

Fig. 25. Young man with headache and stroke-like symptoms. There is a large DVA in the right frontal lobe on SWI (*C*) (*arrowhead*), with a large amount of surrounding edema on FLAIR (*dahsed arrows*) (*D*). DWI (*A*) and ADC map (*B*) show linear restricted diffusion in one of the veins (*white arrows*). There is a filling defect postcontrast (*black arrow*) (*E*).

Cortical Vein Thrombosis

Isolated cortical vein thrombosis without dural venous sinus thrombosis is rare. It is a difficult imaging diagnosis as venous anatomy is variable between patients and not symmetric. A thrombosed vein can be hyperdense (cord sign) on CT. On MRI SWI, it shows more blooming than the other normal veins, which also have a dark signal normally (**Fig. 24**). Abnormal pial enhancement, edema, ischemia, and hemorrhage may also be present. CTV and MRV, particularly contrast MRV, may show a filling defect.

SUMMARY

Vascular causes of headaches range from common to very rare entities, which can result in serious morbidity and mortality if not promptly diagnosed and treated. Clinical presentation and imaging findings are crucial for the diagnosis of many of these entities, and it is important to be familiar with the imaging appearance using different modalities.

CLINICS CARE POINT

- Acute subarachnoid hemorrhage imaging is best done with CT and CTA. Follow up of aneurysms can be performed with a combination of CTA, MRA and DSA.

- Vasculides can be difficult to distinguish on imaging alone and clinical features are often key. A conversation between the neurologist and radiologist can help with problem solving.

- Cerebral venous thrombosis is uncommon but potentially treatable where prompt diagnosis with CTV or MRV is crucial.

DISCLOSURES

L L. Wang: NIH/NINDS NS103824; ENDOLOW Trial, Cerenovus; NIH/NINDS U01NS110772. A. Mahammedi: ENDOLOW Trial, Cerenovus. A.S. Vagal: NIH/NINDS NS103824, NINDS/NIA NS117643, NIH/NINDS NS100417, NIH/NINDS 1U01NS100699, NIH/NINDS U01NS110772, PI, Imaging Core Lab, ENDOLOW Trial, Cerenovus.

REFERENCES

1. de Falco FA. Sentinel headache. Neurol Sci 2004;25(Suppl 3):S215–7.
2. Kassell NF, Torner JC, Jane JA, et al. The international cooperative study on the timing of aneurysm surgery. Part 2: surgical results. J Neurosurg 1990;73(1): 37–47.
3. Sohn CH, Baik SK, Lee HJ, et al. MR imaging of hyperacute subarachnoid and intraventricular hemorrhage at 3T: a preliminary report of gradient echo T2*-weighted sequences. AJNR Am J Neuroradiol 2005;26(3):662–5.
4. McKinney AM, Palmer CS, Truwit CL, et al. Detection of aneurysms by 64-section multidetector CT angiography in patients acutely suspected of having an intracranial aneurysm and comparison with digital subtraction and 3D rotational angiography. AJNR Am J Neuroradiol 2008;29(3):594–602.
5. Westerlaan HE, van Dijk JM, Jansen-van der Weide MC, et al. Intracranial aneurysms in patients with subarachnoid hemorrhage: CT angiography as a primary examination tool for diagnosis–systematic review and meta-analysis. Radiology 2011;258(1):134–45.
6. Guo W, He XY, Li XF, et al. Meta-analysis of diagnostic significance of sixty-four-row multi-section computed tomography angiography and three-dimensional digital subtraction angiography in patients with cerebral artery aneurysm. J Neurol Sci 2014;346(1–2):197–203.
7. Attali J, Benaissa A, Soize S, et al. Follow-up of intracranial aneurysms treated by flow diverter: comparison of three-dimensional time-of-flight MR angiography (3D-TOF-MRA) and contrast-enhanced MR angiography (CE-MRA) sequences with digital subtraction angiography as the gold standard. J Neurointerv Surg 2016;8(1):81–6.
8. Sailer AM, Wagemans BA, Nelemans PJ, et al. Diagnosing intracranial aneurysms with MR angiography: systematic review and meta-analysis. Stroke 2014;45(1): 119–26.
9. Cho YD, Lee JY, Kwon BJ, et al. False-positive diagnosis of cerebral aneurysms using MR angiography: location, anatomic cause, and added value of source image data. Clin Radiol 2011;66(8):726–31.
10. Thompson BG, Brown RD Jr, Amin-Hanjani S, et al. Guidelines for the management of patients with unruptured intracranial aneurysms: a guideline for

healthcare professionals from the american heart association/american stroke association. Stroke 2015;46(8):2368–400.

11. Wang H, Li W, He H, et al. 320-detector row CT angiography for detection and evaluation of intracranial aneurysms: comparison with conventional digital subtraction angiography. Clin Radiol 2013;68(1):e15–20.

12. Bechan RS, van Rooij SB, Sprengers ME, et al. CT angiography versus 3D rotational angiography in patients with subarachnoid hemorrhage. Neuroradiology 2015;57(12):1239–46.

13. Brown RD, Broderick JP. Unruptured intracranial aneurysms: epidemiology, natural history, management options, and familial screening. Lancet Neurol 2014; 13(4):393–404.

14. Wiebers DO, Whisnant JP, Huston J 3rd, et al. Unruptured intracranial aneurysms: natural history, clinical outcome, and risks of surgical and endovascular treatment. Lancet 2003;362(9378):103–10.

15. Soize S, Gawlitza M, Raoult H, et al. Imaging follow-up of intracranial aneurysms treated by endovascular means: why, when, and how? Stroke 2016;47(5): 1407–12.

16. Kassell NF, Torner JC, Haley EC Jr, et al. The international cooperative study on the timing of aneurysm surgery. Part 1: overall management results. J Neurosurg 1990;73(1):18–36.

17. Rinne J, Hernesniemi J, Puranen M, et al. Multiple intracranial aneurysms in a defined population: prospective angiographic and clinical study. Neurosurgery 1994;35(5):803–8.

18. Chason JL, Hindman WM. Berry aneurysms of the circle of Willis; results of a planned autopsy study. Neurology 1958;8(1):41–4.

19. Inagawa T, Hirano A. Autopsy study of unruptured incidental intracranial aneurysms. Surg Neurol 1990;34(6):361–5.

20. Jabbarli R, Pierscianek D, Rölz R, et al. Endovascular treatment of cerebral vasospasm after subarachnoid hemorrhage: more is more. Neurology 2019;93(5): e458–66.

21. de Boysson H, Parienti JJ, Mawet J, et al. Primary angiitis of the CNS and reversible cerebral vasoconstriction syndrome: a comparative study. Neurology 2018; 91(16):e1468–78.

22. Miller TR, Shivashankar R, Mossa-Basha M, et al. Reversible cerebral vasoconstriction syndrome, part 2: diagnostic work-up, imaging evaluation, and differential diagnosis. AJNR Am J Neuroradiol 2015;36(9):1580–8.

23. Chen SP, Wang SJ. Hyperintense vessels: an early MRI marker of reversible cerebral vasoconstriction syndrome? Cephalalgia 2014;34(13):1038–9.

24. Burton TM, Bushnell CD. Reversible cerebral vasoconstriction syndrome. Stroke 2019;50(8):2253–8.

25. Razek AAKA, Alvarez H, Bagg S, et al. Imaging spectrum of CNS vasculitis. RadioGraphics 2014;34(4):873–94.

26. Calabrese LH, Dodick DW, Schwedt TJ, et al. Narrative review: reversible cerebral vasoconstriction syndromes. Ann Intern Med 2007;146(1):34–44.

27. Mandell DM, Matouk CC, Farb RI, et al. Vessel wall MRI to differentiate between reversible cerebral vasoconstriction syndrome and central nervous system vasculitis: preliminary results. Stroke 2012;43(3):860–2.

28. Obusez EC, Hui F, Hajj-Ali RA, et al. High-resolution MRI vessel wall imaging: spatial and temporal patterns of reversible cerebral vasoconstriction syndrome and central nervous system vasculitis. AJNR Am J Neuroradiol 2014;35(8): 1527–32.

29. Roth C, Ferbert A. The posterior reversible encephalopathy syndrome: what's certain, what's new? Pract Neurol 2011;11(3):136–44.
30. Hinchey J, Chaves C, Appignani B, et al. A reversible posterior leukoencephalopathy syndrome. N Engl J Med 1996;334(8):494–500.
31. Bartynski WS. Posterior reversible encephalopathy syndrome, part 2: controversies surrounding pathophysiology of vasogenic edema. AJNR Am J Neuroradiol 2008;29(6):1043–9.
32. Bartynski WS, Boardman JF. Distinct imaging patterns and lesion distribution in posterior reversible encephalopathy syndrome. AJNR Am J Neuroradiol 2007; 28(7):1320–7.
33. Bartynski WS. Posterior reversible encephalopathy syndrome, part 1: fundamental imaging and clinical features. AJNR Am J Neuroradiol 2008;29(6): 1036–42.
34. Singhal AB, Topcuoglu MA, Fok JW, et al. Reversible cerebral vasoconstriction syndromes and primary angiitis of the central nervous system: clinical, imaging, and angiographic comparison. Ann Neurol 2016;79(6):882–94.
35. Pilato F, Distefano M, Calandrelli R. Posterior reversible encephalopathy syndrome and reversible cerebral vasoconstriction syndrome: clinical and radiological considerations. Front Neurol 2020;11:34.
36. Geibprasert S, Pongpech S, Jiarakongmun P, et al. Radiologic Assessment of brain arteriovenous malformations: what clinicians need to know. RadioGraphics 2010;30(2):483–501.
37. Spetzler RF, Martin NA. A proposed grading system for arteriovenous malformations. J Neurosurg 1986;65(4):476–83.
38. Corbelli I, De Maria F, Eusebi P, et al. Dural arteriovenous fistulas and headache features: an observational study. J Headache Pain 2020;21(1):6.
39. Gandhi D, Chen J, Pearl M, et al. Intracranial dural arteriovenous fistulas: classification, imaging findings, and treatment. Am J Neuroradiology 2012;33(6): 1007–13.
40. Borden JA, Wu JK, Shucart WA. A proposed classification for spinal and cranial dural arteriovenous fistulous malformations and implications for treatment. J Neurosurg 1995;82(2):166–79.
41. Cognard C, Gobin YP, Pierot L, et al. Cerebral dural arteriovenous fistulas: clinical and angiographic correlation with a revised classification of venous drainage. Radiology 1995;194(3):671–80.
42. Cornelius JF, Kürten K, Fischer I, et al. Quality of life after surgery for cerebral cavernoma: brainstem versus nonbrainstem location. World Neurosurg 2016; 95:315–21.
43. Triquenot-Bagan A, Lebas A, Ozkul-Wermester O, et al. Brain developmental venous anomaly thrombosis. Acta Neurol Belg 2017;117(1):315–6.
44. Brzegowy K, Kowalska N, Solewski B, et al. Prevalence and anatomical characteristics of developmental venous anomalies: an MRI study. Neuroradiology 2021; 63(7):1001–8.
45. Idiculla PS, Gurala D, Philipose J, et al. Cerebral cavernous malformations, developmental venous anomaly, and its coexistence: a Review. Eur Neurol 2020;83(4): 360–8.
46. Pereira VM, Geibprasert S, Krings T, et al. Pathomechanisms of symptomatic developmental venous anomalies. Stroke 2008;39(12):3201–15.
47. Kiroglu Y, Oran I, Dalbasti T, et al. Thrombosis of a drainage vein in developmental venous anomaly (DVA) leading venous infarction: a case report and review of the literature. J Neuroimaging 2011;21(2):197–201.

48. Assadsangabi R, Mohan S, Nabavizadeh SA. Clinical manifestations and imaging findings of thrombosis of developmental venous anomalies. Clin Radiol 2018;73(11):985.e7-12.
49. Devasagayam S, Wyatt B, Leyden J, et al. Cerebral venous sinus thrombosis incidence is higher than previously thought. Stroke 2016;47(9):2180–2.
50. Canedo-Antelo M, Baleato-González S, Mosqueira AJ, et al. Radiologic clues to cerebral venous thrombosis. RadioGraphics 2019;39(6):1611–28.
51. Ozsvath RR, Casey SO, Lustrin ES, et al. Cerebral venography: comparison of CT and MR projection venography. AJR Am J Roentgenol 1997;169(6):1699–707.
52. Lettau M, Laible M, Barrows RJ, et al. 3-T contrast-enhanced MR angiography with parallel imaging in cerebral venous and sinus thrombosis. J Neuroradiol 2011;38(5):275–82.
53. Leach JL, Fortuna RB, Jones BV, et al. Imaging of Cerebral Venous Thrombosis: Current Techniques, Spectrum of Findings, and Diagnostic Pitfalls. RadioGraphics 2006;26(suppl_1):S19–41.
54. Alper F, Kantarci M, Dane S, et al. Importance of anatomical asymmetries of transverse sinuses: an MR venographic study. Cerebrovasc Dis 2004;18(3):236–9.
55. Dmytriw AA, Song JSA, Yu E, et al. Cerebral venous thrombosis: state of the art diagnosis and management. Neuroradiology 2018;60(7):669–85.
56. Crombé D, Haven F, Gille M. Isolated deep cerebral venous thrombosis diagnosed on CT and MR imaging. A case study and literature review. JBR-BTR 2003;86(5):257–61.

Headache Attributed to Nonvascular Intracranial Disorder

Neoplasms, Infections, and Substance Abuse

Kassie McCullagh, MD*, Mauricio Castillo, MD,
Carlos Zamora, MD, PhD

KEYWORDS

- Brain Tumor • Intracranial infection • Substance abuse • Headache

KEY POINTS

- Approximately 5% of headaches are secondary to other neurologic disorders and can be the initial and only symptom of a serious underlying condition.
- Imaging is appropriate in patients with new or worsening headaches plus at least one of the following: headache related to activity or positional, neurologic deficits, known or suspected cancer, immunocompromised states, pregnancy, age over 50, or head trauma.
- Imaging is usually not indicated in uncomplicated intracranial infection (meningitis) but has a role in evaluating complications such as cerebral abscess, empyema, and ventriculitis.
- Imaging in substance abuse may produce headaches by virtue of injuries related to direct toxicity or secondary to vascular complications such as RCVS, PRES, and intracranial hemorrhage.

INTRODUCTION

Headaches are a common complaint and the majority are primary: migraines, tension-type, cluster headaches (CH), and others (discussed in other chapters). However, 5% of headaches are secondary to other neurologic disorders and can be the initial symptom of a serious underlying condition, including neoplasia and infection.[1] Secondary headaches are more prevalent in tertiary care settings and patients coming to the emergency department.[2] Headaches are also a common presentation in patients with illicit drug use who have a higher prevalence of CH compared with the general population.[3–5] While imaging in substance abuse is often normal or shows nonspecific findings, it has a role in ruling out other serious causes of headaches. Careful

Division of Neuroradiology, Department of Radiology, The University of North Carolina at Chapel Hill, CB 7510 2000 Old Clinic, 101 Manning Drive, Chapel Hill, NC 27599, USA
* Corresponding author.
E-mail address: kassie_mccullagh@med.unc.edu

Neurol Clin 40 (2022) 531–546
https://doi.org/10.1016/j.ncl.2022.02.005
0733-8619/22/© 2022 Elsevier Inc. All rights reserved.

assessment of the headache presentation including onset, evolution, and associated clinical manifestations can help determine the need for further workup and dedicated imaging. Some of the substances which result in characteristic imaging findings are discussed in this article.

DISCUSSION
NEOPLASMS AND HEADACHES

Headaches are frequently the initial and only symptom of primary or metastatic brain tumors. Although the index of suspicion is high in patients with a known primary malignancy who present with a new headache, the diagnosis may be more challenging in other situations. Therefore, careful attention to the characteristics of the headache and a thorough neurologic examination are warranted to determine further workup.

Clinical Presentation

When examining a patient with headaches, certain signs and symptoms increase the likelihood of a serious underlying cause and are considered "red flags."[6–8] While many "red flags" are fairly sensitive, their specificity is more difficult to determine as they are largely based on retrospective studies of patients with known secondary headaches.[2] Other concerning features have been mostly established based on clinical experience.[2] Many of these signs and symptoms are not specific for intracranial tumors but overlap with other serious intracranial pathologies that also warrant further workup. Notably, in patients with unilateral headaches and without elevated intracranial pressure, the laterality of the headache is a reliable predictor of the side of the tumor.[9,10]

The classic "red flags" that warrant further evaluation and imaging are:[2,6–8]

- Early morning headache
- Nocturnal headache
- Exertional headaches (or associated with Valsalva maneuver)
- Headache with fever and/or other systemic symptoms
- Meningismus
- Headache with nausea and vomiting
- Progressive headaches
- Headache with new neurologic signs
- New-onset headaches in children
- New-onset headaches in adults, especially above age 50
- Headache that has changed in nature from prior chronic headaches
- New or changed headaches in patients with cancer
- Papilledema
- Ocular pain with autonomic features (trigeminal autonomic cephalalgia)

Incidence and Prevalence

The most common risk factor for headaches in patients with intracranial tumors is a prior history of a headache disorder. Although headaches occur in roughly 50% of patients with intracranial tumors, the type of headache and clinical characteristics are nonspecific.[11] In the study by Forsyth and Posner, only 17% of patients had symptoms matching the classic description of a brain tumor headache which is severe, worse in the morning, and associated with nausea or vomiting. The most common descriptions in these patients are similar to tension-type headaches, but patients also complain of symptoms, suggesting a focal lesion or increased intracranial pressure. In a different study, migraine-type headaches were present in 4.5% of patients but all had atypical features, emphasizing the importance of accompanying signs and symptoms rather than the quality of the headache.[9]

On the other hand, brain tumors are rare in patients presenting with headaches to primary care providers with a risk of 0.09%.[12] If a patient meets the criteria for a primary headache disorder, the risk is much lower at 0.045%.[12] However, if a specific diagnosis cannot be concluded from the clinical history and physical examination, the risk is 0.15%.[12] If a brain tumor is not diagnosed initially, 74% of them will be discovered within 3 months, and 90% by 6 months.[12]

Patients with cancer are a unique group that warrants a lower threshold to image in the setting of headaches. Several studies have shown that patients with cancer with new or changed headaches have intracranial metastases 32% to 54% of the time.[13,14] Most of the brain metastases are from lung cancers comprising 43% of secondary tumors, followed by breast cancer comprising 8% (**Fig. 1**).[12]

Mechanism

The brain parenchyma is insensitive to pain, however, mechanical stimulation of the dura, pia, and the vasculature secondary to tumor involvement, mass effect, or

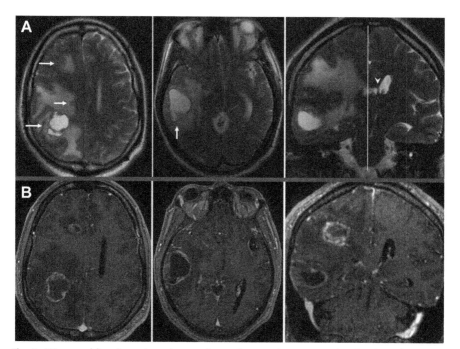

Fig. 1. 56-year-old male undergoing work up of a new lung mass who developed intermittent diffuse headaches for 4 days and subsequently presented when he developed left upper and lower extremity weakness. MRI T2-weighted images (*A*) demonstrate multiple irregular cystic and solid masses (*white arrows*), many located at the gray–white matter junctions. On T1 postcontrast sequences (*B*), there are associated nodular and peripheral enhancing components. The 2 dominant masses in the right temporal and parietal lobes demonstrate extensive vasogenic edema with mass effect and leftward midline shift (best seen on the coronal T2 image whereby the vertical white *line* marks midline and the white *arrowhead* marks the displaced septum pellucidum). Gross total resection of the right temporal mass confirmed lung adenocarcinoma metastasis.

traction also trigger headaches.[15] Pain most commonly occurs along the distribution of the trigeminal nerve which provides most of the innervation to the dura.[15] Additionally, tumors causing elevated intracranial pressure, hydrocephalus, or hemorrhage can lead to headaches (**Fig. 2**).[16,17] Headaches can be associated with edema and rapid growth in the setting of intratumoral hemorrhage or aggressive neoplasia (**Fig. 3**).[18]

Another headache disorder that can be triggered or exacerbated by an intracranial mass is trigeminal autonomic cephalalgia (TAC).[19] While most patients do not have an underlying structural lesion, there are no reliable clinical signs or symptoms to discriminate between primary and secondary TAC and therefore imaging should be obtained in all cases.[2,19] Patients with TAC present with severe, unilateral, and brief headaches with paroxysmal facial autonomic symptoms, which can include ocular pain, lacrimation, rhinorrhea, eyelid edema, facial sweating, miosis, and ptosis.[19] Tumors that have been associated with TAC include pituitary adenoma with cavernous sinus involvement, skull base meningioma, and skull base spread of nasopharyngeal carcinoma.[19] Other non-neoplastic causes include aneurysms, especially of the internal carotid artery, and arteriovenous malformations.[19]

Imaging

According to the American College of Radiology (ACR) Appropriateness Criteria, imaging is appropriate to exclude an underlying serious pathology in patients presenting with a new or progressively worsening headache plus at least one "red flag."[20] The "red flags" to consider per the ACR include headache related to activity or positional, neurologic deficits, known or suspected cancer, immunosuppressed or compromised states, currently pregnant, over the age of 50 years, or subacute head trauma.[20] In these cases, CT without contrast, brain MRI without contrast, or brain MRI without and with contrast are all appropriate.[20] Often, the choice of modality depends on availability, level of suspicion for an underlying etiology, and timeliness of imaging if an acute pathology is of concern. Additionally, per the ACR Appropriateness Criteria, imaging is also recommended when a patient with chronic headaches presents with new features or increasing frequency.[20] In these instances, brain MRI (either without or with contrast), is usually preferred over CT imaging.[19] Patients with large contrast-enhancing tumors associated with midline shift are more likely to have headaches; however, the clinical features of the headache are nonspecific.[9,21]

INTRACRANIAL INFECTIONS AND HEADACHES

Intracranial infections are medical emergencies that warrant timely workup and diagnosis. Because intracranial infections can spread rapidly and cause permanent neurologic damage and even death, prompt diagnosis and initiation of therapy are crucial. Headache is commonly the first symptom of intracranial infection, and therefore, an infection should be considered in the initial differential diagnosis in the appropriate clinical context.

Clinical Presentation

Depending on the site of involvement, all headache types can be observed in intracranial infections.[22] Sites of infection include the epidural and subdural spaces, leptomeninges, parenchyma (focally or diffuse), ventricles, or a combination of these.[23] While a full review of these pathologies is beyond the scope of this article, a common thread of concerning symptoms and signs can lead to the appropriate workup including lumbar puncture and imaging.

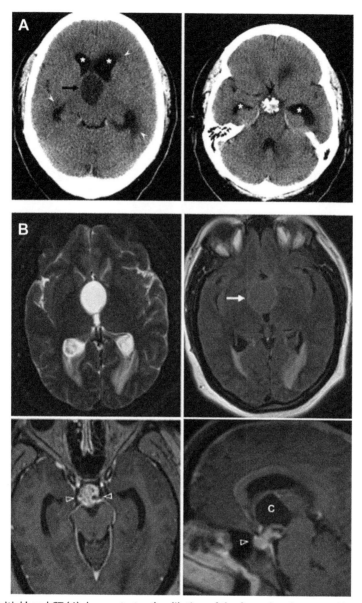

Fig. 2. Initial head CT (*A*) demonstrates the dilation of the frontal and temporal horns of the lateral ventricles (*) with surrounding periventricular hypodensities (white *arrowheads*), compatible with hydrocephalus. The third ventricle is not dilated, but instead obstructed by a cystic lesion that is slightly hyperdense to CSF (*black arrow*). Coarse calcifications are present in the sellar-suprasellar region (black *arrowhead*). Subsequent MRI (*B*) again highlights hydrocephalus with the dilation of the atria and temporal horns of the lateral ventricles and periventricular hyperintense signal on the T2/FLAIR sequences. The cystic component of the mass does not completely suppress on the FLAIR sequence (*white arrow*). T1 postcontrast axial and sagittal sequences demonstrate solid avidly enhancing component in the sellar-suprasellar region (white open *arrowheads*). The sagittal postcontrast sequence also highlights the cystic component (*C*) protruding into and compressing the 3rd ventricle. At surgical resection, this was confirmed to be an adamantinomatous craniopharyngoma.

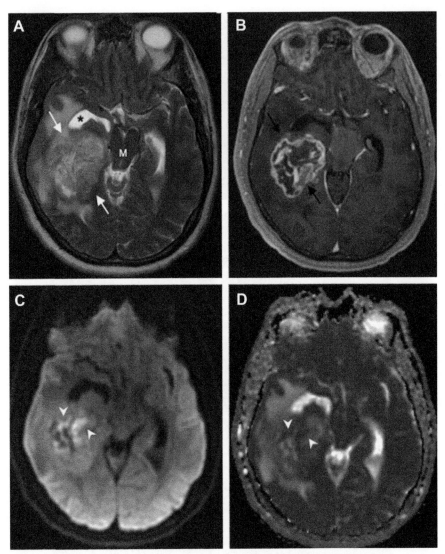

Fig. 3. 34 y.o. male presented with 3 weeks of intractable headaches with associated photophobia, blurry and double vision, nausea, and vomiting. MRI demonstrates a large right frontotemporal heterogenous mass with mixed signal on T2-weighted images (*A, white arrows*). There is a severe mass effect with midline shift and compression of the midbrain (M), obstructive hydrocephalus with the dilation of the temporal horn (*) of the right lateral ventricle, extensive surrounding edema, and infiltrative tumor. On T1 postcontrast sequences (*B*), there is irregular nodular and peripheral enhancement (*black arrows*). DWI (*C*) and ADC (*D*) demonstrate foci of restricted diffusion correlating to the areas of nodular enhancement (white *arrowheads*). Gross total resection was performed, pathology was consistent with glioblastoma (WHO Grade IV), IDH-wildtype, TERT mutated.

Bacterial meningitis is one of the most common intracranial infections and is associated with a diffuse and severe headache. Although patients may present with the classic triad of fever, neck stiffness, and change in mental status, this is only seen in 44% of cases.[24] Notably, 95% of patients have at least 2 of the following: headache, fever, neck stiffness, and altered mental status.[24] Therefore, the absence of all of these manifestations makes a diagnosis of bacterial meningitis highly unlikely. In contrast, patients with viral meningitis commonly present with headaches but signs of meningeal irritation are not as pronounced as with bacterial infection.[25] Patients with viral encephalitis have abnormal cerebral function due to parenchymal involvement, although an overlapping presentation with meningoencephalitis is not uncommon.[26]

Imaging

A lumbar puncture is key in the diagnostic evaluation of patients with suspected intracranial infections. However, due to the potential risk of brain herniation, imaging should be obtained before lumbar puncture in patients who may have elevated intracranial pressure. According to the Infectious Diseases Society of America (IDSA),[27] CT should be obtained first in the following patients:

- Immunocompromised
- History of known CNS disease (mass lesion, stroke, or focal infection)
- New onset of seizure within 1 week of presentation
- Papilledema on fundoscopy
- Abnormal level of consciousness
- Focal neurologic deficit

Although noncontrast head CT is useful to screen for elevated intracranial pressure, it is typically not helpful in the diagnosis of intracranial infection, and in most patients the study is normal. While imaging is usually not indicated in uncomplicated infections, MRI with and without contrast is the best modality for evaluating complications such as abscess and ventriculitis. Salient imaging findings in some of the most common infections will be reviewed.

Pyogenic meningitis

On MRI, meningitis can show failed CSF suppression on FLAIR, restricted diffusion in the sulci, and leptomeningeal enhancement (**Fig. 4**).[28] However, the absence of these findings should not supersede a clinical diagnosis of meningitis as only 50% of patients show leptomeningeal enhancement.[29] Restricted diffusion along the sulci is variable but indicates pyogenic rather than viral infection.[28] Progression of meningitis can lead to cerebritis with a spectrum of findings. This usually starts with an ill-defined T2/FLAIR hyperintense parenchymal signal abnormality on MRI without contrast enhancement. Parenchymal enhancement can occur as the infection evolves and if left untreated will subsequently develop into an organized abscess.[28]

Pyogenic abscess

Brain parenchymal abscess, whether caused by meningitis, hematological dissemination, or direct invasion, has MRI features that help differentiate it from other mass-like lesions. The abscess capsule shows a characteristic pattern on T1 and T2 weighted images, likely due to a combination of hemorrhage, collagen, and free radicals in macrophages.[30] The capsule seems dark on T2 and it is usually mildly bright on T1-weighted images with avid postcontrast enhancement.[30] SWI may show a dual rim with signal dropout peripherally and a hyperintense inner ring, a finding that is absent in necrotic malignancies.[31] The walls of an abscess are relatively smooth but the outer margin may be irregular during the transition stage from cerebritis.[32] On DWI, there is profound central restricted diffusion due to purulent material (**Fig. 5**).

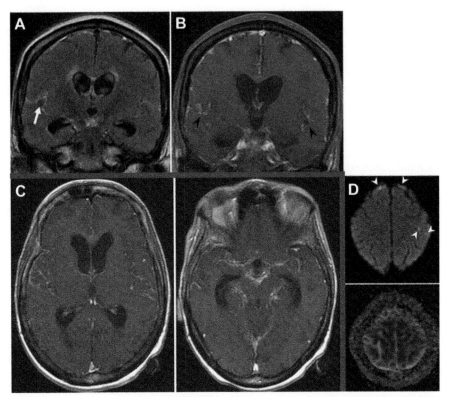

Fig. 4. Coronal FLAIR sequence (*A*) shows failed CSF suppression in the sulci, best seen in the right Sylvian fissure (*white arrow*), as well as mildly dilated ventricles with periventricular hyperintense signal, compatible with hydrocephalus. On the coronal T1-weighted postcontrast sequence (*B*), there is correlating leptomeningeal enhancement (black *arrowheads*). Axial T1-weighted postcontrast sequences (*C*) demonstrate additional areas of leptomeningeal enhancement throughout the cerebral sulci and basilar cisterns. DWI/ADC sequence (*D*) shows a few scattered punctate foci of sulcal restricted diffusion (white *arrowheads*). The constellation of these findings in the appropriate setting is compatible with meningitis.

Ventriculitis

Ventriculitis is a rare but severe complication of meningitis. It is most commonly seen in infants but can occur in adults with certain risk factors including diabetes, head injury, craniotomy, and neurosurgical implants.[33] MRI may show debris layering dependently in the ventricles with restricted diffusion. Ependymal enhancement can be present in immunocompetent patients who can mount an inflammatory response.[29] There may be ependymal thickening and surrounding edema best seen on FLAIR. The most common organisms to cause ventriculitis are Staphylococcus and Enterobacter.[29]

Empyemas

Empyema is another complication of intracranial infections which occurs when the infection spreads to the epidural or subdural space.[28] Because up to one-third of patients with meningitis can develop sterile subdural effusions as a reaction to inflammatory agents, it is important to distinguish between effusions and empyemas on MRI.[29]

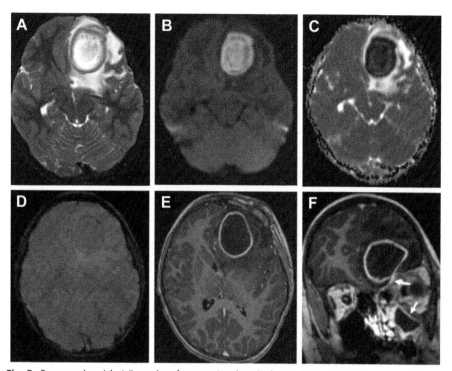

Fig. 5. 8 y.o. male with 1.5 weeks of worsening headache with associated nausea and vomiting. MRI shows a left frontal lobe mass with extensive edema and mass effect with midline shift. There is central hyperintense signal and a hypointense rim on the T2-weighted sequence (*A*). Avid internal restricted diffusion is present on DWI/ADC (*B, C*). The rim also shows a thin line of signal drop out on the SWI image (*D*). There is a relatively thin ring of enhancement on the T1 postcontrast sequences (*E, F*). This is compatible with a parenchymal bacterial abscess, confirmed on surgical evacuation with cultures growing aggregatibacter and Strep anginosus. This was secondary to severe left sided sinus disease (*F, white arrows*).

Empyemas typically need surgical evacuation, while effusions usually resolve over weeks to months.[29] Typically, subdural effusions will have similar signal characteristics to CSF, while empyemas will be hyperintense on FLAIR and maybe slightly hyperintense to CSF on T1-weighted imaging. Another helpful sequence to differentiate between the two is DWI. In empyema, the fluid usually shows restricted diffusion, although this is not always present.[28,34] Because chronic effusions can develop an enhancing fibrin capsule and septations, contrast is not as helpful at distinguishing it from empyema as the pattern of enhancement can look similar.[29]

Fungal infection

There are a variety of intracranial fungal infections which are typically seen in immunocompromised patients, the most common being cryptococcal meningoencephalitis. This is a yeast that has a high tropism for the meninges and preferentially spreads along with the perivascular spaces. Lesions are commonly seen in the basal ganglia, thalami, and cerebellum.[35,36] On MRI, leptomeningeal enhancement may be present depending on the host's capacity to mount an inflammatory response. A distinctive feature is the presence of gelatinous pseudocysts which represent yeast-produced mucoid material expanding the perivascular spaces, frequently seen in the basal ganglia.[28] Hydrocephalus and sustained intracranial hypertension are well-established complications and patients may require serial lumbar punctures or surgical shunting.[37]

Parasitic infection

Numerous parasitic infections can affect the central nervous system (CNS). They vary greatly in prevalence depending on geographic location. In the United States, cysticercosis, toxoplasmosis, and echinococcosis are the three most common parasitic infections, each with unique imaging findings.[28] The first two are more likely to infect the CNS and will be briefly reviewed here.

Cysticercosis is caused by the ingestion of the eggs of taenia solium which is the pork tapeworm. The eggs hatch and the oncosphere (embryo) crosses the intestinal lining to enter the bloodstream where it can spread to the brain and muscles. Early in the disease, patients are often asymptomatic, but headaches are common as the infection progresses (43%).[28] There are various stages of neurocysticercosis, each with unique imaging findings. The vesicular stage is characterized by small nonenhancing cysts often containing a small eccentric nodule representing the scolex. There is no surrounding edema because the cyst wall is intact and there is no localized immune response. This is followed by the colloidal stage, which is marked by the death of the scolex and disruption of the cyst wall with a robust inflammatory response. On MRI the cysts show more proteinaceous signal characteristics, peripheral enhancement, and surrounding edema. In the granular nodular stage, the cysts begin to retract and create a granulomatous nodule, often with surrounding gliosis. Finally, the calcified nodular stage is marked by the development of calcifications. While edema or enhancement may occur at this late stage, this is considered to be an immune response as the infection is quiescent. These stages follow a particular progression, but lesions can be seen at different stages. Another variant of neurocysticercosis is the racemose form with clusters of cysts within the cisterns and Sylvian fissures without scolices or associated enhancement.[38]

Toxoplasmosis is the most common parasitic infection in immunocompromised individuals and is almost always the reactivation of a prior infection. The organisms are disseminated hematogenously and preferentially involve the basal ganglia, thalami, and gray–white matter junction.[39] On MRI lesions may show alternating dark and bright rings on T2/FLAIR due to different layers of edema, hemorrhage, and various types of necrosis.[40] There is usually a significant amount of surrounding vasogenic edema. On postcontrast T1, the presence of ring-enhancing lesions containing an eccentric nodule is highly suggestive of the diagnosis in an immunocompromised individual (**Fig. 6**).[41]

SUBSTANCE ABUSE AND HEADACHES

Assessment of illicit drug use is an important part of a thorough history during the evaluation of a patient with headaches. Patients may not be forthcoming with this information so knowledge of some of the imaging features may help in the diagnostic workup. Some patients may be "self-medicating" while in others the drugs may be the cause of the headaches. Often imaging is negative in these patients, however, some characteristic patterns of brain abnormalities have been described and will be reviewed here.

Clinical Presentation

Headache is not often the main presentation of drug abuse, however, may be an early symptom preceding more serious neurologic complications. Many of the neurologic

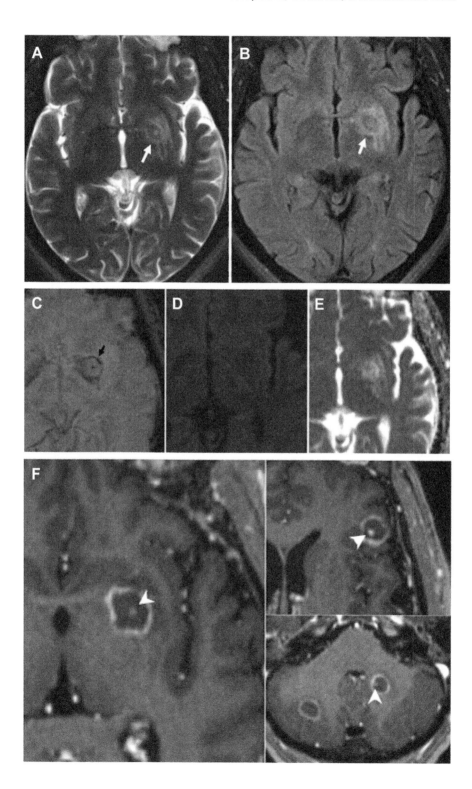

manifestations caused by illicit drugs are related to neurovascular complications or toxic effects primarily affecting the white matter. This can lead to serious neurologic pathologies including ischemic stroke, intracranial hemorrhage, vasculitis, aneurysm, and permanent white matter injury to name a few.[42]

Patients with CH, in particular, have a higher rate of illicit drug use than the general population as documented in several studies.[3–5] Various theories have been proposed to explain this association, including direct effects of the drug on the pathophysiology of CH, use of the drug in an attempt to treat the CH and possible common factors that may predispose patients to both drug abuse and CH.[3–5]

Cocaine

Cocaine has numerous effects on the vascular system including vasoconstriction, vasculitis, platelet aggregation, accelerated atherosclerosis, and cardioembolic events which can result in ischemic infarction. Cocaine also frequently leads to elevated blood pressure which is the primary cause of intraparenchymal hemorrhage in these patients, as well as long-term effects such as aneurysm formation and increased risk for subarachnoid hemorrhage.[42,43] Cocaine has been associated with posterior reversible encephalopathy syndrome (PRES) whereby patients present with headaches, seizures, visual impairment, and altered consciousness.[44] MRI in patients with PRES shows T2/FLAIR hyperintensity involving the cortex and subcortical white matter, cerebellum, and brainstem with intracranial hemorrhage in 15%.[45] Additionally, cocaine has been reported as a potential trigger of reversible cerebral vasoconstriction syndrome (RCVS). Patients with RCVS typically present with recurrent, sudden, and severe headaches. Angiographic imaging shows multifocal intracranial stenoses that resolve on follow-up imaging after the resolution of symptoms.[46] Other drugs that have been associated with RCVS include amphetamine derivatives, lysergic acid diethylamide (LSD), and cannabis. However, except for cannabis (see later in discussion), evidence is scarce to establish a causal link as single precipitating factors.[47]

Heroin

Headaches are a common symptom in heroin addicts and can be seen shortly after drug use.[48] Heroin has both acute and chronic effects on the neurovascular system. Acute ischemic infarcts can be seen with a predisposition to the globus pallidus. Chronic findings are often subclinical, but on imaging, can manifest as chronic ischemic changes in the subcortical and periventricular white matter. These findings are nonspecific but should be considered in the differential diagnosis especially in younger patients whereby small-vessel ischemic changes are unlikely and there is a history of drug abuse.[42]

Fig. 6. 45 y.o. male with intermittent headaches and episodic right-sided weakness. MRI demonstrates multiple lesions with surrounding edema (all are not shown). The representative lesion in the left basal ganglia shows alternating rings of dark and bright signal on the T2-weighted and FLAIR images (*A, B, white arrows*). There is also a thin rim of signal dropout on the SWI sequence, likely from hemorrhage (*C, black arrow*). None of the lesions demonstrated internal or peripheral restricted diffusion on DWI/ADC (*D, E*). On T1 postcontrast sequences (*F*), the lesions show a ring of enhancement with an eccentric nodule (white *arrowhead*). This patient had newly diagnosed AIDS (CD4 count 88 at presentation), and the intracranial lesions were confirmed to be CNS toxoplasmosis.

Another classic pattern of heroin-induced CNS injury is a spongiform leukoencephalopathy seen when the drug is inhaled, the so-called "chasing the dragon." This is due to the vacuolization of the myelin sheath, thought to result from the impurities that can be present in heroin formulations and are activated by heat. While on imaging these features can be nonspecific with diffuse and symmetric involvement of the cerebral white matter, toxicity from heroin inhalation typically involves the cerebellum with relative sparing of the dentate nuclei.[49]

Toluene toxicity

The toxic effects of toluene on the CNS are typically seen with chronic use. Toluene is commonly found in paint thinners, lacquers, and nail polish, and toxicity is seen in individuals who inhale vapors from these compounds. Clinically these patients present with headaches, ataxia, behavioral changes, electrolyte alterations, and euphoria. On imaging, there are changes of demyelination and gliosis in the cerebral and cerebellar white matter and in 30% to 50% of cases there is the involvement of the thalami and basal ganglia.[50]

Cannabis

As cannabis becomes legalized and more readily available, clinicians should be aware of the rare associated neurologic complications. There is emerging data suggesting that cannabis may be a trigger for RCVS.[51] In a study by Wolf and colleagues, cannabis-induced RCVS was more commonly seen in men and the stenoses were predominantly seen in the posterior circulation. Although rare, ischemic strokes have been reported in cannabis use and may be related to RCVS.[50,51] This association may be confounded by concurrent use of tobacco and alcohol in these patients. Additionally, given the rarity of RCVS in cannabis users, there may be a genetic predisposition that places some patients at greater risk of cannabis-induced RCVS, although this needs to be further explored.[51] Conversely, cannabis has been reported as a way to treat headaches. Caution should be used when evaluating the proposed benefits of cannabis in medical use, but there is emerging scientific-based data that may support use as a therapeutic in the appropriate setting.[52]

SUMMARY

Evaluation of secondary headaches is challenging due to overlapping clinical features and the overall prevalence of headaches in the general population. A careful history and neurologic assessment are crucial to determine the need for further workup and imaging. Identifying groups who are at risk for underlying pathology is also important. This includes patients with known or suspected malignancy and those who are immunocompromised with an increased risk for intracranial infections. While CT is helpful in the acute setting and to screen for intracranial hypertension, MRI is the modality of choice for the evaluation of underlying pathologies. Headaches are also common in substance abuse. Imaging has a limited role in this setting but may show patterns of CNS injury that may be directly related to toxicity or secondary vascular effects such as seen with PRES and RCVS.

CLINICS CARE POINTS

- Approximately 5% of headaches are secondary to other neurologic disorders and can be the initial and only symptom of a serious underlying condition.

- Imaging is appropriate in patients with new or worsening headaches plus at least one of the following "red flags": headache related to activity or positional, neurologic deficits, known or suspected cancer, immunocompromised states, pregnancy, age over 50, or head trauma.
- Imaging is usually not indicated in uncomplicated intracranial infection but has a role in evaluating complications such as cerebral abscess, empyema, and ventriculitis.
- In substance abuse, imaging may show injury related to direct toxicity or secondary vascular complications such as RCVS, PRES, and intracranial hemorrhage.

DISCLOSURE

The authors have nothing to disclose.

REFERENCES

1. Bigal ME, Bordini CA, Speciali JG. Etiology and distribution of headaches in two Brazilian primary care units. Headache 2000;40(3):241–7.
2. Do TP, Remmers A, Schytz HW, et al. Red and orange flags for secondary headaches in clinical practice: SNNOOP10 list. Neurology 2019;92(3):134–44.
3. de Coo IF, Naber WC, Wilbrink LA, et al. Increased use of illicit drugs in a Dutch cluster headache population. Cephalalgia 2019;39(5):626–34.
4. Govare A, Leroux E. Licit and illicit drug use in cluster headache. Curr Pain Headache Rep 2014;18(5):413.
5. Ponte C, Giron A, Crequy M, et al. Cluster Headache in Subjects With Substance Use Disorder: A Case Series and a Review of the Literature. Headache 2019; 59(4):576–89.
6. Goffaux P, Fortin D. Brain tumor headaches: from bedside to bench. Neurosurgery 2010;67(2):459–66.
7. Purdy RA. Clinical evaluation of a patient presenting with headache. Med Clin North Am 2001;85(4):847–863, v.
8. Sobri M, Lamont AC, Alias NA, et al. Red flags in patients presenting with headache: clinical indications for neuroimaging. Br J Radiol 2003;76(908):532–5.
9. Forsyth PA, Posner JB. Headaches in patients with brain tumors: a study of 111 patients. Neurology 1993;43(9):1678–83.
10. Suwanwela N, Phanthumchinda K, Kaoropthum S. Headache in brain tumor: a cross-sectional study. Headache 1994;34(7):435–8.
11. Valentinis L, Tuniz F, Valent F, et al. Headache attributed to intracranial tumours: a prospective cohort study. Cephalalgia 2010;30(4):389–98.
12. Kernick DP, Ahmed F, Bahra A, et al. Imaging patients with suspected brain tumour: guidance for primary care. Br J Gen Pract 2008;58(557):880–5.
13. Argyriou AA, Chroni E, Polychronopoulos P, et al. Headache characteristics and brain metastases prediction in cancer patients. Eur J Cancer Care (Engl) 2006; 15(1):90–5.
14. Christiaans MH, Kelder JC, Arnoldus EP, et al. Prediction of intracranial metastases in cancer patients with headache. Cancer 2002;94(7):2063–8.
15. Fontaine D, Almairac F, Santucci S, et al. Dural and pial pain-sensitive structures in humans: new inputs from awake craniotomies. Brain 2018;141(4):1040–8.
16. Kirby S, Purdy RA. Headaches and brain tumors. Neurol Clin 2014;32(2):423–32.
17. Navi BB, Reichman JS, Berlin D, et al. Intracerebral and subarachnoid hemorrhage in patients with cancer. Neurology 2010;74(6):494–501.

18. Sorribes IC, Moore MNJ, Byrne HM, et al. A Biomechanical Model of Tumor-Induced Intracranial Pressure and Edema in Brain Tissue. Biophys J 2019; 116(8):1560–74.

19. Benoliel R. Trigeminal autonomic cephalgias. Br J Pain 2012;6(3):106–23.

20. Douglas AC, Wippold FJ 2nd, Broderick DF, et al. ACR Appropriateness Criteria Headache. J Am Coll Radiol 2014;11(7):657–67.

21. Taylor LP. Mechanism of brain tumor headache. Headache 2014;54(4):772–5.

22. Marchioni E, Minoli L. Headache attributed to infections nosography and differential diagnosis. Handbook Clin Neurol 2010;97:601–26.

23. Foerster BR, Thurnher MM, Malani PN, et al. Intracranial infections: clinical and imaging characteristics. Acta radiologica 2007;48(8):875–93.

24. van de Beek D, de Gans J, Spanjaard L, et al. Clinical features and prognostic factors in adults with bacterial meningitis. New Engl J Med 2004;351(18): 1849–59.

25. Logan SA, MacMahon E. Viral meningitis. BMJ 2008;336(7634):36–40.

26. Kumar R. Understanding and managing acute encephalitis. F1000Res 2020;9.

27. Tunkel AR, Hartman BJ, Kaplan SL, et al. Practice guidelines for the management of bacterial meningitis. Clin Infect Dis 2004;39(9):1267–84.

28. Shih RY, Koeller KK. Bacterial, Fungal, and Parasitic Infections of the Central Nervous System: Radiologic-Pathologic Correlation and Historical Perspectives. Radiographics 2015;140317.

29. Mohan S, Jain KK, Arabi M, et al. Imaging of meningitis and ventriculitis. Neuroimaging Clin N America 2012;22(4):557–83.

30. Villanueva-Meyer JE, Cha S. From Shades of Gray to Microbiologic Imaging: A Historical Review of Brain Abscess Imaging: RSNA Centennial Article. Radiographics 2015;35(5):1555–62.

31. Toh CH, Wei KC, Chang CN, et al. Differentiation of pyogenic brain abscesses from necrotic glioblastomas with use of susceptibility-weighted imaging. AJNR Am J neuroradiology 2012;33(8):1534–8.

32. Smirniotopoulos JG, Murphy FM, Rushing EJ, et al. Patterns of contrast enhancement in the brain and meninges. Radiographics 2007;27(2):525–51.

33. Fukui MB, Williams RL, Mudigonda S. CT and MR imaging features of pyogenic ventriculitis. AJNR Am J neuroradiology 2001;22(8):1510–6.

34. Tsuchiya K, Osawa A, Katase S, et al. Diffusion-weighted MRI of subdural and epidural empyemas. Neuroradiology 2003;45(4):220–3.

35. Franco-Paredes C, Womack T, Bohlmeyer T, et al. Management of Cryptococcus gattii meningoencephalitis. Lancet Infect Dis 2015;15(3):348–55.

36. Charlier C, Dromer F, Leveque C, et al. Cryptococcal neuroradiological lesions correlate with severity during cryptococcal meningoencephalitis in HIV-positive patients in the HAART era. PloS one 2008;3(4):e1950.

37. Cherian J, Atmar RL, Gopinath SP. Shunting in cryptococcal meningitis. J Neurosurg 2016;125(1):177–86.

38. Noujaim SE, Rossi MD, Rao SK, et al. CT and MR imaging of neurocysticercosis. AJR Am J Roentgenol 1999;173(6):1485–90.

39. Lee GT, Antelo F, Mlikotic AA. Best cases from the AFIP: cerebral toxoplasmosis. Radiographics 2009;29(4):1200–5.

40. Mahadevan A, Ramalingaiah AH, Parthasarathy S, et al. Neuropathological correlate of the "concentric target sign" in MRI of HIV-associated cerebral toxoplasmosis. J Magn Reson Imaging 2013;38(2):488–95.

41. Kumar GG, Mahadevan A, Guruprasad AS, et al. Eccentric target sign in cerebral toxoplasmosis: neuropathological correlate to the imaging feature. J Magn Reson Imaging 2010;31(6):1469–72.
42. Tamrazi B, Almast J. Your brain on drugs: imaging of drug-related changes in the central nervous system. Radiographics 2012;32(3):701–19.
43. Toossi S, Hess CP, Hills NK, et al. Neurovascular complications of cocaine use at a tertiary stroke center. J stroke Cerebrovasc Dis 2010;19(4):273–8.
44. Stott VL, Hurrell MA, Anderson TJ. Reversible posterior leukoencephalopathy syndrome: a misnomer reviewed. Intern Med J 2005;35(2):83–90.
45. Hefzy HM, Bartynski WS, Boardman JF, et al. Hemorrhage in posterior reversible encephalopathy syndrome: imaging and clinical features. AJNR Am J neuroradiology 2009;30(7):1371–9.
46. Sattar A, Manousakis G, Jensen MB. Systematic review of reversible cerebral vasoconstriction syndrome. Expert Rev Cardiovasc Ther 2010;8(10):1417–21.
47. Short K, Emsley HCA. Illicit Drugs and Reversible Cerebral Vasoconstriction Syndrome. Neurohospitalist 2021;11(1):40–4.
48. Li L, Yu S. Heroin-induced headache in female heroin addicts. J Int Med Res 2020;48(6). 300060520925353.
49. Bartlett E, Mikulis DJ. Chasing "chasing the dragon" with MRI: leukoencephalopathy in drug abuse. Br J Radiol 2005;78(935):997–1004.
50. Geibprasert S, Gallucci M, Krings T. Addictive illegal drugs: structural neuroimaging. AJNR Am J neuroradiology 2010;31(5):803–8.
51. Wolff V, Armspach JP, Lauer V, et al. Cannabis-related stroke: myth or reality? Stroke; a J Cereb Circ 2013;44(2):558–63.
52. Baron EP. Medicinal Properties of Cannabinoids, Terpenes, and Flavonoids in Cannabis, and Benefits in Migraine, Headache, and Pain: An Update on Current Evidence and Cannabis Science. Headache 2018;58(7):1139–86.

Imaging of Headaches due to Intracranial Pressure Disorders

Jonathon Maffie, MD, PhD[a],*,[1], Eric Sobieski, BS[b],[2],
Sangam Kanekar, MD, DNB[a],[1]

KEYWORDS

- Headache • Intracranial pressure • Idiopathic intracranial hypertension • CSF leak
- Hydrocephalus

KEY POINTS

- Changes in intracranial pressure are an important etiology of headache with specific diagnostic findings in a patient's history, physical exam and imaging.
- Diagnostic imaging, typically CT in the emergent setting and MRI in the outpatient setting, can help to confirm a suspected diagnosis of intracranial hypotension or hypertension and may identify the causative etiology.
- MRI correlates of elevated intracranial pressure include optic nerve sheath dilation, narrowing of the dural venous sinuses, and flattening or protrusion of the optic disc.
- MRI correlates of decreased intracranial pressure include pachymeningeal thickening, subdural hygroma or hemorrhage, dural venous distension, and sagging of the brain stem and cerebellum.

INTRODUCTION

Headaches may be divided into either primary or secondary headaches according to the International Classification of Headache Disorders, whereby primary headaches are those which have no identifiable underlying cause (e.g., tension-type headache, migraine headache), and secondary headaches are those with an underlying cause.[1] In practice, approximately 90% of headaches are primary, and less than 10% are secondary.[2] A subset of secondary headaches are due to disorders affecting intracranial pressure, with both increased and decreased intracranial pressure potentially causing headache. Changes in intracranial pressure may be the result of serious conditions, such as hydrocephalus or a cerebrospinal fluid (CSF) leak, so timely evaluation,

[a] Department of Radiology, Division of Neuroradiology, Penn State Health Milton S. Hershey Medical Center, Hershey, PA, USA; [b] Pennsylvania State College of Medicine, Hershey, PA, USA
[1] 500 University Drive, H066, Room CG533, Hershey, PA 17033-0850, USA.
[2] 500 University Drive, Hershey, PA 17033, USA.
* Corresponding author.
E-mail address: jmaffie@pennstatehealth.psu.edu

Neurol Clin 40 (2022) 547–562
https://doi.org/10.1016/j.ncl.2022.02.006
0733-8619/22/© 2022 Elsevier Inc. All rights reserved.

neurologic.theclinics.com

frequently relying on imaging, is necessary to determine the diagnosis and to direct treatment.

During clinical evaluation, red flags in the patient's history and presentation are often used to determine if a headache is likely due to a secondary cause. Signs and symptoms which may initially suggest the presence of an intracranial pressure disorder include: signs of infection, history of neoplasms, neurologic deficit, positional headache, papilledema, progressive headache, or postpartum timing.[3] Specific elements of clinical evaluation can narrow clinical suspicion (**Table 1**).

Table 1
Clinical Features of conditions causing headaches from intracranial pressure changes

Etiology Category	Condition(s)	Clinical Features Accompanying Headache
Increase pressure		
Noncommunicating Hydrocephalus	Congenital stenosis, hemorrhage, neoplasms, metastasis, cystic lesions, infection	Signs of increased ICP (nausea, vomiting, papilledema, altered mental status), signs of herniation (neurologic deficits)
Communicating Hydrocephalus with Obstruction	Subarachnoid hemorrhage	Initial "thunderclap" headache followed by continued headache or delayed headache, signs of increased ICP
	Leptomeningeal diseases	Cranial nerve deficits, back pain, radicular pain, visual disturbances, diplopia, hearing loss seizures, psychiatric disturbances, cauda equina syndrome
	Meningitis	Fever, meningeal signs (nuchal rigidity, jolt accentuation, Kernig's sign, Brudzinski's sign)
Communicating Hydrocephalus without obstruction	Choroid plexus tumors (CPP, CPC), Villous hypertrophy of the choroid plexus	Diplopia, signs of increased ICP In infants: Increased head of circumference, bulging fontanelles, neurological delay
	Idiopathic intracranial hypertension	Headache worse in the morning and exacerbated by the Valsalva maneuver Pulsatile tinnitus, papilledema, transient visual obscurations, vision loss
Decreased Pressure		
CSF Leak	Postdural puncture headache	Orthostatic headache, nausea, vomiting, dizziness, hearing loss, hypercusis, tinnitus, photophobia, diplopia, neck stiffness, scapular pain Recent epidural or spinal anesthesia, recent LP
	Spontaneous intracranial hypotension	Orthostatic headache, nausea, vomiting, hearing changes, photophobia, visual changes, neck pain or stiffness

Abbreviations: CPC, Choroid plexus carcinoma; CPP, Choroid plexus papilloma; CSF, Cerebrospinal; ICP, Intracranial pressure; LP, Lumbar Puncture; NHL, Non-Hodgkin's lymphoma; NSCLC, Nonsmall cell lung cancer.

Once a pressure-related headache disorder is suspected, diagnostic testing is typically sought if the etiology is not readily apparent. In general, MRI of the brain without contrast is a good starting point for the evaluation of headache suspected to be secondary to changes in intracranial pressure, with the addition of contrast in cases where tumor or infection are suspected, or the addition of MRI venogram if idiopathic intracranial hypotension is suspected. A reasonable place for a clinician to start when considering initial imaging for headache would be the American College of Radiology Appropriateness Criteria. These criteria divide headaches into new-onset headaches and chronic headaches and provide guidance on ordering the most appropriate study. Additionally, they include a variety of common clinical presentations, with suggested studies.[4]

PHYSIOLOGY OF CEREBROSPINAL FLUID DYNAMICS

The majority (80%–90%) of CSF is secreted from the choroid plexus located in the ventricles of the brain. This CSF flows from the lateral ventricles, through the foramen of Monro to the third ventricle, through the cerebral aqueduct to the fourth ventricle, and to the subarachnoid space via the foramen of Magendie and the foramina of Luschka (**Fig. 1**). The remaining 10% to 20% of CSF originates as interstitial fluid produced at the blood–brain barrier, which flows from the interstitial space to the subarachnoid space. CSF likely exits predominantly through the arachnoid villi to the dural venous sinuses; however, exit through the cribriform plate and the cervical lymphatics are hypothesized to be significant alternate pathways.[5] Symptomatic presentation with a headache can be secondary to the disruption of these mechanisms. In the specific disease states, obstruction of normal CSF flow or excess CSF production can lead to pathologic states of increased CSF pressure, accompanied by increased intracranial pressure. Conversely, in the situation whereby CSF leaks from the normal compartment, low intracranial pressure can result in headache as well.

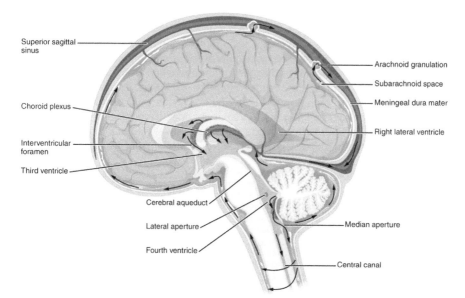

Fig. 1. CSF flow pattern. Diagram showing the flow of CSF from production in the choroid plexus, flow through the ventricles and cisterns, and reabsorption via the arachnoid granulations. (*From* "CSF Circulation" by OpenStax is licensed under CC BY 4.0, https://openstax. org/books/anatomy-and-physiology/pages/13-3-circulation-and-the-central-nervous-system)

INCREASED INTRACRANIAL PRESSURE
Hydrocephalus

Hydrocephalus occurs when there is disruption of normal CSF production, flow, or reabsorption.[6] The prevalence of hydrocephalus is 85 per 100,000 globally, with 88 per 100,000 in pediatrics, 11 per 100,000 in adults, and 175 per 100,000 in the elderly.[7] While hydrocephalus is typically caused by congenital defects in the pediatric population, hydrocephalus in adults is caused by a diverse array of disorders.[8] Because of this, the classification of hydrocephalus has been debated and multiple systems of classification have been proposed.[6,9] For the purposes of this review, categories of hydrocephalus will be divided into noncommunicating, communicating with obstruction, and communicating without obstruction.

Noncommunicating Hydrocephalus

Often referred to as obstructive hydrocephalus, noncommunicating hydrocephalus occurs when the flow of CSF has been impaired enough that intraventricular pressure increases proximal to the point of obstruction. The narrowing usually occurs at anatomic bottlenecks, such as the foramen of Monro, the cerebral aqueduct, and the foramina of Luschka and Magendie. The flow of CSF can be hindered by either extrinsic compression of CSF containing structures or intraventricular blockage, with varied causes such as congenital stenosis/hypoplasia, hemorrhage, neoplasm, metastasis, and infection (**Fig. 2**).[10] The symptoms of hydrocephalus are generally that of increased intracranial pressure, including headache, nausea, vomiting, papilledema, or altered mental status, particularly when the obstruction occurs acutely. This increased intracranial pressure can also result in brain herniation, coma, or rarely death. Additional signs and symptoms vary based on the specific etiology, such as symptoms of infection or metastatic disease, and may be helpful in directing the diagnostic workup.[10]

Imaging is often sought to determine the cause and location of noncommunicating hydrocephalus. In general, ventricular enlargement is seen proximal to the site of obstruction. Because it is fast and readily available, noncontrast CT is the study of choice in the emergent setting to diagnose hydrocephalus. The degree of ventricular dilation and which ventricles are involved can be evaluated, as well as changes in configuration including rounding of the frontal horns and third ventricle, and prominence of the temporal horns (**Fig. 3**A,B). Other changes suggestive of hydrocephalus can be visualized as well, such as hypoattenuation of the white matter adjacent to the frontal horns related to transependymal CSF flow, effacement of sulci from mass effect, and, in extreme cases, brain herniation (see **Fig. 3**C).[10]

MRI can be used to further characterize hydrocephalus or as a more complete initial evaluation in a subacute presentation, as well as potentially identifying a causative lesion. In addition to ventricular enlargement, supportive findings for hydrocephalus on MRI include enlargement of third ventricular recesses, bulging of the third ventricle floor, and T2 hyperintense signal in the paraventricular white matter which represents transependymal CSF flow (see **Fig. 3**D).[11] Normal CSF flow results in a flow-void on T2-weighted turbo spin-echo MR images in the cerebral aqueduct that may not be present if there is reduced flow. CSF flow may be further quantified using phase-contrast MRI techniques. This can be useful in assessing the severity of aqueductal stenosis. High spatial resolution sequences, such as steady-state free precession (SSFP) images, including the widely used 3D-constructive interference in the steady state (3D-CISS), can be valuable in the detection and characterization of thin obstructive structures such as cystic lesions and membranes.[12]

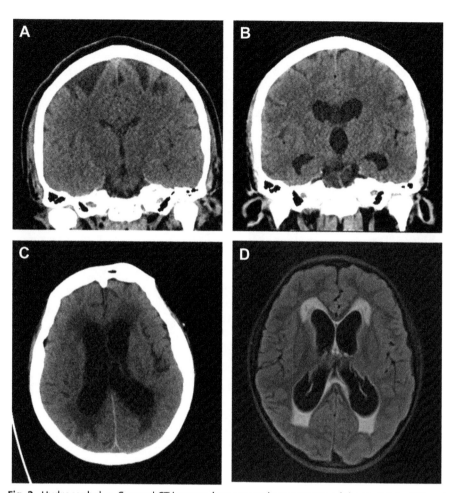

Fig. 2. Hydrocephalus. Coronal CT images show normal appearance of the ventricles (*A*) and dilatation of the bodies and temporal horns of the lateral ventricles and third ventricle, in the same patient, after the development of hydrocephalus (*B*). Axial CT shows dilatation of the lateral ventricles and hypodensity in the periventricular white mater consistent with transependymal CSF flow (*C*). Similarly, axial T2-FLAIR MRI shows dilatation of the ventricles as well as hyperintense signal in the periventricular white matter here demonstrating transependymal flow (*D*).

Imaging is also important in following patients after treatment. Noncontrast CT or MRI may be used to follow the ventricular size and assess treatment success and stability. Flow-sensitive sequences are useful in identifying flow between the prepontine cistern and the third ventricle resulting from CSF flow through a patent third ventriculostomy.[11,13]

Communicating Hydrocephalus with Obstruction

When the point of CSF flow obstruction occurs outside of the ventricles, it is described as communicating hydrocephalus with obstruction. The term "nonobstructive hydrocephalus" is sometimes used to refer to this process, but obstructive processes are likely involved in many cases of communicating hydrocephalus, such as in the case

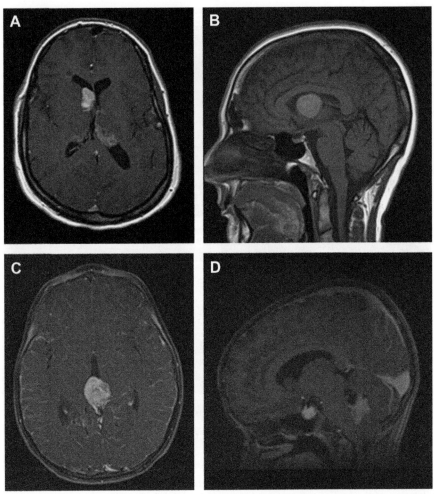

Fig. 3. Example potentially obstructive mass lesions. Axial contrast-enhanced T1 weighted image in a patient with tuberous sclerosis shows an enhancing subependymal giant cell astrocytoma at the right foramen of Monro (*A*). Midline sagittal T1 weighted image shows an intrinsically T1 hyperintense colloid cyst at the level of the foramina of Monro (*B*). Axial contrast-enhanced T1 weighted image shows an enhancing pineoblastoma at risk of obstructing the cerebral aqueduct (*C*). Sagittal contrast-enhanced T1 weighted image shows an enhancing medulloblastoma in the fourth ventricle (*D*).

of subarachnoid hemorrhage.[14–16] For this reason, the term communicating hydrocephalus with obstruction is useful to describe etiologies stemming from the restriction of CSF flow at a point between the basal cisterns and reabsorption. Causes of communicating hydrocephalus with obstruction include subarachnoid hemorrhage, leptomeningeal carcinomatosis, or meningitis.[9] This type of hydrocephalus can also produce dilation of the ventricles, likely related to amplified transient pressure gradients associated with CSF pulsation.

Communicating hydrocephalus with obstruction can occur acutely after subarachnoid hemorrhage or can be a delayed complication presenting weeks or months after the incident. The incidence of hydrocephalus after aneurysmal subarachnoid hemorrhage is estimated to be 20% to 30%.[16] The mechanism of hydrocephalus may be blockage of arachnoid granulations or fibrosis causing blockage of the foramina of Luschka and Magendie.[16]

Diffuse dural metastatic disease may also produce communicating hydrocephalus with obstruction. Leptomeningeal metastatic disease may involve the pia mater, arachnoid mater, and the subarachnoid space. Symptoms vary, but can include cranial nerve deficits, back pain, visual disturbances, seizures, and headache.[17] The proposed mechanisms of these symptoms are increased intracranial pressure, compression and invasion of the brain and spinal cord, ischemia, metabolic competition, and disruption of the blood–brain barrier.[18]

Meningitis is another important etiology of communicating hydrocephalus with obstruction. Generally, in uncomplicated meningitis, imaging is not necessary. CT imaging can be performed when there is clinical concern for increased intracranial pressure before lumbar puncture (LP). LP is safe without prior CT for patients with normal neurologic examination, age less than 60, immunocompetent, no history of CNS disease, and no seizures within 1 week.[19] The cause of CSF flow obstruction is described as both exudates blocking CSF absorption at the arachnoid granulations, as well as increased CSF protein concentration impairing CSF absorption.[20]

Communicating Hydrocephalus without Obstruction

In contrast to hydrocephalus originating from CSF flow obstruction, communicating hydrocephalus without obstruction occurs as a result of over production of CSF. When the rate of CSF production overwhelms the ability of the body to reabsorb it, the result is increased intraventricular pressure and dilation of the ventricles, causing hydrocephalus. Increased CSF production can be a result of choroid plexus tumors, along with more rare conditions including hypertrophy of the choroid plexus and villous hyperplasia of the choroid.[9,21–24] Choroid plexus tumors have an incidence of 0.05 per 100,000 in the general US population and a pediatric incidence of 0.1 per 100,000.[25] Clinically, choroid plexus tumors can present with headache, diplopia, or signs of increased intracranial pressure, such as nausea and vomiting.[26] In infants, increased head circumference, bulging fontanelles, and neurologic delay can occur, with these symptoms of hydrocephalus often being the presenting symptom.[27,28] Choroid plexus papilloma (CPP) represents the more common type of choroid plexus tumor, with choroid plexus carcinoma being more rare.[29]

On CT, CPP is often isodense or hyperdense in comparison to gray matter, with a slightly irregular border, and a minority of tumors contain calcifications. On T1-weighted MRI CPP appears as a large heterogeneously enhancing lobulated mass (**Fig. 4**). T2-weighted imaging can show heterogenous hyperintensity. Imaging, however, cannot reliably distinguish between malignant and benign choroid plexus neoplasms.[29]

Villous hypertrophy of the choroid plexus is very rare. Imaging findings include equal and diffuse enlargement of the choroid plexus of both lateral ventricles, evident on both MRI and CT. Histologic examination of choroid tissue shows normal choroid plexus structure, which can help to differentiate villous hypertrophy of the choroid plexus from CPP.[22,29]

Idiopathic Intracranial Hypertension

Idiopathic intracranial hypertension (IIH) has an incidence of approximately 3 per 100,000 in women, which is ten times greater than the incidence in men. Recently, rates of IIH have been increasing. There is a strong correlation between increased IIH incidence and increased obesity rates, with the incidence of IIH in obese women being

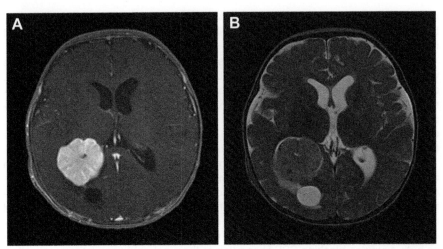

Fig. 4. Choroid plexus papilloma. Contrast-enhanced T1 weighted (*A*) and T2 weighted (*B*) axial images show an enhancing choroid plexus papilloma located in the trigone of the right lateral ventricle and enlargement of the lateral ventricles.

approximately 22 per 100,000.[30] Unlike many other causes of headache associated with increased intracranial pressure, IIH is not associated with hydrocephalus, and its etiology remains unclear. Some hypotheses propose CSF hypersecretion or CSF outflow obstruction as the cause of increased intracranial pressure, as is the case in communicating hydrocephalus both with and without obstruction, though the lack of hydrocephalus in IIH makes these hypotheses less likely. Sinus stenosis at the transverse-sigmoid sinus junction is also associated with IIH, and stenting has been shown to alleviate symptoms in some cases, suggesting an association between these conditions (**Fig. 5**).[31,32] These and other proposed causes are reviewed elsewhere.[33]

Headache is present in 84% of patients with IIH and is often a presenting symptom.[34] This headache is typically global and worsens with maneuvers that increase ICP, such as the Valsalva maneuver. Headaches are often worse in the mornings and can be associated with nausea and vomiting. More than half of patients also experience pulsatile tinnitus,[34] which is likely secondary to turbulent flow across stenotic transverse sinuses.[35] Papilledema is also common, and can be the only presenting finding.[36] Transient visual obscurations occur in 68% of patients with IIH and are associated with worse degrees of papilledema.[34,37] The feared consequence of IIH is irreversible vision loss.

MRI is the preferred test for an initial evaluation in suspected IIH. MRI can rule out other causes of increased intracranial pressure when IIH is suspected, as well as identify findings indicative of IIH.[38,39] Many of the imaging findings in IIH are MRI correlates of elevated intracranial pressure. These include concavity of the superior margin of the pituitary deformity with partially empty sella turcica (**Fig. 6**A), enlarged Meckel's caves (see **Fig. 6**B), optic nerve sheath dilation (see **Fig. 6**C), optic nerve tortuosity, and narrowing of the dural venous sinuses (see **Fig. 6**E).[40,41] Posterior globe flattening or protrusion of the optic disc (see **Fig. 6**D) on MRI has been reported in IIH,[41,42] though a more recent study suggests that this finding may have little diagnostic utility because its sensitivity is significantly lower than clinical fundoscopic examination.[40] MR venography can be used to evaluate for venous sinus stenosis in IIH.[32] In one study, high degrees of stenosis were found to be 94.7% sensitive and 93.5% specific for IIH, making MRV a diagnostically significant method for evaluating IIH (see **Fig. 5**A).[43]

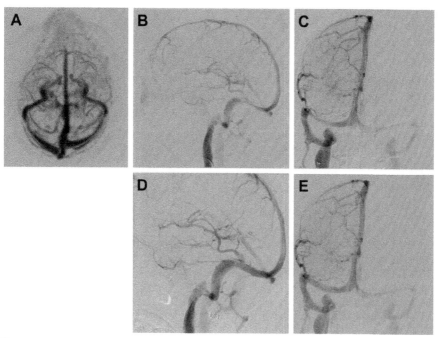

Fig. 5. Transverse sinus stenosis in idiopathic intracranial hypertension. Axial, maximum intensity projection of a dynamic, contrast-enhanced MRI venogram shows stenosis of the distal bilateral transverse sinuses (A). Images from catheter angiogram show stenosis of the distal transverse sinus before stenting (B) and (C) and with widely patent sinus after stent placement (D) and (E).

DECREASED INTRACRANIAL PRESSURE

When decreased intracranial pressure occurs, it is usually because of a CSF leak. This loss of CSF results in an orthostatic headache, where the headache improves with recumbency and worsens when upright. The pathophysiology of headache caused by decreased intracranial pressure is unclear, though it is hypothesized to be from traction on structures sensitive to pain when upright, as reduced CSF volume may provide less support for the brain.[44–46] Alternatively, cerebral venous dilation may occur secondary to reduce intracranial pressure, resulting in pain from the distention of these veins.[44,46,47] The source of the CSF leak may be due to spontaneous leaks, trauma, or iatrogenic injury. This can occur at any location within the neuroaxis, although CSF leak within the spine is much more likely to present with headache than CSF leak in the head. Trauma causing an opening through the dura, such as in the case of brachial plexus avulsion may result in intracranial hypotenion.[48] Similarly, procedures that penetrate the dura can lead to iatrogenic CSF leaks, such as LP, unintentional dural puncture during epidural injection or surgery, intrathecal catheters, or excessive CSF shunting.[44] We will focus on postdural puncture headache (PDPH) and spontaneous intracranial hypotension, both of which share imaging findings consistent with intracranial hypotension.[49]

Several imaging findings can support suspected intracranial hypotension. Pachymeningeal thickening and enhancement, that is smooth thickened dura circumferentially surrounding the brain and along the interhemispheric falx, with no signs of

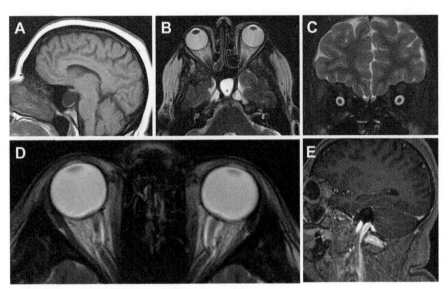

Fig. 6. Imaging findings in intracranial hypertension. Sagittal T1 weighted image showing the expansion of the sella turcica with small, flattened pituitary along the floor of the sella (*A*). Axial T2 weighted image showing prominence of Meckel's caves as well as prominent CSF in the sella (*B*). Coronal high-resolution T2 weighted image through the orbits shows the prominence of CSF space surrounding the optic nerves (*C*). Axial T2 weighted image shows bulging of the optic nerve heads with the indentation of the posterior contour of the globes, imaging correlate of papilledema (*D*). Sagittal postcontrast T1 weighted image shows narrowed concave appearance of the transverse sinus (*E*).

neoplastic disease such as nodular enhancement, is a classic finding (**Fig. 7**C).[50] On unenhanced MRI, T2 and FLAIR hyperintense pachymeningeal thickening (see **Fig. 7**A) can evolve into similarly T2 hyperintense and FLAIR hypointense subdural hygroma and even subdural hemorrhage with long standing intracranial hypotension.[49] The venous distension sign, where there is spinal and cerebral venous engorgement, has been described as both sensitive (94%) and specific (94%) for intracranial hypotension (see **Fig. 7**D).[51] This venous distension is best evaluated at the inferior margin of the dominant transverse sinus on T1 weighted sagittal MRI, which becomes convex when intracranial hypotension is present.[51] Other findings indicative of intracranial hypotension include caudal displacement of the brain and contents of the posterior fossa, effacement of the basal cisterns around the brainstem, and inferior displacement of the cerebellar tonsils which may be mistaken for a Chiari I malformation (see **Fig. 7**B).[49,52] Pituitary enlargement has also been reported with varying frequency (see **Fig. 7**B),[53–55] These findings are not always present, but in combination with the appropriate clinical history are supportive of intracranial hypotension.[56]

Postdural Puncture Headache

Postdural puncture headache (PDPH) is not uncommon, particularly after epidural anesthesia in obstetric patients. In this population, there is about a 1.5% risk of accidental dural puncture during epidural insertion, with PDPH occurring in 52% of those with an accidental dural puncture.[57] Dural puncture with spinal needles, used in LPs and spinal anesthesia procedures, can also lead to PDPH. The incidence of PDPH

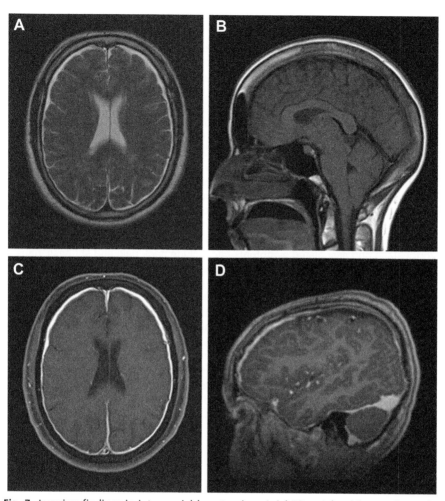

Fig. 7. Imaging findings in intracranial hypotension. Axial T2 weighted image shows the expansion of the extra-axial space (*A*). Sagittal T1 weight image shows sagging and inferior displacement of the brainstem, flattening of the belly of the pons with the effacement of the prepontine cistern, and herniation of the cerebellar tonsils. This image also shows expansion with superior convex margin of the pituitary (*B*). Axial enhanced T1 weighted image shows pachymeningeal enhancement (*C*). Sagittal enhanced T1 weighted image shows budging of the transverse sinus (*D*).

in a study of spinal needles used for spinal anesthesia was 4.6% overall, with a possible reduction in incidence to 2.8% to 3.1% when atraumatic needles were used.[58] Other studies have shown a larger effect of atraumatic needles in LP.[59] In addition to the hypothesized pathophysiology of low-pressure headaches mentioned above (Section 4.0), some have argued that puncture at the lumbar portion of the dura can lead to increased dural compliance, which may cause headache.[60] Symptoms associated with PDPH can more rarely include vestibular symptoms such as nausea, vomiting, or dizziness; cochlear symptoms such as hearing loss, hyperacusis, or tinnitus; ocular symptoms such as photophobia or diplopia; and musculoskeletal symptoms such as neck stiffness or scapular pain.[61]

While PDPH is usually diagnosed based on characteristic symptoms and a recent history of dural puncture,[46] development of focal neurologic signs, loss of the positional nature of the headache, or persistence of the headache are indications for neuroimaging.[62] In these cases, imaging can be used to evaluate for subdural hematoma, which is a rare but serious complication of dural puncture.[62,63]

Spontaneous Intracranial Hypotension

Spontaneous intracranial hypotension is a condition of CSF leakage arising without apparent precipitating dural injury. Incidence has been estimated as 1 per 50,000.[64] While the etiology of spontaneous intracranial hypotension is not well understood, there is an association with connective tissue disorders such as Marfan's syndrome and Ehlers–Danlos syndrome. This suggests that underlying structural weakness of the dura may predispose some patients to spontaneous CSF leaks. Other etiologies, including an association with degenerative disc disease, whereby irregular osteophytes have been hypothesized to tear the thecal sac, are reviewed elsewhere.[65] Like in PDPH, the headache associated with spontaneous intracranial hypotension is orthostatic and associated symptoms can include neck pain and stiffness, nausea and vomiting, hearing changes, and visual changes.[66]

Neuroimaging in spontaneous intracranial hypotension can be normal, but often shows typical signs of intracranial hypotension (Section 4.0).[45] In addition to MRI examination of the head and spine, other techniques have been used to detect and localize a site of CSF leak. These include techniques such as CT and MR myelography, dynamic myelography under fluoroscopy, and radioisotope cisternography. Detection of a leak may be a real diagnostic challenge. In one study, CT myelographic evidence of CSF leaks was found in only 55% of patients with spontaneous intracranial hypotension.[67] Conversely, when a large leak is present CT or MR myelography may provide critical information to localize the leak and guide surgical treatment. Radioisotope cisternography is useful in limited situations such as when cribriform plate or mastoid leak is suspected.[68,69]

SUMMARY

Headaches caused by changes in intracranial pressure are an important category of headache with specific clinical and imaging features. Understanding the major causes of altered intracranial pressure, including the clinical presentation and the role of imaging in each diagnosis is critical to guide the diagnostic evaluation of these patients. Elements of a patient's history and clinical presentation may indicate a headache is related to changes in intracranial pressure as well as differentiate those with increased or decreased intracranial pressure. These headaches often require diagnostic imaging. Specific imaging findings may confirm the relationship of the headache to changes in intracranial pressure and suggest a causative etiology. In certain cases, additional specialized neuroimaging, including MR venography, dynamic myelography, nuclear medicine, and advanced MRI sequences may add additional diagnostic power in identifying the underlying etiology and directing clinical management.

CLINICS CARE POINTS

- Signs and symptoms which may initially suggest the presence of an intracranial pressure disorder include: neurologic deficit, positional headache, papilledema, progressive headache, signs of infection or history of cancer.

- LP is generally safe without prior CT for immunocompetent patients with normal neurologic examination, age less than 60, no history of CNS disease, and no seizures within 1 week.
- The American College of Radiology Appropriateness Criteria is an evidence-based resource to aid selection of the best imaging study for a wide variety of clinical scenarios.

REFERENCES

1. Headache Classification Committee of the International Headache Society (IHS) The International Classification of Headache Disorders, 3rd edition. Cephalalgia 2018;38(1):1–211.
2. Ravishankar K. WHICH headache to investigate, WHEN, and HOW? Headache 2016;56(10):1685–97.
3. Do TP, Remmers A, Schytz HW, et al. Red and orange flags for secondary headaches in clinical practice. Neurology 2019;92(3):134–44.
4. Whitehead MT, Cardenas AM, Corey AS, et al. ACR Appropriateness Criteria: Headache. J Am Coll Radiol 2019;16(11S):S364–77.
5. Bothwell SW, Janigro D, Patabendige A. Cerebrospinal fluid dynamics and intracranial pressure elevation in neurological diseases. Fluids Barriers CNS 2019; 16(1):9.
6. Rekate HL. A contemporary definition and classification of hydrocephalus. Semin Pediatr Neurol 2009;16(1):9–15.
7. Isaacs AM, Riva-Cambrin J, Yavin D, et al. Age-specific global epidemiology of hydrocephalus: Systematic review, metanalysis and global birth surveillance. PLoS One 2018;13(10):e0204926.
8. Bir SC, Patra DP, Maiti TK, et al. Epidemiology of adult-onset hydrocephalus: institutional experience with 2001 patients. Neurosurg Focus 2016;41(3):E5.
9. Agarwal A, Bathla G, Kanekar S. Imaging of communicating hydrocephalus. Semin Ultrasound CT MRI 2016;37(2):100–8.
10. Maller VV, Gray RI. Noncommunicating Hydrocephalus. Semin Ultrasound CT MRI 2016;37(2):109–19.
11. Hodel J, Rahmouni A, Zins M, et al. Magnetic resonance imaging of noncommunicating hydrocephalus. World Neurosurg 2013;79(2, Supplement):S21.e9–12.
12. Dinçer A, Kohan S, Ozek MM. Is all "communicating" hydrocephalus really communicating? Prospective study on the value of 3D-constructive interference in steady state sequence at 3T. AJNR Am J Neuroradiol 2009;30(10):1898–906.
13. Hoffmann KT, Lehmann TN, Baumann C, et al. CSF flow imaging in the management of third ventriculostomy with a reversed fast imaging with steady-state precession sequence. Eur Radiol 2003;13(6):1432–7.
14. Rekate HL. A consensus on the classification of hydrocephalus: its utility in the assessment of abnormalities of cerebrospinal fluid dynamics. Childs Nerv Syst 2011;27(10):1535.
15. Chen S, Luo J, Reis C, et al. Hydrocephalus after Subarachnoid Hemorrhage: Pathophysiology, Diagnosis, and Treatment. Biomed Res Int 2017;2017: e8584753.
16. Germanwala AV, Huang J, Tamargo RJ. Hydrocephalus after aneurysmal subarachnoid hemorrhage. Neurosurg Clin N Am 2010;21(2):263–70.
17. Nayar G, Ejikeme T, Chongsathidkiet P, et al. Leptomeningeal disease: current diagnostic and therapeutic strategies. Oncotarget 2017;8(42):73312–28.
18. Le Rhun E, Taillibert S, Chamberlain MC. Carcinomatous meningitis: leptomeningeal metastases in solid tumors. Surg Neurol Int 2013;4(Suppl 4):S265–88.

19. Hasbun R, Abrahams J, Jekel J, et al. Computed tomography of the head before lumbar puncture in adults with suspected meningitis. N Engl J Med 2001;345(24): 1727–33.

20. Hughes DC, Raghavan A, Mordekar SR, et al. Role of imaging in the diagnosis of acute bacterial meningitis and its complications. Postgrad Med J 2010;86(1018): 478–85.

21. Ceddia A, Di Rocco C, Carlucci A. [Hypersecretive congenital hydrocephalus due to choroid plexus villous hypertrophy associated with controlateral papilloma]. Minerva Pediatr 1993;45(9):363–7.

22. Hirano H, Hirahara K, Asakura T, et al. Hydrocephalus due to villous hypertrophy of the choroid plexus in the lateral ventricles. Case report. J Neurosurg 1994; 80(2):321–3.

23. Britz GW, Kim DK, Loeser JD. Hydrocephalus secondary to diffuse villous hyperplasia of the choroid plexus: case report and review of the literature. J Neurosurg 1996;85(4):689–91.

24. Aziz AA, Coleman L, Morokoff A, et al. Diffuse choroid plexus hyperplasia: an under-diagnosed cause of hydrocephalus in children? Pediatr Radiol 2005; 35(8):815–8.

25. Ostrom QT, Gittleman H, Farah P, et al. CBTRUS statistical report: primary brain and central nervous system tumors diagnosed in the United States in 2006-2010. Neuro-Oncol 2013;15(Suppl 2):ii1–56.

26. Crea A, Bianco A, Cossandi C, et al. Choroid plexus carcinoma in adults: literature review and first report of a location into the third ventricle. World Neurosurg 2020;133:302–7.

27. Hart S, Avery R, Barron J. Late recurrence of choroid plexus carcinoma. Childs Nerv Syst 2020;36(8):1601–6.

28. Pascual-Castroviejo I, Villarejo F, Perez-Higueras A, et al. Childhood choroid plexus neoplasms. A study of 14 cases less than 2 years old. Eur J Pediatr 1983;140(1):51–6.

29. Guermazi A, De kerviler E, Zagdanski A-M, et al. Diagnostic imaging of choroid plexus disease: pictorial review. Clin Radiol 2000;55(7):503–16.

30. Kilgore KP, Lee MS, Leavitt JA, et al. Re-evaluating the incidence of idiopathic intracranial hypertension in an era of increasing obesity. Ophthalmology 2017; 124(5):697–700.

31. Dinkin MJ, Patsalides A. Venous sinus stenting in idiopathic intracranial hypertension: results of a prospective trial. J Neuroophthalmol 2017;37(2):113–21.

32. Farb RI, Vanek I, Scott JN, et al. Idiopathic intracranial hypertension: the prevalence and morphology of sinovenous stenosis. Neurology 2003;60(9):1418–24.

33. Markey KA, Mollan SP, Jensen RH, et al. Understanding idiopathic intracranial hypertension: mechanisms, management, and future directions. Lancet Neurol 2016;15(1):78–91.

34. Wall M, Kupersmith MJ, Kieburtz KD, et al. The idiopathic intracranial hypertension treatment trial: clinical profile at baseline. JAMA Neurol 2014;71(6):693–701.

35. Thurtell MJ. Idiopathic intracranial hypertension. Contin Minneap Minn 2019; 25(5):1289–309.

36. Galvin JA, Van Stavern GP. Clinical characterization of idiopathic intracranial hypertension at the Detroit Medical Center. J Neurol Sci 2004;223(2):157–60.

37. Wall M, Falardeau J, Fletcher WA, et al. Risk factors for poor visual outcome in patients with idiopathic intracranial hypertension. Neurology 2015;85(9):799–805.

38. Hoffmann J, Mollan SP, Paemeleire K, et al. European Headache Federation guideline on idiopathic intracranial hypertension. J Headache Pain 2018; 19(1):93.
39. Friedman DI, Liu GT, Digre KB. Revised diagnostic criteria for the pseudotumor cerebri syndrome in adults and children. Neurology 2013;81(13):1159–65.
40. Hoffmann J, Huppertz H-J, Schmidt C, et al. Morphometric and volumetric MRI changes in idiopathic intracranial hypertension. Cephalalgia 2013;33(13): 1075–84.
41. Agid R, Farb RI, Willinsky RA, et al. Idiopathic intracranial hypertension: the validity of cross-sectional neuroimaging signs. Neuroradiology 2006;48(8):521–7.
42. Brodsky MC, Vaphiades M. Magnetic resonance imaging in pseudotumor cerebri. Ophthalmology 1998;105(9):1686–93.
43. Carvalho GB da S, Matas SL de A, Idagawa MH, et al. A new index for the assessment of transverse sinus stenosis for diagnosing idiopathic intracranial hypertension. J Neurointerventional Surg 2017;9(2):173–7.
44. Schievink WI, Deline CR. Headache secondary to intracranial hypotension. Curr Pain Headache Rep 2014;18(11):457.
45. Friedman DI. Headaches due to low and high intracranial pressure. Contin Lifelong Learn Neurol 2018;24(4):1066.
46. Peralta F, Devroe S. Any news on the postdural puncture headache front? Best Pract Res Clin Anaesthesiol 2017;31(1):35–47.
47. Grant R, Condon B, Hart I, et al. Changes in intracranial CSF volume after lumbar puncture and their relationship to post-LP headache. J Neurol Neurosurg Psychiatry 1991;54(5):440–2.
48. Hébert-Blouin M-N, Mokri B, Shin AY, et al. Cerebrospinal fluid volume-depletion headaches in patients with traumatic brachial plexus injury. J Neurosurg 2013; 118(1):149–54.
49. Forghani R, Farb RI. Diagnosis and temporal evolution of signs of intracranial hypotension on MRI of the brain. Neuroradiology 2008;50(12):1025–34.
50. Fedder SL. Pachymeningeal gadolinium enhancement of the lumbar region secondary to neuraxis hypotension. Spine 1999;24(5):463–4.
51. Farb RI, Forghani R, Lee SK, et al. The venous distension sign: a diagnostic sign of intracranial hypotension at MR imaging of the brain. AJNR Am J Neuroradiol 2007;28(8):1489–93.
52. Messori A, Simonetti BF, Regnicolo L, et al. Spontaneous intracranial hypotension: the value of brain measurements in diagnosis by MRI. Neuroradiology 2001;43(6):453–61.
53. Shimazu N, Oba H, Aoki S, et al. [Pituitary enlargement in spontaneous intracranial hypotension on MRI]. Nihon Igaku Hoshasen Gakkai Zasshi 1998;58(7): 349–52.
54. Alvarez-Linera J, Escribano J, Benito-León J, et al. Pituitary enlargement in patients with intracranial hypotension syndrome. Neurology 2000;55(12):1895–7.
55. Ferrante E, Savino A, Sances G, et al. Spontaneous intracranial hypotension syndrome: report of twelve cases. Headache 2004;44(6):615–22.
56. Corbonnois G, O'Neill T, Brabis-Henner A, et al. Unrecognized dural puncture during epidural analgesia in obstetrics later confirmed by brain imaging. Ann Fr Anesth Reanim 2010;29(7–8):584–8.
57. Choi PT, Galinski SE, Takeuchi L, et al. PDPH is a common complication of neuraxial blockade in parturients: a meta-analysis of obstetrical studies. Can J Anesth 2003;50(5):460–9.

58. Vallejo MC, Mandell GL, Sabo DP, et al. Postdural puncture headache: a random-ized comparison of five spinal needles in obstetric patients. Anesth Analg 2000; 91(4):916–20.

59. Lavi R, Yernitzky D, Rowe JM, et al. Standard vs atraumatic Whitacre needle for diagnostic lumbar puncture: a randomized trial. Neurology 2006;67(8):1492–4.

60. Levine DN, Rapalino O. The pathophysiology of lumbar puncture headache. J Neurol Sci 2001;192(1):1–8.

61. Lybecker H, Djernes M, Schmidt JF. Postdural puncture headache (PDPH): Onset, duration, severity, and associated symptoms: An analysis of 75 consecu-tive patients with PDPH. Acta Anaesthesiol Scand 1995;39(5):605–12.

62. Cuypers V, Van de Velde M, Devroe S. Intracranial subdural haematoma following neuraxial anaesthesia in the obstetric population: a literature review with analysis of 56 reported cases. Int J Obstet Anesth 2016;25:58–65.

63. Kale A, Emmez H, Pişkin Ö, et al. Postdural puncture subdural hematoma or post-dural puncture headache?: two cases report. Korean J Anesthesiol 2015;68(5): 509–12.

64. Schievink W, Roiter V. Epidemiology of cervical artery dissection. Handb Cereb Artery Dissection 2005;20:12–5.

65. Graff-Radford SB, Schievink WI. High-pressure headaches, low-pressure syn-dromes, and CSF leaks: diagnosis and management. Headache J Head Face Pain 2014;54(2):394–401.

66. Schievink WI. Misdiagnosis of Spontaneous Intracranial Hypotension. Arch Neu-rol 2003;60(12):1713–8.

67. Kranz PG, Tanpitukpongse TP, Choudhury KR, et al. Imaging signs in sponta-neous intracranial hypotension: prevalence and relationship to CSF Pressure. AJNR Am J Neuroradiol 2016;37(7):1374–8.

68. Mokri B. Radioisotope cisternography in spontaneous CSF leaks: interpretations and misinterpretations. Headache J Head Face Pain 2014;54(8):1358–68.

69. Monteith TS, Kralik SF, Dillon WP, et al. The utility of radioisotope cisternography in low CSF/volume syndromes compared to myelography. Cephalalgia 2016; 36(13):1291–5.

Headache Attributed to Disorder of the Cranium and Base of the Skull

Amit Agarwal, MD[a],*, Sangam Kanekar, MD, DNB[b]

KEYWORDS

- Skull base • Calvarium • CT • MRI • Radionuclide • Tumor • Infection
- Inflammation

KEY POINTS

- Section 11 of the International Classification of Headache Disorders (ICHD-3) provides "Headache or facial pain attributed to disorder of the cranium, neck, eyes, ears, nose, sinuses, teeth, mouth or other facial or cervical structure."
- Includes new headaches occurring for the first time in a characterization distribution and pattern or could be preexisting with significant worsening in close temporal relationship to the anatomic regions mentioned earlier.
- Main diagnostic criterion for these headaches relies on clinical, laboratory, and/or imaging evidence of lesion in these regions and not attributed to another ICHD-3 code.
- Imaging evaluation plays an important role in identification of structural lesion in this class of headaches, unlike primary headaches and many other subtypes of secondary causes.

INTRODUCTION AND TERMINOLOGY

The International Headache Society (IHS) released the third edition of the International Classification of Headache Disorders (ICHD-3) in 2018. The basic segregation of primary and secondary headaches was preserved from the prior editions. Primary headache includes conditions where headache itself was the problem and not a symptom of any underlying condition. The list of cases for secondary headaches is much more diverse and exhaustive, with wide range of conditions with further subtype classifications.[1] This article elaborates on secondary headaches attributed to disorders of the cranium and base of skull (**Table 1**), including headaches attributed to disorders of the ear, which is a part of the calvarium. There is strong clinical overlap with headaches attributed to cervicogenic causes and retropharyngeal tendonitis, which are

[a] Department of Radiology, Mayo Clinic, Jacksonville, FL, USA; [b] Radiology Research, Division of Neuroradiology, Penn State Health, Penn State College of Medicine, Mail Code H066 500 University Drive, Hershey, PA 17033, USA
* Corresponding author. 8613 Homeplace Drive, Jacksonville, FL 32256.
E-mail address: amitmamc@gmail.com

Neurol Clin 40 (2022) 563–589
https://doi.org/10.1016/j.ncl.2022.03.001
0733-8619/22/© 2022 Elsevier Inc. All rights reserved.

Table 1
Headache or facial pain attributed to disorder of the cranium, neck, eyes, ears, nose, sinuses, teeth, mouth, or other facial or cervical structure

11.1 Headache attributed to disorder of cranial bone (including skull base)	Headache has developed or significantly worsened in temporal relation to the onset of the cranial bone disorder	Imaging evaluation with CT and MRI occasionally commonly indicated
11.4 Headache attributed to disorder of the ears	Headache caused by an inflammatory, neoplastic, or other disorder of 1 or both ears, with involvement of mastoids and petrous bones	Clinical diagnosis in most cases with imaging (CT) reserved when suspicion of petrous, mastoid, or intracranial complications
11.2.1 Cervicogenic headache	Headache causally associated with cervical myofascial pain sources, including upper cervical facets, muscles, and dura of the upper cervical cord	Imaging evaluation with radiographs and MRI commonly done for work-up
11.2.2 Headache attributed to retropharyngeal tendonitis	Headache caused by inflammation or calcification in the retropharyngeal soft tissues	Clinical diagnosis with characteristic imaging findings on CT
11.7 Headache attributed to temporomandibular joint	Headache caused by a disorder involving structures in the temporomandibular region, including joint disorders	Clinical diagnosis with increasing role and utilization of imaging (radiographs and MRI)

Adapted from Headache Classification Committee of the International Headache Society (IHS) The International Classification of Headache Disorders, 3rd edition. Cephalalgia. 2018;38(1):1-211. https://doi.org/10.1177/0333102417738202; with permission

briefly discussed here, although classified separately in the ICHD manual. All of these conditions are included in section 11 of the ICHD-3 listed as "Headache or facial pain attributed to disorder of the cranium, neck, eyes, ears, nose, sinuses, teeth, mouth or other facial or cervical structure." These headaches could be new disorders occurring for the first time in a characterization distribution and pattern or could be preexisting with significant worsening in close temporal relationship to the anatomic regions mentioned earlier. This section excludes headaches secondary to trauma, which might still conform to these anatomic regions. The main diagnostic criterion for these headaches relies on clinical, laboratory, and/or imaging evidence of lesion in these regions and not attributed to another ICHD-3 code. Imaging evaluation plays an important role in identification of structural lesion in this class of headaches, unlike primary headaches and many other subtypes of secondary causes.

Table 1 describes the common calvarial structural lesions presenting with secondary headaches where imaging plays a vital role in diagnosis. Significant clinical overlap exists with cervicogenic disorders, also discussed in this article. Ear disorders, although classified as a separate subset, have significant imaging and clinical overlap with the cranial causes.

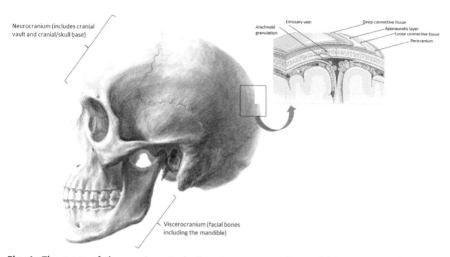

Fig. 1. The parts of the cranium, including the neurocranium, which encases and protects the brain, and the viscerocranium, which includes the facial bones, including the mandible. The scalp consists of numerous layers (*inset*), with the pericranium being particularly sensitive to pain sensation.

The ICHD-3 separately classifies facial pain and painful lesions of the cranial nerves under section 13 and includes trigeminal neuralgia and glossopharyngeal neuralgia; however in many cases the difference from the cranial bone cause is subtle. Facial pain may be the primary feature of many structural lesions of the calvarium and skull base given the proximity of these cranial nerves. Often, 2 different subtypes of headache may be attributed to a single patient given the anatomic proximity.

ANATOMY AND PATHOPHYSIOLOGY OF HEADACHE IN CRANIAL LESIONS

The term cranium is derived from the Greek term kranion and includes the neurocranium, which encases and protects the brain, and the viscerocranium, which includes the facial bones, including the mandible (**Fig. 1**). The embryology of these structures is different and, in general practice, the term cranium is usually used for neurocranium or the calvarium and includes the cranial vault and the cranial base (simply referred to as skull base). The cranial vault consists of flat bones developing from the membranous neurocranium with intramembranous ossification and no intervening cartilage and includes the frontal, parietal, occipital and squamous temporal bone.[2] The cartilaginous neurocranium has endochondral ossification and forms the skull base, including the sphenoid, petrous, and mastoid portion of the temporal bone. The ossification pattern is like the facial bones.[3] The skull base has a complex anatomy and is broadly divided into 3 zones: anterior, middle, and posterior cranial fossas with numerous foramina for vessels and nerves (**Fig. 2**).The posterior margins of the lesser wing of sphenoid, the anterior clinoid processes, and tuberculum sellae demarcate the anterior from middle (central) cranial fossas. The superior part of the petrous temporal and the dorsum sellae separate the middle and posterior skull base.[4,5] The sensory innervation of meninges and their related blood vessels are the major intracranial pathway for primary and secondary headaches. The extracranial origin of headaches is primarily through the calvarium periosteum. The nerves that innervate the scalp skin have collaterals through the galea aponeurotica and terminate in the calvarium periosteum,

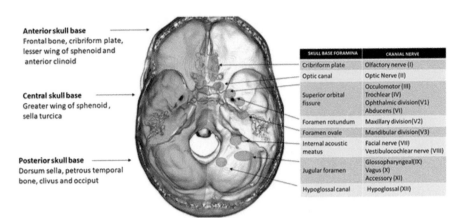

Fig. 2. The 3 compartments of the cranial base (anterior, central, and posterior) and their boundaries along with the prominent foramina and the exiting nerve roots.

which forms the major pathway for extracranial headache. Other deep cephalic tissues, including the pericranial muscles and arteries such as the superficial temporal artery, might also be sources of headache, but their role as the main pathway remains uncertain. Although the intracranial and extracranial sensory pathways have traditionally been considered to be separate, there is increasing evidence to support sharing and overlap of these innervations. Apart from extracranial, the calvarium periosteum likely has intracranial trajectories resulting in recent significant increase in therapies aimed at superficial nerve blockage for treatment of intracranial and extracranial headaches. Many lesions of the skull are, surprisingly, not associated with headache, given the limited sensitivity of the bones of the skull to pain. The periosteum is the main sensory pathway for extracranial headaches, and skull lesions primarily cause headaches by periosteal involvement. Cranial lesions most likely to result in headache include inflammatory lesions, rapidly expansile lesions such as Paget disease, or lesions with high osteoclastic activity such as multiple myeloma. Inflammatory lesions such as skull-base osteomyelitis (SBO) are more likely to cause headache than neoplastic lesions such as intraosseous hemangiomas. The mastoid and petrous bones are commonly involved in inflammatory conditions, such as otomastoiditis, and have numerous lesions resulting in headaches.[6–8] Many lesions of the skull, such as hemangiomas, are usually incidental findings on imaging and should not be considered as the cause of headache if other criteria are not fulfilled.

IMAGING APPROACH TO SKULL-BASE AND CALVARIAL LESIONS

Imaging is not recommended for most headaches, which usually resolve spontaneously. Imaging is usually not appropriate for headaches (new or chronic) with classic clinical features of primary causes such as migraine and tension headaches. Chronic headache with new features or increasing frequency or change in pattern may prompt imaging work-up, which may be appropriate in certain clinical settings. The American College of Radiology came out with the appropriateness criteria categorizing conditions from usually appropriate to usually not appropriate. However, given the rapid availability and ease of access of imaging modalities, the threshold to get imaging is very low. The American Board of Internal Medicine (ABIM) started the Choosing Wisely campaign, which seeks to advance a national dialogue on avoiding unnecessary

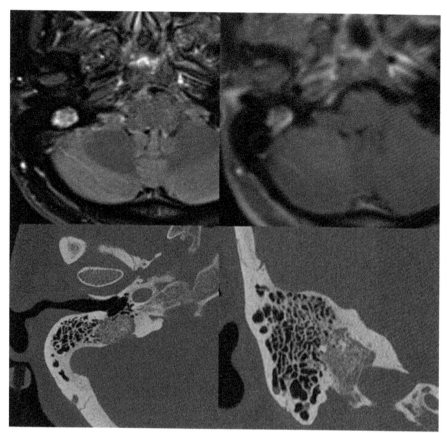

Fig. 3. Enhancing T2 hyperintense lesion along the right posterior skull-base (top row) with indeterminate findings on MRI seen as focal enhancing lesion within the petromastoid bone. Axial and coronal CT (bottom row) shows trabeculated well-circumscribed lesion classic of intraosseous hemangioma. This case serves as an example as to how CT is the modality of choice for most cranial osseous lesions.

medical tests, treatments, and procedures. The appropriate category included sudden or new unexplained headaches, neurologic deficit, or other red flags such as visual symptoms, history of malignancy, or immunocompromise. Although imaging for headache is unnecessary in most cases, it is of utmost importance to know what the best modality is when neuroimaging is indicated.[9,10] As with other conditions, a one-size-does-not-fit-all approach is important, and what may be appropriate for sudden-onset acute headache might not be the best examination for headaches with mastoid tenderness. The primary imaging modality for evaluation of cranial lesions is computed tomography (CT), with MRI reserved for a smaller subset. Radionuclide scans are increasingly being used for calvarial and skull-base inflammatory lesions and as a part of the work-up for systemic conditions such as metastasis and myeloma.

Unenhanced CT is the first line of imaging in most headaches with suspected cranial (osseous) lesions. High-resolution submillimeter multiplanar reconstruction can be created from single acquisition with excellent cortical and trabecular details. CT

Table 2 Prototype skull-base MRI protocol		
Routine brain sequences	• T1-weighted sagittal • T2 FLAIR axial	One set of non–fat-saturated T1-weighted images is necessary because it provides excellent anatomic details
Dedicated skull-base sequences	• T2-weighted (fat saturated) axial and coronal • Contrast-enhanced T1-weighted (fat-saturated Dixon) axial and coronal • 3D spoiled gradient (acquired in axial with sagittal and coronal reformations)	Dixon sequence based on chemical shift is now the preferred technique for fat suppression with higher uniformity, lesser artifacts
Diffusion sequences (part of routine brain imaging)	• Nonechoplanar (EPI) diffusion sequences (DWI) preferred to multishot or single-shot EPI for skull-base disorder	Non-EPI sequences provide higher resolution, up to 2 mm, with significantly lower skull-base susceptibility artifacts compared with EPI and DWI

Abbreviations: DWI, diffusion-weighted imaging; EPI, echoplanar imaging; FLAIR, fluid-attenuated inversion recovery.

temporal bones can provide even better details if the clinical suspicion is for skull-base or ear disorder. Contrast-enhanced CT is usually not needed because any significant lesion on the noncontrast scan is invariably further worked up with contrast-enhanced MRI. Vascular complications such as venous sinus involvement can be evaluated with CT/magnetic resonance (MR) angiogram or venogram studies. MR has definite superiority over CT when looking for intracranial complications and soft-tissue details; however, when the suspicion is for an osseous lesion, CT usually provides a quick answer and is sufficient. In fact, many lesions that might look concerning or equivocal between benign and malignant can be easily be demarcated by a simple noncontrast CT scan (**Fig. 3**).[11] The single most important prognostic factor for cranial lesions is the presence or absence of dural invasion, which determines the surgical approach and risk of postoperative neurologic deficits. Extradural surgical lesions can be approached through an endoscopic-endonasal approach; however, once the dura has been transgressed, a combined craniofacial approach is needed.

A dedicated skull-base MRI protocol is now available at most centers, which can be tailored to patients depending on the clinical history and prior imaging. This approach includes standard brain sequences apart from additional sequences, noted in **Table 2**. Routine contrast-enhanced brain MRI is usually sufficient for lesions of the cranial vault. With continued advancement in MR pulse sequences, these protocols are continuously updated.

Diffusion-weighted sequences, especially the non–echoplanar imaging (EPI) diffusion weighted imaging (DWI) sequences, is very helpful in skull-base disorders and in demarcation of infectious lesions, such as osteomyelitis, from neoplasm. Conventional single-shot EPI-DWI sequences are prone to substantial susceptibility artifacts

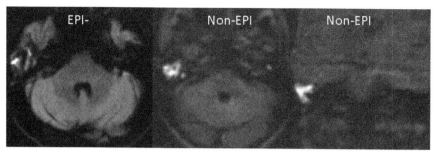

Fig. 4. Recurrent right middle ear cholesteatoma. Single-shot EPI-DWI is the more widely available standard DWI technique; however, it is prone to susceptibility artifacts, geometric distortion, and low spatial resolution (5 mm) as seen here. Non-EPI sequences (such as HASTE) have excellent motion insensitivity, are less prone to susceptibility artifacts and geometric distortion, with better spatial resolution (2 mm).

and are limited for evaluation of small skull-base lesions. However, there has been continuous advancement in MRI pulse sequences, with non-EPI sequences using turbo-spine techniques (half-Fourier acquisition single-shot turbo spin echo [HASTE]) or readout-segmented multi-shot EPI (RESOLVE; Siemens) DWI providing superior imaging of skull-base lesions such as recurrent cholesteatoma (**Fig. 4**).[12] Major advancements in CT include dual-energy CT (multispectral CT), which is becoming increasingly popular in clinical practice. This technique uses 2 separate x-ray photon energy spectra with demarcation of similar-looking lesions (such as blood and calcium) with different attenuation properties and offers huge advantages compared with conventional single-energy CT. The US Food and Drug Administration (FDA) recently approved photon-counting detector CT, which is revolutionary with huge potential to overcome the limitation of current CT by providing very high spatial resolution with minimal noise and significantly lower radiation dose.[13]

Although nuclear medicine studies are less common than CT/MRI for cranial lesions, they do offer complimentary information with functional (physiologic) and molecular details. These studies are also helpful in cases of diagnostic dilemma such as differentiation of infectious and noninfectious inflammatory and neoplastic conditions. Simultaneous PET and CT (PET-CT) is a well-established technology that combines the anatomic superiority of CT with physiologic information obtained from PET using 18F-fluorodeoxyglucose (FDG) as the metabolic tracer. PET-MRI is a new emerging technology that offers greater anatomic details than PET-CT and capitalizes on the inherent advantages of MRI, including better soft tissue contrast and no radiation exposure. However, there is limited availability of PET-MRI systems in the United States, compared with widespread availably of PET-CT. At present, there are around 50 PET-MRI units in the country compared with more than 1600 PET-CT units. PET-CT with FDG tracer is routinely used for diagnosis, staging, and to monitor treatment response in skull-base malignances, including nasopharyngeal squamous cell carcinomas and sinonasal carcinomas; however, the anatomic details are missing in these studies, necessitating additional MRI or contrast-enhanced CT. Initial literature regarding the use of simultaneously acquired PET and MRI data for the evaluation of skull-base tumors (**Fig. 5**) has been promising because of the added value of soft-tissue details and diffusion (DWI) characteristics of the lesions. Apart from commonly used FDG tracer, somatostatin receptors such as 68Ga-DOTA-TATE and 68Ga-DOTA-TOC are beneficial for skull-base lesions such as paragangliomas and

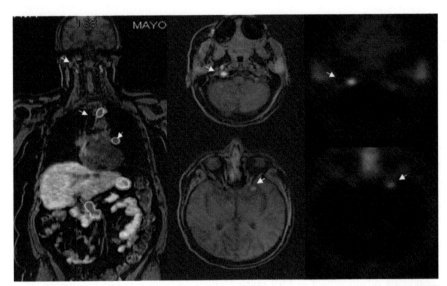

Fig. 5. PET-MRI in metastatic small bowel neuroendocrine tumor using Ga-68 DOTA-TATE. Fusion images on the left show multiple metastatic lesions in the thorax and few along the skull base (*arrows*) with good anatomic details. PET-only images on the left provide functional details, but with no anatomic localization.

meningiomas, and more so in postsurgical cases where scars and fibrous tissue limits confident segregation on MRI (see **Fig. 5**).[14]

Three-dimensional (3D) printing technology has seen an exponential surge in variety of medical and surgical specialties as the costs have significantly declined. This technology can quickly and accurately recreate models of complex anatomic structures and is helpful in surgical planning, particularly so in complex anatomic regions such as skull base and heart. The 3D printing laboratory performs virtual surgical planning with 3D-printed sterilizable biocompatible osteotomy cutting guides and is especially useful for multicompartment skull-base lesions (**Fig. 6**). Everything from imaging and segmentation is planned before going to the operating room and is printed on-site in biocompatible resins that can be autoclaved. Extracranial soft-tissue involvement of skull-base tumors, most importantly the orbital and carotid sheath vessel involvement, is vital for surgical planning because orbital involvement is another important issue in surgical planning because orbital apex involvement by a skull-base lesion usually requires orbital exenteration with sacrifice of the optic nerve. Three-dimensional printing has also evolved as a useful tool to improve patient understanding, informed patient consent, and imaging interpretation by trainees.[15]

HEADACHES ATTRIBUTED TO DISORDER OF CALVARIUM AND SKULL BASE

Inflammatory lesions of the calvarium (infectious and noninfectious): osteomyelitis of the cranial vault and skull base are usually seen as a complication of otomastoiditis, otitis externa, or sinusitis in diabetic and immunocompromised individuals. Typical SBO occurs as a complication of middle ear, external ear, or mastoid infection, usually by *Pseudomonas aeruginosa*. Atypical SBO occurs as a complication of sinus inflammatory disease or may be caused by hematogenous bacterial or fungal seeding, classically involving the central skull base. Gram-positive bacteria, including

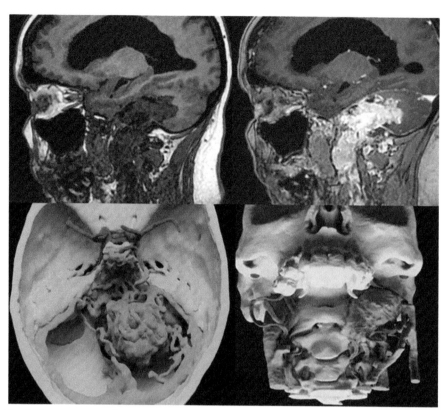

Fig. 6. Pre-contrast and post-contrast MRI images (top row) reveal an avidly enhancing mass extending through the destroyed jugular foramen with extensive vascularity seen as flow voids consistent with paraganglioma (Glomus Jugulare). 3D printed models (bottom row) with excellent depiction the mass (green) and overlying vasculature including the venous sinuses (blue) and arteries (red), used for surgical planning, patient consent and education. (*Courtesy of* Dr Jonathan Morris MD, Department of Radiology, Mayo Clinic, Rochester).

Staphylococcus species, are more common than *Pseudomonas* in atypical SBO.[5] Osteomyelitis of the cranial vault is uncommon and invariably results as a complication of intervention or a complication of scalp infection. Early on during the course, the clinical presentation includes headaches and fever with cranial neuropathies (frequently multiple) as the disease progresses. Facial nerve is usually the first cranial nerve to be involved, with involvement of other lower (IX–XII) cranial nerves as the disease progresses. Upper cranial innerves can be involved as the infection spreads into the cavernous sinuses. Biopsy, usually under imaging guidance, is needed for cultures and to rule out neoplastic causes such as nasopharyngeal carcinoma. However, once empiric antibiotics has been started, the sensitivity for cultures deceases significantly. MRI and CT provide complimentary roles in diagnosis and follow-up of SBO. MRI can detect changes earlier with marrow edema and soft tissue inflammation (**Fig. 7**). CT eventually picks up these details, but the disease must be more advanced for cortical bone erosion or trabecular demineralization. These osseous changes are classically seen at bony external auditory canal, mastoid tip, and petrous apex. MRI is superior for detecting small abscesses, especially with the use of non-EPI DWI,

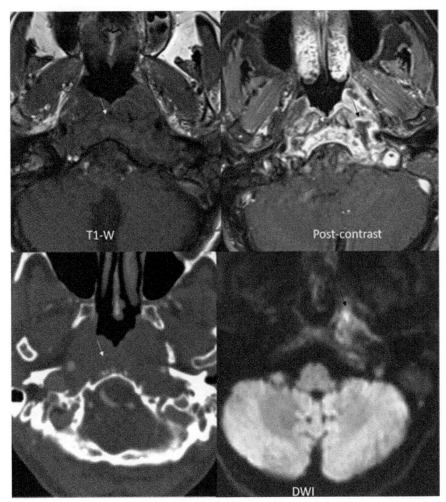

Fig. 7. Atypical SBO. Soft tissue inflammatory changes with marrow edema within the central skull base showing subtle loss of cortical definition on CT (*white arrows*). Rim-enhancing abscess with restricted diffusion along the left with extensive surrounding soft tissue enhancement. Marrow edema is much more pronounced than changes seen on CT. T1-W, T1 weighted.

which has better skull-base inhomogeneity artifacts compared with conventional EPI-DWI. Abscesses show rim enhancement with central contents appearing bright on diffusion imaging. MRI is also superior to CT for diagnosing intracranial complications, including subdural empyema, meningitis, and cerebritis. Given the proximity to the carotid sheath vessels, a high index of suspicion should be kept for vascular complications, including carotid arteritis and venous sinus thrombosis. Nuclear medicine scans such as technetium Tc99m methylene diphosphonate (Tc99m MDP) provide functional information showing increased tracer uptake with sensitivity near 100%. However, these scans have limited specificity and cannot differentiate noninfectious inflammation or neoplasm. Note that imaging lags behind clinical findings by few weeks for diagnosis and in monitoring the treatment response.[16,17]

Typical SBO usually has classic temporal course, being predated by otitis externa or mastoiditis, and is easier to diagnose than atypical SBO. Numerous neoplasms and noninfectious inflammatory conditions can affect the skull base, and it is the latter group that is a bigger diagnostic dilemma given the overlap in radiographic and clinical findings. Neoplasms mimicking SBO include nasopharyngeal carcinoma, chondrosarcoma, and chordoma, and are discussed in detail later. Noninfectious inflammatory conditions are commonly mislabeled as SBO given the stark similarity on imaging. These conditions include a wide range of granulomatous diseases, such as sarcoidosis, granulomatosis with polyangiitis (Wegner), idiopathic skull-base inflammatory disease, and immunoglobulin G4 (IgG4)–related disease. Soft tissue enhancement with marrow edema and osseous erosive changes can be seen in all these diseases; however, none of them results in abscess formation, characteristically seen in advanced-stage SBO. Although there is increased T2 signal in most of the inflammatory (infectious and noninfectious) conditions, some conditions, such as inflammatory pseudotumor, show characteristic low signal intensity because of the fibrotic contents. Image-guided or endoscopic biopsy should be done in a timely manner to avoid rapid progression of infection and rule out the differentials.[5,16–18]

Benign Calvarial Lesions

Most of the calvarial lesions are benign and discovered incidentally on imaging for other indications. Even if the indication of the examination is headaches, caution should be exercised in falsely attributing an incidental benign lesion as the underlying cause. Even when presenting clinically as palpable lumps, they can still be incidental without headaches. CT is the preferred modality for most of these lesions, usually showing well-defined margins with narrow zone of transition and no extraosseous soft tissue component. **Table 3** provides a summary of the common benign and malignant neoplastic conditions of the calvarium along with common systemic diseases affecting the cranium.

Venous vascular malformation, also commonly known as intraosseous hemangiomas, are the most common benign lesion of the calvarium, accounting for up to 10% of all benign calvarial lesions. These lesions are not true neoplasms and are usually intradiploic dilated vascular spaces with intervening trabecular thickening resulting in characteristic sunburst appearance. Bony expansion is frequently seen, usually with preserved margins, sclerotic changes, and less commonly with dehiscence of the cortical tables and extraosseous soft-tissue components. Even with bony expansion, these lesions are usually asymptomatic, requiring no further treatment. The MRI appearance of these lesions is variable depending on the extent of fat and hemorrhagic contents. Most of these lesions do have some T1-hyperintense (fat) contents, which suppress on fat-saturated images and show diffuse contrast enhancement. If there is ambiguity on MRI, CT usually provides a confident diagnosis (see **Fig. 3**); however, the reverse is usually not true. These lesions do not show restricted diffusion which can be helpful in demarcating them from epidermoid cysts.[11,19,20]

Epidermoid and dermoid cysts are slow-growing lesions that may be congenital or acquired secondary to prior surgery or trauma. They are incidental lesions, nontender, and usually not a cause for headaches. These lesions are ectoderm-lined inclusion cysts that differ in complexity with epidermoids lined by squamous epithelium with cholesterol and keratin contents, whereas dermoids also contain epidermal appendages such as sebaceous gland and hair follicles. Both these lesions appear as well-defined intradiploic lytic lesions usually without internal matrix or trabeculations with frequent remodeling and expansion of the cortical table. Epidermoids have fluid

Table 3
Imaging characteristic of common benign and malignant lesions of cranium

Lesion	CT	MRI
Venous vascular malformation (commonly known as hemangioma)	Modality of choice: well-defined lytic lesion with trabecular thickening resulting in characteristic sunburst appearance	Variable depending on the extent of fat and hemorrhagic contents. Most of these lesions do have some T1-hyperintense (fat) contents
Epidermoid cyst	Complimentary role: well-circumscribed lytic lesion with sclerotic margins	Complimentary role: characteristic restricted diffusion within the lesion. Low signal on T1-weighted imaging with heterogenous bright signal on T2 and FLAIR
Dermoid cyst	Modality of choice: midline expansile lytic lesion with or without soft tissue component	MR is usually not indicated. Lesion invariably shows predominant fat signal with heterogenous T2 contents
Fibrous dysplasia	Modality of choice: ground-glass expansile sclerotic area is characteristic, but cystic appearance is common	Heterogenous T1 and T2 signal caused by mineralization and fibrotic contents. Lesion may look aggressive on MR and caution should be exercised before moving to biopsy
Paget disease	Modality of choice: findings variable depending on the stage of the disease, with early active lytic stage to late inactive sclerotic phase	Variable depending on the stage, with most common pattern being heterogeneously T1-bright signal representing fat. Lesion may enhance and look aggressive on MR
Intraosseous meningioma	Complimentary role: nonspecific, with ~65% being osteoblastic whereas ~35% are osteolytic	Complimentary role: differentiate hyperostotic changes from dural meningiomas because intraosseous meningiomas have enhancing components with restricted diffusion within the bone
Multiple myeloma	Complimentary role: osteoporosis or numerous lytic punched-out lesions. Whole-body low-dose CT is more accurate than a skeletal survey	Complimentary role: MRI is more sensitive than CT or radiographs. Variable appearance including normal marrow, diffuse involvement, focal

(continued on next page)

Table 3
(continued)

Lesion	CT	MRI
		lesions, or a combination of both
Metastasis	Complimentary role: lytic, blastic, or a combination. CT can assess the risk of pathologic fracture	Complimentary role: MRI is more sensitive for early marrow replacing lesions with no cortical involvement and to assess extraosseous extension
Chordoma	Midline well-circumscribed lytic lesion with associated hyperdense soft tissue mass with intratumoral calcification	Modality of choice: midline clival mass with very high T2 signal, heterogeneous enhancement, with a honeycomb appearance
Chondrosarcoma	Modality of choice: lytic lesion with endosteal scalloping and matrix calcification, classically as rings and arcs	Paramedian mass with very high T2 signal, such as chordomas, with heterogenous enhancement pattern

(low T1 and high T2) signal on MR with no enhancement and characteristic diffusion restriction with low apparent diffusion coefficient (ADC) values (**Fig. 8**). Dermoids almost always have macroscopic T1 hyperintense fat contents, which signal suppression on fat-saturated sequences. These lesions have heterogenous internal matrix and thick peripheral contrast enhancement with no restricted diffusion. Combination of CT and MRI can confidently demarcate these benign cystic lesions of the calvarium.[11,21,22]

Fibrous dysplasia (FD) is a localized progressive disorder of the bone with defects in osteoblastic differentiation and maturation resulting in abnormal proliferation of fibrous tissue within bone. FD can be monostotic (single bone) or polystotic (multiple bones) and is usually sporadic, seen predominantly in children and young adults. The monostotic form is the mildest and most common form (approximately 70% of cases), usually involving the ribs and craniofacial bones. Polyostotic FD has an earlier onset, usually presenting before the age of 10 years with more severe craniofacial involvement. McCune-Albright syndrome, although uncommon, is the best example of syndromic FD and is associated with short stature, endocrinal dysfunction, and pigmented skin lesions. Headache and facial pain are the most common clinical symptoms. The mechanism of pain in FD is extremely complex and multifactorial, ranging from periosteal involvement, cytokine overproduction, to encroachment on the neural foramina. The radiographic appearance is variable, ranging from lytic/cystic lesions to a homogeneous ground-glass sclerotic appearance. Bony expansion is the hallmark of this disease, with loss of normal corticomedullary differentiation and extension across the suture lines resulting in facial asymmetry. MRI appearance is even more heterogeneous with variable T1 and T2 signal and may give the false appearance of an aggressive disorder. As in most cranial osseous lesions, CT is the examination of choice and diagnosis can confidently be made in most cases. Paget disease and intraosseous meningiomas are general imaging differential considerations, the former being much more common in incidence.

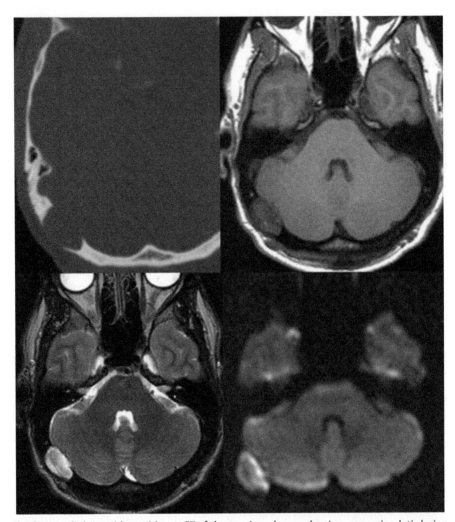

Fig. 8. Intradiploic epidermoid cyst. CT of the cranium shows a benign-appearing lytic lesion within the right occiput with bony expansion and loss of cortex. Lesion shows no macroscopic fat on T1-weighted image, and shows heterogeneously bright T2 signal with restricted diffusion, which is characteristic of epidermoid cyst. T1-hyperintense signal representing fat is almost always seen in dermoids, which are usually midline. Other differentials on CT include histiocytosis, although these do not restrict diffusion.

Paget disease is a common osseous disorder seen in the older age group, characterized by excessive bone remodeling and usually affecting the spine, skull, pelvis, and long bones, with common polyostotic involvement. As in FD, the imaging appearance can be variable depending on the stage of the disease, with an early active lytic stage to late inactive sclerotic phase. Early stages are characterized by large lytic areas involving the outer table with sparing of the inner table (osteoporosis circumscripta) with eventual extensive involvement of the inner table and bony expansion. These features are in sharp contrast to FD, where the inner table is generally spared (**Fig. 9**). CT is the best imaging modality for diagnosis, with mixed lytic and sclerotic areas resulting in the classic cotton-wool appearance. Platybasia and basilar invagination are common complications secondary to weakening of the bony trabeculae.[11,23,24] Intraosseous meningiomas are a form of primary extradural meningiomas that can be purely extracalvarial (type I), purely calvarial (type II), or mixed calvarial with extracalvarial extension (type III). These lesions are rare and arise from ectopic meningeal cells or arachnoid cap cells trapped in the cranial sutures. The most common locations for these tumors include the frontoparietal and orbital regions, commonly presenting as sclerotic lesions, less commonly with lytic or mixed sclerotic morphology. CT is excellent to assess the extent of tumor, especially in the common sclerotic type, along with assessment of cortical involvement. However, because these are often associated with the extraosseous soft tissue component, MRI is usually needed and provides complimentary information. Intraosseous meningiomas show avid enhancement with restricted diffusion of the intradiploic component, which contrasts with primary intradural meningioma, where no enhancement is noted within the reactive, usually densely sclerotic, osseous changes.[24,25]

Malignant Calvarial Neoplasms

Osseous metastases are the most common malignant bone lesions, with breast and lung cancers being the most common primary. Other common primary tumors include prostate, renal, and thyroid cancers. Skull metastasis is seen across all age groups, although the incidence increases with age. New skull-base osseous lesion in older adults should always raise the suspicion for metastasis and prompt further work-up to diagnose the underlying primary, if not already known. In the pediatric age group, neuroblastoma is the most common primary, with a tendency to be located along

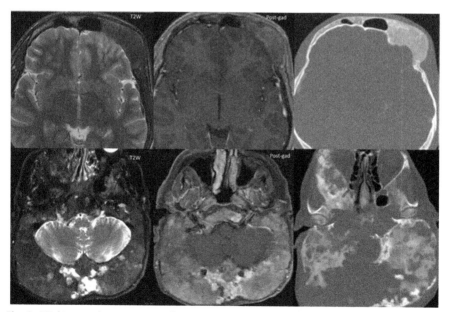

Fig. 9. FD (*top row*) versus Paget disease (*bottom row*). Although the MRI findings can be variable for FD and Paget, with heterogenous signal and enhancement pattern mimicking aggressive lesions, the CT findings are classic, as seen here. Homogeneous expansion with ground-glass density seen in FD and extensive lytic sclerotic areas seen in Paget with characteristic sparing of inner table in FD. T2W, T2 weighted.

suture lines. Skull metastasis can be seen in 20% to 30% of patients with breast, lung, or prostate cancer who undergo nuclear bone scan, and skull may be the only site of bony metastasis in up to around 12% of patients. Diagnostic umbrella includes whole-body bone scan, CT, and MRI. Metastasis may be lytic, mixed, or sclerotic depending on the underlying primary and the stage. Breast and lung metastases are usually lytic or mixed, presenting as frank lytic lesions on CT, whereas prostate classically has dense sclerotic metastasis. Focal metastasis is much more common than diffuse calvarial metastasis. The latter is occasionally seen in hematological malignancies such as leukemia and lymphoma, often presenting with diffuse loss of marrow fat signal on T1-weighted images, where demarcation with increased hematopoietic activity is not possible on imaging. DWI is helpful in detection of lytic metastasis where the lesions appear bright because of increased cellular contents of these tumors compared with low diffusion-weighted signal of adjacent normal skull bones. Extracalvarial and intra-calvarial extradural soft tissue components are frequently seen, but transgression of the thick dural layer is infrequent.[23,26–28]

Multiple myeloma (MM) is the most common primary bone tumor classically seen in adults more than 40 years of age, with a predilection for men. As per the World Health Organization (WHO) classification of tumors of hematopoietic and lymphoid tissues, it is called plasma cell myeloma and is a monoclonal gammopathy with proliferation of plasma cells in red marrow and a wide range of radiographic changes. This condition classically presents with bone pain and anemia with serologic findings including anemia, hypercalcemia, high erythrocyte sedimentation rate with normal C-reactive protein, and high total level of serum protein with a low albumin to globulin ratio. MM involves the axial skeleton, with vertebrae being the most common site, followed by ribs and skull. The pattern ranges from disseminated diffuse to disseminated focal, solitary plasmacytoma and osteosclerosing fibroma. Disseminated diffuse presents as osteoporosis and may not be picked up on imaging, whereas disseminated focal presents as punched-out lesions with sharp nonsclerotic margins and endosteal scalloping. Whole-body low-dose CT (WBLDCT) has become popular with the advent of low-dose CT protocols and has higher sensitivity than skeletal survey; however, it is still limited in sensitivity for early disease and the extraosseous component. MRI has high sensitivity for the early detection of marrow infiltration by myeloma cells as compared to WBLDCT, which only detects lytic changes representing secondary effects of myeloma. DWI characterizes tumor cellularity and has significantly higher sensitivity to detect focal myeloma lesions and background marrow infiltration. Whole-body MRI with DWI (**Fig. 10**) is becoming increasing popular for MM, because it detects disease at an earlier stage before bone destruction, is helpful to differentiate between smoldering and active myeloma given the difference in plasma cell percentage, and also provides a quick screening for cord compromises. Bone scintigraphy has limited utility given the lack of osteoblastic activity, wherein the lesions may appear cold or normal. FDG-PET/CT can assess the extent of both osseous and extramedullary disease, but has limited spatial resolution and has lower sensitivity than whole-body DWI for the diffuse form of MM. FDG-PET allows differentiation between active and treated lesions and is currently the gold-standard method for evaluating and monitoring response to therapy.[29]

Although MM is the most common primary bone tumor of the cranial vault, chordoma and chondrosarcoma form the most common primary bone malignancies arising from the skull base. Both these chondroid tumors have similar clinical features, often presenting with headaches and cranial nerve deficit, with chordomas centered on the clivus and chondrosarcomas along the petro-occipital fissure. Chordomas arise from notochordal remnants and vary in mitotic activity, which is low in typical chordomas and high in

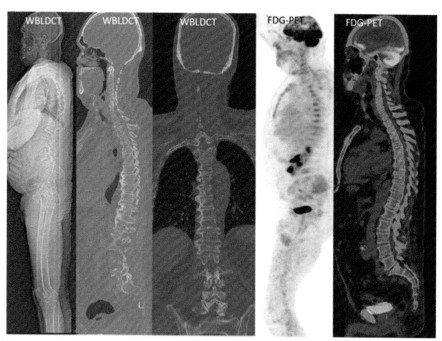

Fig. 10. Multiple myeloma with diffuse osteoporosis, multiple compression fractures on CT, with no active lesion on FDG-PET. Whole-body low-dose CT (WBLDCT) has become popular with the advent of low-dose CT protocols and has higher sensitivity than skeletal survey; however, it is still limited in sensitivity for early disease and extraosseous component. FDG-PET allows differentiation between active and treated lesion and is currently the gold standard method for evaluating and monitoring response to therapy.

poorly differentiated variants. These lesions are relatively evenly distributed along the skull base and sacrococcygeal region, with a smaller proportion seen in the vertebral bodies. Chondrosarcoma is composed of atypical chondrocytes and graded from low to high depending on the mitotic activity. CT and MRI have complementary roles in evaluation of these tumors, with CT depicting expansile destructive soft tissue mass with intratumoral classification in both with characteristic ring and arc pattern in chondrosarcomas. MRI depicts characteristically very high T2 signal with heterogenous enhancement. The soft tissue component in chordomas is disproportionately larger than the osseous component. Despite the difference in location, there is significant overlap between these entities as the tumor grows, and lesions may be indistinguishable on imaging (**Fig. 11**).[11,30] Diffusion imaging has been shown to be helpful in differentiating these tumors (see **Fig. 10**). Chondrosarcomas are associated with the highest ADC values (mean ADC: $2051 \pm 261 \times 10^{-6}$ mm^2/s), followed by classic chordoma ($1474 \pm 117 \times 10^{-6}$ mm^2/s) and poorly differentiated chordoma ($875 \pm 100 \times 10^{-6}$ mm^2/s) secondary to the cartilaginous stroma, with free extracellular water in the former and cellular matrix in the latter.[31] Other less common bone tumors include sarcomas (Ewing, osteosarcoma) and lymphoma, which can involve any part of the calvarium. Apart from the primary osseous neoplasm, a wide range of extraosseous tumors arise from the adjacent soft tissues with involvement of skull base, discussed in detail later.

Extraosseous Skull-base Neoplasms

Most of the primary osseous lesions, such as benign fibro-osseous lesions, sarcomas (Ewing, osteosarcoma), lymphoma, and metastasis, can be seen anywhere along the skull base. However, the 3 compartments of the skull base have anatomic proximity to varying soft tissue structures, resulting in a variable but predictable morphology of tumor involvement. The anterior skull base is commonly involved by sinonasal malignancies, and the posterior skull base is commonly involved by neurogenic tumors. Apart from the extracranial tumors, the skull base can be involved by intracranial tumors such as meningioma (all 3 compartments) or pituitary macroadenoma (central skull base). Because the middle and posterior skull have numerous foramina, neurogenic tumors and vascular lesions are commonly seen in these compartments with secondary osseous changes. **Table 4** provides an overview of the common lesions in the 3 compartments.

Nasopharyngeal carcinoma (NPC) arises from the nasopharyngeal mucosa just below the skull base and frequently presents with erosion of the skull base and involvement of cranial nerves secondary to its infiltrating nature. These changes are seen in around one-third of patients and range from fine erosive changes to frank intracranial extension, the latter signifying poor prognosis and higher chance of recurrence. NPC are subdivided into T3 and T4 stages according to the severity of osseous erosion, cranial nerve involvement, and intracranial extension. CT and MRI play complimentary roles, with the former being used to detect osseous erosion and MRI providing excellent delineation of perineural tumor spread and intracranial extension. As in other skull-base tumors, transgression of dura is uncommon; however, when seen, it correlates with poor survival.[32]

The central skull base shaping the middle cranial fossa is formed predominantly by the sphenoid and temporal bones and houses the pituitary gland and has numerous foramina, most prominently the foramen ovale.[5] Consequently, this part of the skull base may be involved by pituitary neoplasms and tumors of neurogenic origin, apart from a wide range of osseous skull base neoplasms described earlier. Pituitary and neurogenic tumors in this region are usually benign and slow growing, and are commonly associated with involvement of the neurovascular structures in the cavernous sinus. Common middle cranial fossa locations of meningioma include parasellar (cavernous sinus) and sphenoid ridge. Pituitary macroadenomas usually extend into the suprasellar and parasellar compartment, presenting with visual pathway

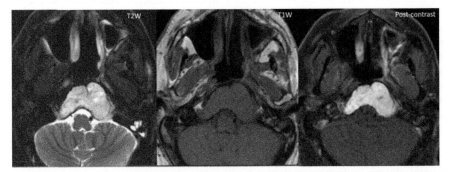

Fig. 11. Chondrosarcoma of the central skull base, which shows very high T2 signal with avid enhancement. Chordoma was kept as the first possibility on imaging; however, the disorder showed classic features of chondrosarcoma. Although chondrosarcomas are more paramedian, they can be indistinguishable from chordomas on imaging, as seen here.

compressive symptoms, cavernous sinus neuropathies, along with headaches. Expansion of the sellar floor is commonly seen with macroadenomas, whereas destruction of the skull base and extension into the sphenoid sinus and nasal cavity is only seen in a small percentage of invasive macroadenomas. Imaging demarcation between pituitary adenomas and meningiomas is straightforward, with the latter showing homogeneous enhancement, dural tail, and restricted diffusion. Although both tumors can encase the internal carotid artery (ICA), pituitary adenomas are soft and friable and almost never result in luminal narrowing (**Fig. 12**), unlike meningiomas.[33,34]

The jugular foramen is the largest skull-base foramen after the foramen magnum. The anteromedial pars nervosa has the glossopharyngeal nerve (cranial nerve IX), and the larger posterolateral pars vascularis transmits the sigmoid sinus and the vagus (X) and accessory (XI) spinal nerves. Parasympathetic paragangliomas make up 80% of jugular foramen neoplasms arising from the branches of the glossopharyngeal and vagus nerve. Other common lesions from the jugular foramen include schwannomas and meningiomas. Apart from headaches, these lesions are associated with numerous cranial nerve palsies, including Vernet syndrome (motor paralysis of cranial nerves IX, X, and XI), Collet-Sicard syndrome (Vernet syndrome with additional involvement of cranial nerve XII), and Horner syndrome. Imaging differentiation of these 3 common tumors is fairly straightforward in most cases, given the difference in T1/T2 signal, enhancement pattern, and adjacent osseous changes. Paragangliomas, also known as glomus tumors, may be sporadic or multicentric, the latter associated with inherited syndromes linked to pathogenic variations of succinate dehydrogenase (SDH) enzyme, multiple endocrine neoplasia types 2A and 2B (MEN2), neurofibromatosis type 1 (NF1), and von Hippel Lindau (VHL). These lesions have the characteristic salt-and-pepper appearance on MRI secondary to numerous intralesional flow voids from high vascularity. Like other neuroendocrine tumors, paragangliomas show high uptake on 111In-labeled octreotide nuclear scan. Glomus tumors result in permeative destruction of the skull base (see **Fig. 6**), compared with the smooth remodeling seen with benign neurogenic tumors and hyperostotic reactive changes seen with meningiomas.[34–36]

Ear and Petrous Inflammatory Disorders

Headache attributed to disorder of the ears are classified in section 11.4 of the ICHD-3, but are described here given the significant overlap in clinical and imaging findings with skull-base disorders. This condition is described in the ICHD code as "Headache caused by an inflammatory, neoplastic or other disorder of one or both ears."[1] One of the most common indications for CT of the temporal bones is inflammatory (noninfectious) and infectious diseases of the external ear, otomastoid, the inner ear, and the petrous apex. These conditions are also common causes of imaging in the emergency room, presenting with headaches, fever, and otalgia. Necrotizing external otitis, a complication of otitis externa, previously called malignant otitis externa, is an inflammatory disease usually seen in diabetics and immunocompromised patients. This disease is most commonly caused by *P aeruginosa*, which can spread through the fissures of Santorini and the tympanomastoid suture to the osseous structures, including mastoid and petrous. Imaging is usually needed in advanced stages of the disease to assess for extent and to rule out intracranial complications. Soft tissue swelling within the external auditory canal, erosion at the petrotympanic fissure, and stranding of the retrocondylar fat is seen in almost all cases.[37,38]

Otomastoiditis implies inflammation of the mastoid and middle ear and entails 2 different entities (otitis and mastoiditis) with acute or chronic manifestation. Acute

Table 4
Common neoplasms (osseous and extraosseous) in the 3 compartments of the skull base

Compartment	Foramen and Canals	Adjacent Structures	Common neoplasms
Anterior skull base	Cribriform plate, foramen cecum	Nasal cavity, paranasal sinuses orbits	Sinonasal malignancy Epithelial: inverted papilloma, nasal polyposis, nasopharyngeal carcinoma Nonepithelial: olfactory neuroblastoma, juvenile nasopharyngeal angiofibroma
Central skull base	Optic canal (CNII), superior orbital fissure (CN III, IV, V1, VI), inferior orbital fissure (CN V2); foramen rotundum, CN V2; Vidian canal (vidian nerve); foramen ovale (CN V3); foramen spinosum (middle meningeal artery)	Pterygopalatine fossa, masticator space, parotid space, carotid space, middle and external ear, temporomandibular joints, cavernous sinuses	Sellar and parasellar: pituitary adenoma craniopharyngioma, cavernous sinus meningioma Pteryogopalatine fossa: juvenile nasopharyngeal angiofibroma Nasopharynx: nasopharyngeal carcinoma Nerve foramina: benign neurogenic tumors, perineural tumors spread
Posterior skull base	Internal auditory canal (CN VII and VIII), jugular foramen, pars nervosa (CN IX), Jacobson nerve), pars vascularis (CN X and XI, hypoglossal canal (CN XII), foramen magnum	Mastoid air cells, labyrinth, jugular fossa, prevertebral space, cerebellopontine angle	Jugular foramina: paraganglioma, schwannoma Cerebellopontine angle tumors: schwannoma, meningioma, endolymphatic sac tumors, chordoma Foramen magnum: meningioma

Abbreviation: CN, cranial nerve.

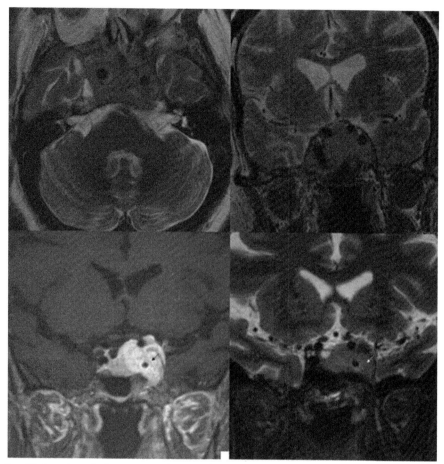

Fig. 12. Invasive pituitary macroadenoma (*top row*) versus parasellar meningioma (*bottom row*). Heterogenous T2 signal pituitary mass (macroadenoma) with complete encasement of cavernous ICA but with no narrowing, compared with moderate narrowing of ICA (*arrows*) by avidly enhancing left parasellar meningioma seen in the bottom row.

otomastoiditis is usually seen in children, is bacterial in origin, and is most frequently caused by *Streptococcus pneumoniae*. Although middle ear inflammation is known as otitis media and mastoid inflammation is mastoiditis, it is important to remember that mild mastoid inflammation is technically present in nearly all cases of acute otitis media and the condition is better described as otomastoiditis. This condition characteristically presents with postauricular tenderness, otalgia, and fever. Eventually, as inflammation persists, there is resorption of mastoid septa resulting in coalescent mastoiditis, a diagnosis made on imaging. Coalescent mastoiditis is complicated by subperiosteal soft tissue inflammation or abscess in almost half of the patients. CT is the best imaging modality to assess for mastoid cortical integrity and formation of soft tissue subperiosteal abscess, which requires an aggressive treatment approach. Less common extracranial complications include Bezold abscess, characterized by abscess medial to the attachment of the sternocleidomastoid muscle, labyrinthitis,

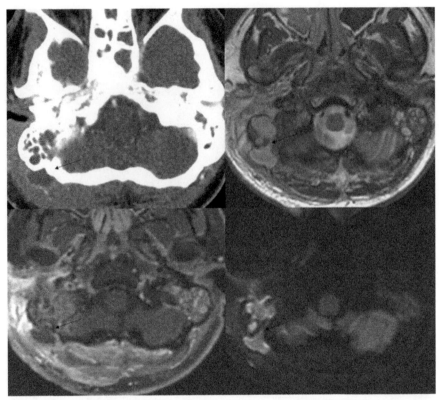

Fig. 13. Otomastoiditis with Bezold abscess. Enhanced CT and multiple MR images show complete opacification of mastoid with cortical erosion (*arrows*) and Bezold abscess. The soft tissue abscess shows characteristic restricted diffusion.

and petrous apicitis (**Fig. 13**). Intracanal complications, although uncommon, include subdural empyema, cerebral abscess, and sinus thrombosis.[39,40]

Chronic otomastoiditis is a separate entity, largely secondary to eustachian tube dysfunction resulting in persistent or recurrent inflammation of the middle ear (chronic otitis media) lasting for more than 3 months and frequently resulting in permanent tympanic membrane perforation. Although tympanic membrane changes can be seen on imaging, the role of CT is basically to evaluate for ossicular changes and extent of mastoid inflammation, and to rule out inner ear involvement. It is also important to remember that, although ossicular chain erosion is much more commonly seen with cholesteatomas, it can frequently also be seen with granulation tissue secondary to chronic inflammation. Erosive changes classically involve the long and lenticular processes of incus and the stapes, less frequently involving the malleus and incus body. Although the ossicles can be seen accurately with high-resolution temporal bone CT, a limitation exists to detect early erosive changes. The FDA recently approved photon-counting CT, which provides substantially better delineation of fine anatomy for the temporal bones and has the potential to replace conventional CT for skull-base and ear imaging.[17] Because CT cannot differentiate between different types of middle ear with opacification (fluid, fibrotic tissue, granulation tissue, or cholesteatoma), there is heavy reliance on detection of classic erosive changes involving structures that define cholesteatoma. Osseous structures involved early in the erosive process include the scutum (lateral epitympanic wall), the lateral semicircular canal, tegmen, and the facial nerve canal wall. Postinflammatory ossicular fixation is a common complication of otomastoiditis resulting in conductive hearing loss. However, CT is currently limited in making a definitive diagnosis and demarcating fibrous tissue from cholesteatoma. DWI is now increasingly being used to detect cholesteatoma and to follow up for recurrence after surgery. Different single-shot and multishot echo-planar and nonechoplanar diffusion techniques have been described. Nonecho-planar images have higher resolution (up to 2 mm), significantly less susceptibility arti-fact, and is becoming the technique of choice at most centers (see **Fig. 4**). Contrast-enhancement MRI is also helpful in differentiating cholesteatoma (which does not enhance) from granulation and fibrous tissues (enhancement present). Petrous apicitis or inflammation of the petrous apex is seen as a complication of otomastoiditis or sec-ondary to infection of pneumatized petrous apex. This condition presents with otor-rhea, abducens nerve (VI) palsy, and retroorbital pain, classically described as Gradenigo syndrome, but has become increasingly rare after the advent of antibiotics.[41,42]

Labyrinthitis refers to inflammation of the inner ear presenting with headache and a wide range of cochlear and vestibular symptoms, including dizziness, vertigo, and sensorineural hearing loss. It is usually infective in origin, although autoimmune causes are increasingly being identified. This condition may be secondary to bacterial menin-gitis, where it is usually bilateral or unilateral tympanogenic secondary to adjacent oto-mastoid inflammation. CT imaging is limited in the acute and fibrotic stages of the disease, but the late (ossificans) stage is picked up easily with mild haziness to high-density bone deposition within the membranous labyrinth, depending on the severity of disease. Enhancement of the membranous labyrinth on MRI is a fairly spe-cific and sensitive finding in the acute phase, but is not seen with the fibrotic or chronic ossific stages. The later stages present with loss of normal fluid signal on MRI on the heavily T2-weighted sequences.[43,44]

CERVICOGENIC HEADACHES

Headaches attributed to disorder of the neck are described under section 11.2 of the ICHD-3 code and include cervicogenic headache, headache attributed to retrophar-yngeal tendonitis, and headache attributed to craniocervical dystonia.[1] A brief discus-sion is included in this article because there is significant overlap in the clinical characteristic of these headaches with those secondary to skull-base and cranial vault lesions. Cervicogenic headaches are usually myofascial secondary to inflammatory (including degenerative) diseases of the upper cervical facets, C2 to C3 intervertebral disc, and dura matter of the upper spinal cord. Diagnosis requires clinical and/or im-aging evidence of a lesion in these anatomic regions. Because degenerative changes in the cervical spine are almost universally seen beyond a certain age, imaging findings should not be falsely determined to be the cause for headaches. The evidence of causation must be established by evidence of causation shown by at least 2 of the following: (1) headache has developed in temporal relation to the onset of the cervical disorder or appearance of the lesion; (2) headache has significantly improved or resolved in parallel with improvement in or resolution of the cervical disorder or lesion; (3) cervical range of motion is reduced and headache is made significantly worse by provocative maneuvers, and headache is abolished following diagnostic blockade of a cervical structure or its nerve supply.[1] Cervicogenic headaches arise primarily from musculoskeletal abnormality in the upper 3 cervical segments, with acute degeneration-related inflammatory changes being the most common cause in this group. This condition is characterized by marrow edema at the occipitoatlantal or atlantoaxial junction with joint effusion. Rheumatoid arthritis is the most common non-degenerative inflammatory condition of the upper cervical spine, manifesting as erosive changes within the odontoid frequently associated with pannus formation. Pannus represents inflammatory synovial mass classically described with rheumatoid arthritis; however, it also seen in other inflammatory conditions. These conditions should be differentiated from degenerative retrodental ligamentous thickening or calcium deposition disease. Calcium pyrophosphate dihydrate (CPPD) disease or pseudogout of the cervical spine presents with calcified retrodental pseudomass with remodeling of the adjacent bone, but with the absence of the erosive changes seen in pannus. Enhancement is usually seen within the pannus and is absent in degenerative ligamentous hypertrophy and CPPD. Calcium deposition can frequently occur in the longus colli muscles, resulting in an inflammatory response known as calcific tendinitis (acute or chronic). This condition is classified as retropharyngeal tendonitis under the ICHD-3 code and is characterized by amorphous calcifications in the superior fibers of the longus colli muscle tendons at the C1 to C2 level, frequently associated with retropharyngeal space effusions. This condition can present acutely with headaches, fever, dysphagia, and neck stiffness and should not be misdiagnosed as retropharyngeal abscess, because the treatments of these 2 conditions are completely different. Longus colli tendinitis is managed conservatively with aspirin or other pain killers and usually resolves within a couple of weeks.[45,46]

SUMMARY

The article describes the approach to imaging that clinicians should adopt in cases of headaches suspected to be secondary to cranial vault or skull-base disorder. As a rule, CT is superior to MR for most of the osseous lesions and lesions of the middle and external ear. MR provides a complimentary role to CT and is the modality of choice in a few conditions such as extraosseous neoplasms of the skull base. Photon-counting CT and ultra-high-field MR are now both approved by the FDA for clinical usage and provide substantial improvement in imaging of skull-base lesions. Imaging protocols are becoming more and more specific and tailored to the suspected cause and patient's need, and a good knowledge of various imaging protocols is helpful in early diagnosis, avoiding unnecessary examinations and eventually lowering the cost of health care in imaging evaluation of headaches.

CLINICS CARE POINTS

- Headache or facial pain attributed to disorder of the cranium, neck, eyes, ears, nose, sinuses, or teeth forms a separate classification subset in the International Classification of Headache Disorders (ICHD-3)
- Diagnosis based on clinical, laboratory, and/or imaging evidence of lesion in these regions
- Imaging evaluation plays an important role in identification of structural lesion

DISCLOSURE

The authors have nothing to disclose.

REFERENCES

1. Headache Classification Committee of the International Headache Society (IHS) The International Classification of Headache Disorders, 3rd edition. Cephalalgia 2018;38(1):1–211.
2. Jin SW, Sim KB, Kim SD. Development and Growth of the Normal Cranial Vault : An Embryologic Review. J Korean Neurosurg Soc 2016;59(3):192–6.
3. Caetano-Lopes J, Canhão H, Fonseca JE. Osteoblasts and bone formation. Acta Reumatol Port 2007;32:103–10.
4. Dixon AD, Hoyte DA, Ronning O. Fundamentals of craniofacial Growth. New York: CRC Press; 1997. p. 101–2.
5. Janez F, Barriga A, Inigo T, et al. Diagnosis of Skull Base Osteomyelitis. Radiographics 2001;41(1):156–73.
6. Zhao J, Levy D. The sensory innervation of the calvarial periosteum is nociceptive and contributes to headache-like behavior. Pain 2014;155(7):1392–400.
7. Schueler M, Messlinger K, Dux M, et al. Extracranial projections of meningeal afferents and their impact on meningeal nociception and headache. Pain 2013; 154(9):1622–31.
8. Göbel H. Headache from Cranial Bone. In: Gebhart GF, Schmidt RF, editors. Encyclopedia of pain. Berlin: Springer; 2013. p. 94–268.
9. Callaghan BC, Kerber KA, Pace RJ, et al. Headaches and neuroimaging: high utilization and costs despite guidelines. JAMA Intern Med 2014;174(5):819–21.
10. Whitehead MT, Cardenas AM, Corey AS, et al. Expert Panel on Neurologic Imaging. ACR Appropriateness Criteria: Headache. J Am Coll Radiol 2019;16(11S): S364–77.
11. Gomez CK, Schiffman SR, Bhatt AA. Radiological review of skull lesions. Insights Imaging 2018;9(5):857–82.
12. Benson JC, Carlson ML, Lane JI. Non-EPI versus Multishot EPI DWI in cholesteatoma detection: correlation with operative findings. AJNR Am J Neuroradiol 2021; 42(3):573–7.
13. Zhou W, Lane JI, Carlson ML, et al. Comparison of a Photon-Counting-Detector CT with an Energy-Integrating-Detector CT for Temporal Bone Imaging: A Cadaveric Study. AJNR Am J Neuroradiol 2018;39(9):1733–8.
14. Nensa F, Beiderwellen K, Heusch P, et al. Clinical applications of PET/MRI: current status and future perspectives. Diagn Interv Radiol 2014;20(5):438–47.
15. Huang X, Fan N, Wang Hj, et al. Application of 3D printed model for planning the endoscopic endonasal transsphenoidal surgery. Sci Rep 2021;11:5333.
16. Chapman PR, Choudhary G, Singhal A. Skull Base Osteomyelitis: A Comprehensive Imaging Review. AJNR Am J Neuroradiol 2021;42(3):404–13.
17. Chandler JR, Grobman L, Quencer R, et al. Osteomyelitis of the base of the skull. Laryngoscope 1986;96(3):245–51.
18. Jain N, Jasper A, Vanjare HA, et al. The role of imaging in skull base osteomyelitis - Reviewed. Clin Imaging 2020;67:62–7.
19. Politi M, Romeike BF, Papanagiotou P, et al. Intraosseous hemangioma of the skull with dural tail sign: radiologic features with pathologic correlation. AJNR Am J Neuroradiol 2005;26(8):2049–52.
20. Bastug D, Ortiz O, Schochet SS. Hemangiomas in the calvaria: imaging findings. AJR Am J Roentgenol 2013;164(3):683–7.
21. Arana E, Martí-Bonmati L. CT and MR imaging of focal calvarial lesions. AJR Am J Roentgenol 1999;172:1683–8.

22. Younghee Y, Woon-JinM, Hyeong SA, et al. Imaging findings of various calvarial bone lesions with a focus on osteolytic lesions. J Korean Soc Rad Iol 2016;74(1): 43–54.
23. Yalçin Ö, Yildirim T, Kizilkiliç O, et al. CT and MRI findings in calvarial non-infectious lesions. Diagn Interv Radiol 2007;13:68–74.
24. Razek AA. Imaging appearance of bone tumors of the maxillofacial region. World J Radiol 2011;3(5):125–34.
25. Agrawal V, Ludwig A, Agrawal A, et al. Intraosseous intracranial meningioma. AJNR Am J Neuroradiol 2007;28(2):314–5.
26. Mitsuya K, Nakasu Y, Horiguchi S, et al. Metastatic skull tumors: MRI features and a new conventional classification. J Neurooncol 2011;104(1):239–45.
27. Stark AM, Eichmann T, Mehdorn HM. Skull metastases: clinical features, differential diagnosis and review of the literature. Surg Neurol 2003;60(3):219–25.
28. Messiou C, Hillengass J, Delorme S, et al. Guidelines for Acquisition, Interpretation, and Reporting of Whole-Body MRI in Myeloma: Myeloma Response Assessment and Diagnosis System (MY-RADS). Radiology 2019;291(1):5–13.
29. Dimopoulos MA, Hillengass J, Usmani S, et al. Role of magnetic resonance imaging in the management of patients with multiple myeloma: a consensus statement. J Clin Oncol 2015;33(6):657–64.
30. Oot RF, Melville GE, New PF, et al. The role of MR and CT in evaluating clival chordomas and chondrosarcomas. AJR Am J Roentgenol 1988;151(3):567–75.
31. Yeom KW, Lober RM, Mobley BC, et al. Diffusion-weighted MRI: distinction of skull base chordoma from chondrosarcoma. AJNR Am J Neuroradiol 2013; 34(5):1056–61.
32. Roh JL, Sung MW, Kim KH, et al. Nasopharyngeal carcinoma with skull base invasion: a necessity of staging subdivision. Am J Otolaryngol 2004;25(1):26–32.
33. Borges A. Imaging of the central skull base. Neuroimaging Clin N Am 2009;19(4): 669–96.
34. Quirk B, Connor S. Skull base imaging, anatomy, pathology and protocols. Pract Neurol 2020;20(1):39–49.
35. Chaljub G, Van Fleet R, Guinto FC Jr, et al. MR imaging of clival and paraclival lesions. AJR Am J Roentgenol 1992;159(5):1069–74.
36. Vogl TJ, Bisdas S. Differential diagnosis of jugular foramen lesions. Skull Base 2009;19(1):3–16.
37. Harnsberger HR, MBBS CMG, Michel MA et-al. Diagnostic Imaging Head and Neck. Lippincott Williams & Wilkins. 2010. p. 1304-22. ISBN:1931884781.
38. Trojanowska A, Drop A, Trojanowski P, et al. External and middle ear diseases: radiological diagnosis based on clinical signs and symptoms. Insights Imaging 2012;3(1):33–48.
39. Kwon BJ, Han MH, Oh SH, et al. MRI findings and spreading patterns of necrotizing external otitis: is a poor outcome predictable? Clin Radiol 2006;61(6): 495–504.
40. Mafee MF, Singleton EL, Valvassori GE, et al. Acute otomastoiditis and its complications: role of CT. Radiology 1985;155(2):391–7.
41. Vazquez E, Castellote A, Piqueras J, et al. Imaging of complications of acute mastoiditis in children. Radiographics 2003;23(2):359–72.
42. Mafee MF, Aimi K, Kahen HL, et al. Chronic otomastoiditis: a conceptual understanding of CT findings. Radiology 1986;160(1):193–200.
43. Verbist B. Imaging of sensorineural hearing loss: a pattern-based approach to diseases of the inner ear and cerebellopontine angle. Insights Imaging 2011; 3(2):139–53.

44. Taxak P, Ram C. Labyrinthitis and labyrinthitis ossificans - a case report and re-
    view of the literature. Radiol Case 2020;14(5):1–6.
45. Chang EY, Lim WY, Wolfson T, et al. Frequency of atlantoaxial calcium pyrophos-
    phate dihydrate deposition at CT. Radiology 2013;269(2):519–24.
46. Shi J, Ermann J, Weissman BN, et al. Thinking beyond pannus: a review of retro-
    odontoid pseudotumor due to rheumatoid and non-rheumatoid etiologies. Skel-
    etal Radiol 2019;48(10):1511–23.

Imaging of Cranial Neuralgias

Samika Kanekar, MS[a], Manal Saif, DO[b], Sangam Kanekar, MD, DNB[c],*

KEYWORDS

- Cranial neuralgia • Trigeminal neuralgia
- Constructive interference steady state (CISS) • Glossopharyngeal nerve

KEY POINTS

- Cranial neuralgia (CN) is caused by an inflammatory, infectious, or structural abnormality along the path of a cranial nerve that can cause debilitating symptoms, often seen in the trigeminal or occipital nerve dermatomes, and less commonly in the glossopharyngeal nerve dermatome.
- Diagnostic imaging plays a key role in diagnosing CN and identifying the underlying cause, specifically in identifying neurovascular abnormality or secondary causes such as demyelinating lesions, aneurysm, tumor, infection, or intracranial hemorrhage.
- Constructive interference steady state and fast imaging employing steady-state acquisition MRI sequences and 3D time-of-flight MR angiography are used to optimally diagnose nerve deviation, distortion, groove formation, and atrophy.
- Microvascular decompression surgery is the most curative treatment option for both trigeminal and glossopharyngeal neuralgia.

INTRODUCTION

Cranial neuralgia (CN) is defined as pain along the distribution of a cranial or cervical nerve.[1,2] Symptoms are described as brief, paroxysmal, and often triggered lancinating pain within a specific nerve dermatome. At times, this pain is sharp, stabbing, electric shock-like, or very rarely continuous. Clinically, CN needs to be distinguished from cranial neuropathy, the latter of which is a sensory deficit within the nerve distribution with persistent neuropathic pain. CN may be encountered along the branches of multiple cranial nerves or along the terminal branches of the upper cervical nerves. The most encountered neuralgias include trigeminal, postherpetic trigeminal, and occipital neuralgias. Less common neuralgias include facial, glossopharyngeal, superior laryngeal, auriculotemporal, and nervus intermedius neuralgias. The clinical course of these neuralgias may be monophasic, relapsing and remitting, or chronic.

[a] Warren Alpert Medical School, Brown University, 222 Richmond Street, Providence, RI 02903, USA; [b] Department of Radiology, Penn State Health, Penn State College of Medicine, Mail Code H066 500 University Drive, Hershey, PA 17033, USA; [c] Radiology Research, Division of Neuroradiology, Penn State Health, Penn State College of Medicine, Mail Code H066 500 University Drive, Hershey, PA 17033, USA
* Corresponding author.
E-mail address: skanekar@pennstatehealth.psu.edu

Neurol Clin 40 (2022) 591–607
https://doi.org/10.1016/j.ncl.2022.02.008
0733-8619/22/© 2022 Elsevier Inc. All rights reserved.

neurologic.theclinics.com

Abbreviations	
MRI	Magnetic resonance imaging (MRI)
MRA	MR angiography (MRA)
REZ	Root Entry Zone
DWI	Diffusion-weighted imaging
FLAIR	Fluid-attenuated inversion recovery
CN V	Cranial Nerve V
3D-TOF-MRA	3D-Time of flight Magnetic resonance angiography
TGN	Trigeminal neuralgia
ON	occipital neuralgia
MPRAGE	Magnetization Prepared - RApid Gradient Echo

The clinical evaluation of a patient with CN begins with the localization of the cranial nerve based on symptom distribution. Identifying triggering factors, whether the pain is unilateral or bilateral, and if there are any other associated findings that are important components of clinical history. Additionally, evaluation must distinguish between primary and secondary neuralgias based on clinical clues to develop an appropriate diagnostic and therapeutic plan. Diagnostic imaging, specifically MRI, plays an important role in distinguishing primary from secondary neuralgias by evaluating the underlying structural, inflammatory, or infectious process along the length of the nerve. When the specific cause of neuralgia is not found on imaging or other investigations, the neuralgia is termed as idiopathic CN and treated accordingly.

TRIGEMINAL NEURALGIA

Trigeminal neuralgia (TN), or tic douloureux, is the most common CN. TN is defined as a "disorder characterized by recurrent unilateral brief electric shock-like pains, abrupt in onset and termination, limited to the distribution of one or more divisions of the trigeminal nerve, and triggered by innocuous stimuli".[2] Incidence rate of TN is around 4 to 13 per 100,000 people annually, with man-to-woman prevalence ratio of 1 to 1.5 to 1 to 1.7.[3] Majority of the cases of the TN are seen after the age of 50.[3,4] The diagnosis of TN in a young person should raise suspicion for secondary cause such as multiple sclerosis (MS) or neoplasm.

The *International Classification of Headache Disorders*, Third Edition (ICHD-3)[2] classified the TN depending on the causes into three types: classic TN, secondary TN, and idiopathic TN. The term classic TN is applied when imaging shows neurovascular compression of the trigeminal nerve. When the TN is due to causes such as a MS, petrous apex meningioma or metastasis leading to compression of the nerve, TN is termed as secondary TN. When there is no cause identified on the imaging and the electrophysiological tests are normal, the diagnosis is labeled as idiopathic TN. Idiopathic and classic TN are further subclassified into groups with purely paroxysmal pain or with concomitant continuous pain by pain phenotype.

Most commonly, the vascular compression is from the superior cerebellar artery, but compression due to other vessels such as the anterior inferior cerebellar artery, trigeminal vein, and superior petrosal vein may be responsible for TN.

Pathophysiology

Trigeminal nerve (CN V) is the largest cranial nerve, with mixed motor and sensory functions. It originates in and exits the pons laterally and traverses the prepontine cistern before it enters Meckel cave [**Fig. 1**]. Meckel cave houses the Gasserian

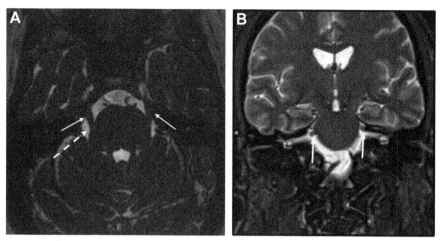

Fig. 1. Axial CISS (*A*) and coronal T2 (*B*) thin sections show cisternal segment of the trigeminal nerve (*arrows*). Nerve root entry zone (*dashed arrow*) is segment of the trigeminal nerve a few millimeters from where it enters the pons.

ganglion, which trifurcates into ophthalmic (V1), maxillary (V2), and mandibular (V3) branches. V1 exits from the superior orbital fissure, and V2 exits from foramen rotundum and V3 exits through the foramen ovale [**Figs. 2** and **3**]. V1 division innervates the forehead and orbital region. V2 enters the pterygopalatine fossa and supplies sensory information to the midface region from the eye to the upper lip. V3 is the largest branch of the trigeminal nerve, and it supplies motor innervation to the masticator muscles and sensory innervation to the lower face, ear, and temporomandibular regions.

The exact pathophysiology of the TN is not clearly understood. The most widely accepted theory for the classic TN is that the nerve shows morphologic changes such as interstitial neuritis, neural fiber demyelination, and perineural and endoneural

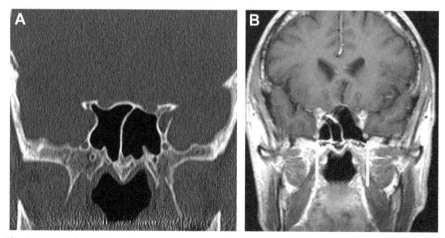

Fig. 2. Coronal CT (*A*) and coronal T1 postcontrast (*B*) images at the level of sphenoid sinus show foramen rotundum (*red arrows*) through which the maxillary division (V2) of the trigeminal nerve exits.

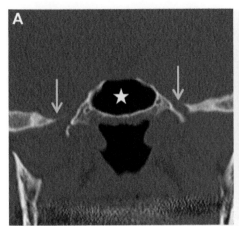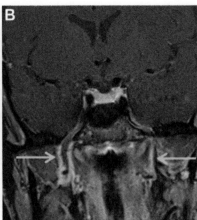

Fig. 3. Coronal CT (*A*) and coronal T1 postcontrast (*B*) images of foramen ovale on CT (*green arrows*) at the level of the sphenoid sinus (yellow star) and the mandibular division (V3) of the trigeminal nerve exiting through foramen ovale to enter the masticator space.

sclerosis of the trigeminal nerve at the nerve root entry zone (NREZ) from vascular compression.[5] This leads to atrophy or hypertrophy of peripheral axons with damage to both Schwann cells and the peripheral myelin.[3,5–7] NREZ, is a segment of the trigeminal nerve a few millimeters from where it enters the pons. The transition of peripheral Schwann cell myelination to central oligodendroglia myelination within the zone is hypothesized to make the entry zone particularly susceptible to pressure.[3,7] This theory is well supported by documentation of the demyelination, dysmyelination, and remyelination, and direct apposition of demyelinated axons on the biopsy segment obtained from the compressed region.[3,6–8] It is well established that demyelinated afferents tend to become hyperexcitable and capable of generating ectopic impulses manifesting as spontaneous pain. It is further hypothesized that the ephaptic connections between demyelinated Aβ (pain generation) and Aδ fibers (fibers mediating light touch) might provide the mechanism for touch-evoked pain called short connection theory.[6–8] The intense, near-explosive pain has been hypothesized to be due to trigeminal ganglion cell somata developing touch-evoked prolonged discharges, which spread from 1 cell to another. In addition, the fibers transmitting light touch and pain are in closest proximity with REZ and cause paroxysmal pain provoked by cutaneous stimuli making the region most vulnerable. Mere documentation of the neurovascular contact is not enough for the diagnosis of TN. Neurovascular contact is commonly in the asymptomatic patients or in the asymptomatic side of the symptomatic patients. This indicates that the neurovascular contact may be a normal anatomic variant. Neurovascular conflict in an appropriate clinical context clinches the diagnosis of the classic TN. Idiopathic TN is thought to be due to neuronal voltage-gated ion channel gain-of-function mutations and/or neural inflammation.[8]

Clinical Examination and Diagnosis

Diagnosis of TN is largely clinical and is based on the ICHD criteria.[2] The physical and neurologic examinations are generally normal in patients with classic or idiopathic TN. Any abnormal neurologic findings should raise the suspicion of secondary TN. Main criteria used for the diagnosis of the TN include the pain along at least one trigeminal nerve division without associated neurologic deficit; pain not radiating beyond the distribution of the trigeminal nerve; and pain showing a classic pattern of sharp, electric, shock-like, or stabbing in quality, which is abrupt in onset and termination, limited to the distribution of one or more divisions of the trigeminal nerve, and triggered by innocuous stimuli.[9] The pain of TN is usually in a unilateral maxillary or mandibular distribution; the ophthalmic division alone is involved in less than 5% of cases.[9] The pain may be triggered by innocuous mechanical stimuli such as light touch, talking, chewing, tooth brushing, and washing the face.[4] Most patients have several trigger factors located in the nasolabial area, upper and lower lip, chin, cheek, and alveolar gingiva. On physical examination, palpation of trigger zones may precipitate an attack.

Imaging

Once the diagnosis is confirmed clinically, neuroimaging, especially high-resolution MRI, is recommended to establish the etiologic subclassification of clinically identified TN, so that the appropriate treatment may be initiated. High-resolution MRI with and without contrast remains the investigation of choice in suspected cases of TN. The main objective of the imaging is to document the neurovascular conflict [**Fig. 4**] or to identify the secondary causes such as demyelinating lesions, aneurysms, tumors, and intracranial hemorrhage or infection [**Fig. 5**].

Besides axial FLAIR and DWI images through the brain, for better visualization of the trigeminal and adjacent areas, three-dimensional (3D) constructive interference steady state/fast imaging employing steady-state acquisition (CISS/FIESTA) and 3D time-of-flight MR angiography along with postcontrast 3D T1-weighted fast spoiled gradient recalled echo are performed through the pons and along the divisions (V1, V2, and V3) of the trigeminal nerve.[10,11] CISS/FIESTA is currently the sequence of choice for visualizing cranial nerves at the skull base. On these sequences, on the background of hyperintense CSF, traversing trigeminal nerve and vessels are hypointense and are clearly identified. 3D CISS/FIESTA combined with 3D-TOF-MRA makes it easy to identify the responsible vessels. A meta-analysis indicated that the sensitivity and specificity of 3D-TOF-MRA for neurovascular contact are 95% and 77%, respectively.[12] The main disadvantage of 3D-TOF-MRA is the suboptimal display of the vessels with slow flow due to inflow enhancement effects.

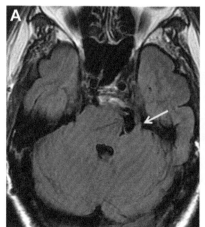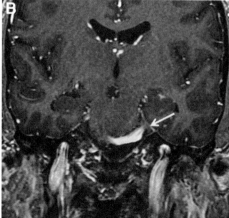

Fig. 4. A 49-year-old man presents with TN. Axial FLAIR (*A*) and postcontrast thin coronal MPRAGE (*B*) images show ectatic basilar artery (*red arrows*) causing significant displacement of the trigeminal nerve and indentation of the nerve root zone (*yellow arrows*).

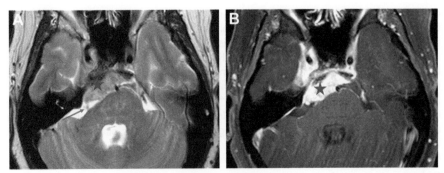

Fig. 5. A 41-year-old woman with TN. Axial T2 (*A*) and axial postcontrast T1-weighted (*B*) images show avidly enhancing mass (*red star*) involving the prepontine cistern, right petrous apex and ipsilateral Meckel cave and cavernous sinuses, also showing encasement of the right trigeminal nerve (*blue arrow*).

Multiplanar oblique reconstructions and fusion of 3D T2-weighted sequences with the corresponding TOF images or 3D T1-weighted gadolinium-enhanced images are very useful in the preoperative context. Nerve deviation, distortion, groove formation, and atrophy can be clearly diagnosed on high-resolution MR imaging [**Fig. 6**]. Atrophic changes in trigeminal nerve are shown to correlate with severity of compression and may help to predict long-term prognosis after vascular decompression. MRI is also very sensitive in identifying the secondary cause such as cerebral aneurysms, tumors, demyelinating plaque, and intracranial hemorrhage.

Neuroimaging of the Peripheral Segments

When no significant abnormality is detected in the brain stem and in the prepontine cistern along the course of trigeminal nerve, special attention is paid to the cavernous sinus, pterygopalatine fossa, superior orbital fissure, and neurovascular foramen for visualization of peripheral branches. On imaging, the affected nerve may show irregular or smooth thickening and enhancement, and/or occlusion of the fat pad in the

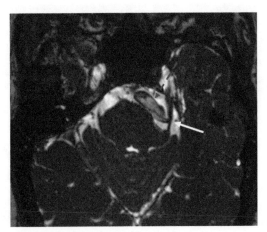

Fig. 6. Axial CISS image shows dolichoectasia of the basilar artery (*red dotted arrow*) causing lateral displacement, stretching, and thinning (*white arrow*) of the left trigeminal nerve.

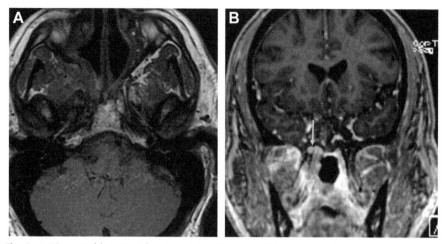

Fig. 7. A 59-year-old man with squamous cell cancer of the paranasal sinuses presents with maxillary distribution of pain 3 months following surgery. Axial T1 (*A*) and postcontrast T1 coronal (*B*) images show recurrent tumor along the posterior margin of the sinuses and perineural invasion along the right V2 division of the trigeminal nerve (*orange arrow*).

foramen. Except for herpes zoster (HZ), V1 TN is rare.[4] Rarely it may be seen due to facial fractures, bacterial or fungal sinusitis, or nerve sheath tumors.

The V2 division of the trigeminal nerve exits the cranial cavity through the foramen rotundum and may be affected in infection, trauma, and tumors. Infection and tumors of the maxilla, temporal bone, and paranasal sinuses can track along the branches of V2 involving the foramen rotundum, infraorbital canal, palatal foramen, or pterygopalatine fossa.[4,13,14] Thin coronal or axial fat sat T1-weighted precontrast and postcontrast images show loss of normal fat signal, nerve enhancement. Perineural invasion of the V2 division presenting as TN is not rare [**Fig. 7**]. This is seen as smooth enhancement along the nerve along with primary neoplasm in the sinus.

TN along the V3 division is common, with this segment usually involved due to direct tumor extension, perineural spread of odontogenic infection, or following a fracture. CT and MRI remain complimentary to each other in the diagnosis of the odontogenic infection. CT may show ill-defined lytic areas, cortical destruction, periosteal reactions, or an abscess formation in close proximity to the mandible. Soft tissue extension and nerve enhancement are better depicted on the combination of T2/FLAIR and postcontrast fat sat T1-weighted images.[4,13,14] In a suspected case of tumor [**Fig. 8**] or perineural spread, MRI with and without contrast remains the modality of the choice. Mandibular division may show nerve thickening, widening of the neural foramen, loss of fat surrounding the nerve and abnormal contrast enhancement along the course of the nerve. Perineural spread is most commonly seen in squamous cell carcinoma of the oral cavity, adenoid cystic carcinoma, mucoepidermoid carcinoma of the salivary gland, basal cell cancer, and melanoma [**Fig. 9**].

Diffusion tensor imaging (DTI) with tractography may be used in selected cases of clinically suspected TN with normal conventional MRI imaging. DTI has a unique advantage in demonstrating the microstructural damage by quantifying the amount of nonrandom water diffusion within the tissue. Fractional anisotropy was found to decrease significantly in the involved side of the trigeminal nerve, with corresponding increase in the radial diffusivity and unchanged axial diffusivity, confirming that the pathologic basis of affected TGN is demyelination without obvious axonal injury.[15,16]

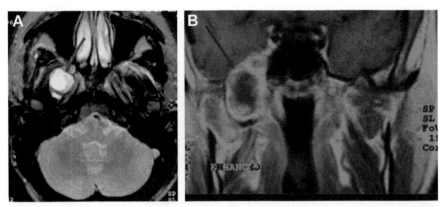

Fig. 8. A 41-year-old woman presents with right TN and numbness. Axial T2 (*A*) and post-contrast T1 coronal (*B*) images show cystic mass from the V3 division of the right fifth nerve, which biopsy revealed as cystic neurofibroma.

Treatment

Treatment options of TN largely depend on the causes, pathophysiology, clinical presentation, age, and comorbidities. The initial treatment of choice for classic and idiopathic TN is always medical pharmacotherapy. Medications such as anticonvulsants and tricyclic antidepressants (TCAs) remain the mainstream treatment. The antiepileptic drugs such as carbamazepine and oxcarbazepine are the first drug of choice for long-term treatment of TN.[17,18] If carbamazepine and oxcarbazepine are ineffective or poorly tolerated, lamotrigine, gabapentin, botulinum toxin type A, pregabalin, baclofen, or phenytoin could be used, either as add on or as monotherapy.[17,18]

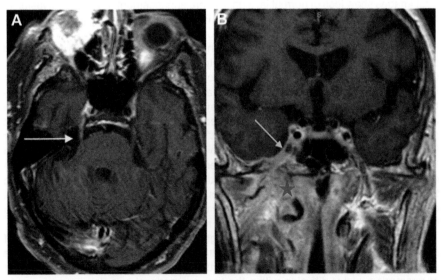

Fig. 9. A 62-year-old man with nasopharyngeal carcinoma (*red star*) with trigeminal neuralgia along the V3 division due to perineural invasion. Postcontrast T1 axial (*A*) and coronal (*B*) images show enhancement along the V3 division (*green arrow*) in the right foramen ovale and the cisternal segment (*white arrow*) of the right trigeminal nerve.

Surgical management for TN patients is reserved for those who do not tolerate or fail medical management or who have suffered relapse of symptoms. Surgical options, including microvascular decompression (MVD) and rhizotomy or ablative treatments using radiofrequency thermocoagulation, mechanical (compression by a balloon), or chemical (injection of glycerol).[17] In the MVD, the vascular loop compressing one or more trigeminal nerve roots or divisions is separated from the nerve using a gelatin sponge pledget inserted between the vessel and the nerve. MVD is the surgical treatment of choice in patients with classic TN. Among all the surgical procedures, MVD is the most invasive surgical procedure, but potentially, more curative. Ninety percent of patients obtain pain relief immediately after the surgery, more than 80% will still be pain free at 1 year, 75% at 3 years, and 73% at 5 years.[17,19]

Noninvasive stereotactic radiosurgery (gamma knife) is the only noninvasive but destructive technique, which aims a focused beam of radiation at the trigeminal root entry zone. Radiosurgery is an alternative approach to patients with poor surgical candidates with comorbidities, high-risk medical illness, or pain refractory to prior surgical procedures.[20,21] High doses of 70 to 80 Gy of submillimeter radiation beams focused at the trigeminal nerve either at root entry zone close to the brainstem or just proximal to the trigeminal ganglion or the ganglion itself. The goal is to induce the focal axonal degeneration. Unlike MVD, the pain-relieving effects of stereotactic radiosurgery are not immediate and can take up to 8 weeks. After 1 year, close to 70% of patients remain pain-free, but this decreases to about 50% at 3 years.[20,21] Rarely postgamma knife complications such as focal hemorrhage, weakness along the trigeminal distribution, or mild atrophy of the trigeminal nerve is seen [**Fig. 10**].

PAINFUL TRIGEMINAL NEUROPATHIES

The painful trigeminal neuropathies listed under the ICHD-3 classification include acute HZ infection, postherpetic, posttraumatic, MS plaque, and neoplasm.[2]

PAINFUL TRIGEMINAL NEURALGIA AND HERPES ZOSTER INFECTION

HZ is an acute, localized self-limiting infection caused by the varicella zoster virus (VZV), characterized by a severe painful skin rash in the corresponding dermatome, most often on the face or chest wall. It is most common along the ophthalmic division of the trigeminal nerve (V1) as opposed to the classic TN, which is more common in V2 and V3. The dermatomal pain may persist long after the rash has cleared, giving rise to a chronic painful condition known as postherpetic neuralgia (PHN).[2,22]

In the acute reactivation, varicella zoster presents with unilateral vesicular eruptions with acute, stabbing radiating pain, confined mostly to the V1 dermatome. This pain in the acute phase of HZ is thought to be due to VZV-induced vasoconstriction and ischemic nerve damage from ganglionitis and neuritis in the sensory ganglia and in the peripheral sensory nerves.[2,23]

Majority of the time, diagnosis is made from the clinical presentation and the classic appearance of the rash. In the absence of rash or when in dilemma, a positive assay for varicella-zoster antigen direct immunofluorescence or varicella-zoster viral polymerase chain reaction will confirm the diagnosis.[22,23] Acute herpetic infection should always raise the question of immunocompromise either by infection, such as human immunodeficiency virus, or by cancer. Once a diagnosis of acute HZ is established, the patient is treated with antiviral medication and antiepileptic drugs (AEDs), specifically gabapentin and pregabalin or TCAs, such as amitriptyline and nortriptyline for neuralgic pain.[22,24]

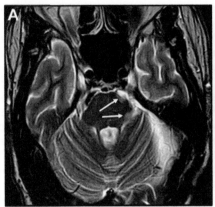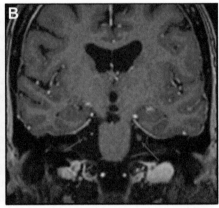

Fig. 10. Postgamma knife complications. Axial T2 image (*A*) shows tiny focal hyperintensities (*arrows*) involving the anterior and lateral aspects of the pons possibly from postradiation damage. Postcontrast MPRAGE coronal images (*B*) obtained 8 months after the gamma knife therapy for TN. Patient presents with weakness along the trigeminal distribution; images showing mild atrophy of the right trigeminal nerve compared with the left.

POSTHERPETIC TRIGEMINAL NEUROPATHY

Postherpetic neuralgia (PHN) is the most frequent chronic complication of HZ infection and may involve any of the cranial nerves. When the pain along the trigeminal division persists beyond 3 months from a herpes infection, it is labeled as postherpetic neuropathy (PHN). About 10% to 15% of the patients with HZ will develop PHN, which is most seen in patients older than 60 years.[25,26] The ophthalmic division of the trigeminal nerve is the commonly affected nerve and is called HZ ophthalmicus. It is also seen that the patient with more intense mucocutaneous eruptions of HZ and the acute herpetic neuritis pain during the acute phase of HZ, have the greater frequency and intensity of the PHN. PHN pain is characterized by allodynia and hyperalgesia in response to nonnoxious mechanical and thermal stimuli. Pain is described as burning, sharp, shooting, or electric shock-like along the affected nerve. Ganglionitis, neuritis, and ischemic nerve damage during the acute phase of the infection cause both peripheral and central sensitization characterized by downregulation of central pain inhibitory pathways, alterations in the expression of genes encoding neuropeptides, and expansion of receptive fields.[25,26] This results in hyperexcitability of dorsal horn neurons with the capacity to fire spontaneously. Treatment of PHN is primarily symptomatic. In some patients, pain may persist for years or even for life, which requires prolonged medication.

PAINFUL POSTTRAUMATIC TRIGEMINAL NEUROPATHY

Painful posttraumatic trigeminal neuropathy (PTTN) is defined as oral or facial pain, secondary to injury to the peripheral branches of the trigeminal nerve. These are commonly seen following orthognathic surgery, facial trauma, tooth avulsions, or endodontic treatments. Pain classically presents as burning, pricking, crushing, or electric shock-like pain, often associated with mechanical allodynia or hypoesthesia. Pain is often due to lingual nerve and inferior alveolar nerve injuries, accounting for up to 90% of all cases of PTTN. PTTN may interfere with daily activities such as eating and drinking, shaving, kissing, tooth brushing, and applying make-up, thus mandating long-term treatment.

Following trauma, an inflammatory response is seen within the injured nerve. If the proximal stump survives, healing involves disorganized sprouting of nerve fibers leading to neuroma formation that often depends on the degree of nerve damage.[27] Milder injuries, such as nerve constriction or compression, may also cause neuroma formation and focal demyelination. These changes lead to the ectopic discharges.

TRIGEMINAL NEUROPATHY ATTRIBUTED TO MULTIPLE SCLEROSIS PLAQUE

Secondary TN accounts for around 15% of TN patients and the diagnosis is usually made on cross-sectional imaging, specifically MRI.[28] One of the most frequent secondary TN is due to MS. MS patients have a 20-fold increased risk of developing TN. Clinically, patients present very similarly to the classic and idiopathic TN, characterized by a sudden, usually unilateral, brief, stabbing or electrical shock-like, recurrent pain along one or more divisions of the fifth cranial nerve. Clinically, it is very challenging to distinguish MS-induced TN from idiopathic/classic TN. However, MS-related TN is more common in women, has early age of onset in the fourth or fifth decade, is more common on the right side and may have associated sensory deficits.

MRI remains the investigation of choice for the diagnosis of TN secondary to MS. Axial FLAIR/T2-weighted images show demyelinating plaques in the intrapontine segment of the trigeminal nerve, an area centered in the ventrolateral pons between the trigeminal root entry zone and the trigeminal nuclei, which is along the intrapontine trigeminal primary afferents [**Fig. 11**]. Due to demyelination, the axons tend toward a depolarization level, making them hyperexcitable, which in turn, produces ectopic excitation, high-frequency discharges, and ephaptic transmission from neighboring, healthy nerve fibers.[29,30] Once a diagnosis of MS is established, the treatment is empiric with possible benefit by adding AEDs including gabapentin, carbamazepine, topiramate, and lamotrigine.

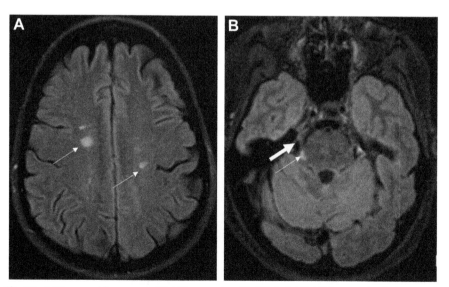

Fig. 11. A 31-year-old woman with MS presents with TN. Axial FLAIR images (*A,B*) show multiple demyelinating plaques in the centrum semiovale (*thin arrows*). Axial image at the pons shows demyelinating plaque (*fine arrow*) at the nerve root entry zone of the right fifth nerve (*thick arrow*).

GLOSSOPHARYNGEAL NEURALGIA

The glossopharyngeal nerve (CN IX) exits the medulla posterior to the olivary sulcus, along with the cranial nerves X and XI nerve root complex [**Fig. 12**]. After traversing the cistern, it exits the skull through the jugular foramen. It is responsible for general somatic sensation, visceral sensation, brachial motor innervation, and parasympathetic innervation. It provides general somatic sensation of touch, pain, and temperature to the posterior one-third of the tongue, pharynx, middle ear, and the area near the external auditory meatus. It also supplies motor innervation to stylopharyngeal muscle, which is responsible for elevation of pharynx and contributes to the gag reflex.

Glossopharyngeal neuralgia (GPN) is a rare CN characterized by paroxysms of excruciating pain in the sensory distribution of the auricular and pharyngeal branches of glossopharyngeal (IX) and vagus (X) cranial nerves. The estimated incidence of GPN is 0.2% to 1.3% of the facial pain syndromes and occurs most frequently in the fifth or sixth decades of life.[31] Patient usually presents with unilateral paroxysmal electrical shock–like pain affecting the posterior tongue, pharynx, tonsillar fossa, deep in the ear, and/or beneath the angle of the jaw. GPN is commonly provoked by swallowing, yawning, coughing, or sometimes even talking. Approximately 10% of attacks are associated with autonomic symptoms referable to vagal dysfunction including bradycardia, hypotension, syncope, seizures, and even cardiac arrest.[32] Some clinicians term it as vagoglossopharyngeal neuralgia; however, this term is not included in the ICHD-3. Based on the distribution of pain, GPN has been clinically divided into tympanic, which predominantly affects the ear along the auricular branch of the vagus nerve, and the oropharyngeal, which affects the oropharyngeal area along the pharyngeal branches of the vagus nerve.[22,33]

Most of GPN cases are idiopathic, which is mostly due to neurovascular compression of the glossopharyngeal nerve.[31] Similar to TN, secondary GN can be due to compression or injury of the glossopharyngeal nerve by tumors from the cerebellopontine angle or the oropharynx, trauma, infection, carotid aneurysm, and demyelinating lesions at the root entry zone, and elongated styloid process, or ossification of the styloid ligament known as Eagle syndrome.[22,31,33] Most cases are thought to be due to compression of the nerve by a vessel because it exits from the medulla and travels through the subarachnoid space to the jugular foramen [**Fig. 13**].

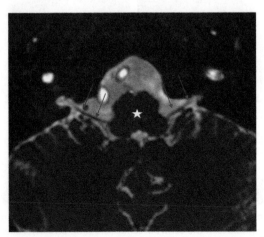

Fig. 12. Axial CISS image at the level of medulla (*yellow star*) shows normal IX, X, and XI nerve complex arising from the post-olivary sulcus, and coursing toward the jugular foramen.

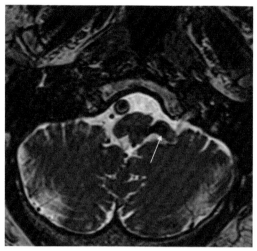

Fig. 13. A 61-year-old hypertensive woman presenting with left glossopharyngeal neuralgia. Axial T2 image shows ectatic left vertebral artery (*yellow arrow*) causing severe indentation and displacement of the left IX-XI nerve complex.

GPN is a clinical diagnosis mostly established by the characteristic distribution of the pain. Otherwise, no significant findings are noted on the clinical examination in idiopathic GN. Imaging plays an important role in diagnosis of the secondary GN, documentation of the vascular compression, or exclusion of other secondary causes.[34] High-resolution MRI or CT imaging remains the imaging of choice in a suspected case of GPN. Imaging should cover the region of the brainstem to reveal the presence of vascular compression or intra or axial mass within the posterior fossa and should extend up to the lower neck to exclude base of the skull, neck masses including elongated styloid process.

CISS sequence on MRI is very sensitive in documenting the vascular pathologies crossing the IX, X, and XI nerve complex within the cistern. Axial FLAIR, thin T2, DWI, and postcontrast images are usually used for the evaluation of other lesions such as MS, tiny infarctions, or to rule out base of the skull lesions [**Fig. 14**]. Contrast-enhanced CT scan of the neck is important when the cause of the GN is suspected in the base of the skull and below.

Treatment

Similar to TN, the first-line of treatment of GN is pharmacologic, which includes carbamazepine or oxcarbazepine, gabapentin, pregabalin, and phenytoin. Surgical MVD remains an option in a patient with pharmaco-resistant GN.[35,36] The main aim of MVD for GPN is to separate the offending vessel, most commonly the posterior inferior cerebellar artery or the vertebral artery from the ninth and tenth cranial nerve complex. MVD has the highest initial and long-term success rate. Gamma knife radiotherapy is also an option for the management of GPN, especially in patients without evident of neurovascular conflict on imaging or with pain recurrence after MVD.[35,36] The intracisternal glossopharyngeal nerve is targeted with radiation dose usually ranges from 55 to 90 Gy delivered in a single fraction. Of note, patients who are treated with stereotactic radiosurgery have higher recurrence rates compared with those treated with MVD.

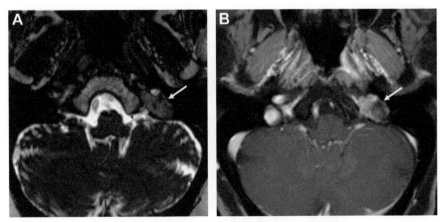

Fig. 14. A 54-year-old woman with known case of left jugular foramen meningioma presenting with left glossopharyngeal neuralgia. Axial T2 (*A*) and axial postcontrast T2-weighted (*B*) images show cranial nerve IX (*red arrows*) encased by the enhancing jugular foramen meningioma (*yellow arrow*).

OCCIPITAL NEURALGIA

Occipital neuralgia is defined by sharp, electrical, paroxysmal pain, occasionally throbbing in quality, originating from the occiput and extending along the posterior scalp, skull base, and radiating toward the vertex.[2] Pain is distributed along the greater occipital nerve, which originates from the dorsal ramus of C2, and the lesser occipital nerve, which originates from C2 and C3 in the cervical plexus.[37] The pain is unilateral in 85% of patients with distribution along the greater occipital nerve in 90%, and lesser occipital nerve in 10% of cases. Occipital neuralgia has been reportedly caused by irritation or compression of the occipital nerves by muscular entrapment, vascular anomalies, vascular inflammation, primary or metastatic tumors, myelitis, MS, cervical degenerative disease or callus formation and secondary to scalp biopsy and whiplash injury.[37–39] The usual cause of greater occipital neuralgia is entrapment along the path from C2 to the trapezius aponeurosis. On examination, tenderness may be elicited over the occipital nerve region while palpating, but it is a nonspecific sign. Imaging, most commonly CT scan of the brain is performed to eliminate the secondary causes such as neoplasm, infection, vascular malformations, giant cell arteritis, or Chiari malformations.[37–39]

Initial conservative treatment includes warm or cold compress, massage, and physical therapy directed to improve posture. Nonsteroidal anti-inflammatory medications, muscle relaxants, TCAs, and anticonvulsants have proven to be helpful. Local anesthetic injection can both confirm the diagnosis and provide temporary pain relief. Surgical management should be reserved only for intractable cases.

Surgical interventions for ON is an option in patients who are refractory to pharmacologic treatment. These surgical treatment options include both ablative procedures and chronic electrical stimulation.[37–39] Ablative therapy includes neurectomies and neurolysis at several anatomic levels of the greater, lesser, or third occipital nerves, including the C2 ganglion via ganglionectomy and high cervical dorsal roots. Nerve block over the occipital notch may also be considered. Occipital nerve stimulation is a newer treatment option for the ON [**Fig. 15**]. Peripheral stimulation of sensory afferents inhibits nociceptive activity in c-fibers and a-delta fibers thus reducing the pain.

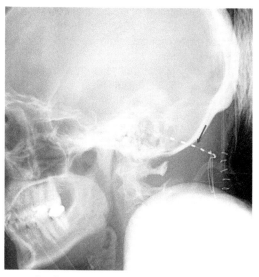

Fig. 15. Occipital nerve stimulators as a neuromodulation therapy for chronic refractory headache and occipital neuralgia. Lateral radiograph of the skull shows the occipital nerve stimulation electrodes and leads (*arrow*) placed superficially in the region of the greater occipital and lesser occipital nerves.

CLINICS CARE POINTS

- CN is a pain along the distribution of a cranial or cervical nerve. Clinically, CN needs to be distinguished from cranial neuropathy, the latter of which is a sensory deficit within the nerve distribution with persistent neuropathic pain.

- The most encountered neuralgias include trigeminal, postherpetic trigeminal, and occipital neuralgias. The evaluation is mainly targeted to distinguish between primary and secondary neuralgias based on clinical clues to develop an appropriate diagnostic and therapeutic plan.

- Diagnostic imaging, specifically MRI, plays an important role in distinguishing primary from secondary neuralgias by evaluating the underlying structural, inflammatory, or infectious process along the length of the nerve.

REFERENCES

1. Robertson C. Cranial Neuralgias Continuum (Minneap Minn) 2021;27(3):665–85.
2. Headache Classification Committee of the International Headache Society (IHS). The international classification of headache disorders, 3rd edition (beta version). Cephalalgia 2018;38(1):1–211.
3. Gambeta E, Chichorro JG, Zamponi GW. Trigeminal neuralgia: an overview from pathophysiology to pharmacological treatments. Mol Pain 2020;16. https://doi.org/10.1177/1744806920901890. 1744806920901890.
4. Maarbjerg S, Gozalov A, Olesen J, et al. Trigeminal neuralgia—a prospective systematic study of clinical characteristics in 158 patients. Headache 2014;54(10):1574–82.
5. Peker S, Kurtkaya O, Uzün I, et al. Microanatomy of the central myelin-peripheral myelin transition zone of the trigeminal nerve. Neurosurgery 2006;59:354–9.

6. Maarbjerg S, Wolfram F, Gozalov A, et al. Significance of neurovascular contact in classical trigeminal neuralgia. Brain 2015;138(pt 2):311–9.

7. Love S, Coakham HB. Trigeminal neuralgia: pathology and pathogenesis. Brain 2001;124(pt 12):2347–60.

8. DevorM Amir R, Rappaport ZH. Pathophysiology of trigeminal neuralgia: the ignition hypothesis. Clin J Pain 2002;18(1):4–13.

9. Cruccu G, Finnerup NB, Jensen TS, et al. Trigeminal neuralgia: new classification and diagnostic grading for practice and research. Neurology 2016;87(2):220–8.

10. Leal PR, Hermier M, Souza MA, et al. Visualization of vascular compression of the trigeminal nerve with high-resolution 3T MRI: a prospective study comparing preoperative imaging analysis to surgical findings in 40 consecutive patients who underwent microvascular decompression for trigeminal neuralgia. Neurosurgery 2011;69:15–25.

11. Leal PR, Froment JC, Sindou M. MRI sequences for detection of neurovascular conflicts in patients with trigeminal neuralgia and predictive value for characterization of the conflict (particularly degree of vascular compression) [in French]. Neurochirurgie 2010;56:43–9.

12. Cai J, Xin ZX, Zhang YQ, et al. Diagnostic value of 3D time-of-flight MRA in trigeminal neuralgia. J Clin Neurosci 2015;22(8):1343–8.

13. Cassetta M, Pranno N, Pompa V, et al. High resolution 3-TMR imaging in the evaluation of the trigeminal nerve course. Eur Rev Med Pharmacol Sci 2014;18(2):257–64.

14. Graff-Radford S, Gordon R, Ganal J, et al. Trigeminal neuralgia and facial pain imaging. Curr Pain Headache Rep 2015;19(6):19.

15. Dessouky R, Xi Y, Zuniga J, et al. Role ofMR Neurography for the diagnosis of peripheral trigeminal nerve injuries in patients with prior molar tooth extraction. AJNR Am J Neuroradiol 2018;39(1):162–9.

16. Liu Y, Li J, Butzkueven H, et al. Microstructural abnormalities in the trigeminal nerves of patients with trigeminal neuralgia revealed by multiple diffusion metrics. Eur J Radiol 2013;82(5):783–6.

17. Bendtsen L, Zakrzewska JM, Abbott J, et al. European Academy of Neurology guideline on trigeminal neuralgia. Eur J Neurol 2019;26(6):831–49.

18. Di Stefano G, Truini A, Cruccu G. Current and innovative pharmacological options to treat typical and atypical trigeminal neuralgia. Drugs 2018;78(14):1433–42.

19. Heinskou TB, Rochat P, Maarbjerg S, et al. Prognostic factors for outcome of microvascular decompression in trigeminal neuralgia: a prospective systematic study using independent assessors. Cephalalgia 2019;39:197–208.

20. Tuleasca C, Régis J, Sahgal A, et al. Stereotactic radiosurgery for trigeminal neuralgia: a systematic review. J Neurosurg 2018;130(3):733–57.

21. Park SH, Chang JW. Gamma knife radiosurgery on the trigeminal root entry zone for idiopathic trigeminal neuralgia: results and a review of the literature. Yonsei Med J 2020;61(2):111–9.

22. Tepper SJ. Cranial Neuralgias. Continuum (Minneap Minn) 2018;24(4, Headache):1157–78.

23. Lovell B. Trigeminal herpes zoster: early recognition and treatment are crucial. BMJ Case Rep 2015;2015. https://doi.org/10.1136/bcr-2014-208673. pii: bcr2014208673.

24. Klasser GD, Ahmed AS. How to manage acute herpes zoster affecting trigeminal nerves. J Can Dent Assoc 2014;80:e42.

25. di Luzio Paparatti U, Arpinelli F, Visonà G. Herpes zoster and its complications in Italy: an observational survey. J Infect 1999;38(2):116–20.

26. Oaklander AL. The density of remaining nerve endings in human skin with and without postherpetic neuralgia after shingles. Pain 2001;92:139–45.

27. Benoliel R, Kahn J, Eliav E. Peripheral painful traumatic trigeminal neuropathies. Oral Dis 2012;18(4):317–32.

28. B Foley PL, Vesterinen HM, Laird BJ, et al. Prevalence and natural history of pain in adults with multiple sclerosis: systematic review and meta-analysis. Pain 2013; 154(5):632–42.

29. MS Di Stefano G, Maarbjerg S, Truini A. Trigeminal neuralgia secondary to multiple sclerosis: from the clinical picture to the treatment options. J Headache Pain 2019;20(1):20.

30. Sarlani E, Grace EG, Balciunas BA, et al. Trigeminal neuralgia in a patient with multiple sclerosisand chronic inflammatory demyelinating polyneuropathy. J Am Dent Assoc 2005;136:469–76.

31. Blumenfeld A, Nikolskaya G. Glossopharyngeal neuralgia. Curr Pain Headache Rep 2013;17(7):343.

32. Wallin BG, Westerberg CE, Sundlöf G. Syncope induced by glossopharyngeal neuralgia: sympathetic outflow to muscle. Neurology 1984;34(4):522–4.

33. Son KB. The glossopharyngeal nerve, glossoPharyngeal neuralgia and the Eagle's syndrome-Current concepts and management. Singapore Med J 1999;40: 659–65.

34. Truini A, Colonnese C, Manfredi M. Glossopharyngeal nerve contrast enhancement in recent-onset glossopharyngeal neuralgia. Neurology 2015;84(12):1283.

35. Zhao H, Zhang X, Zhu J, et al. Microvascular decompression for glossopharyngeal neuralgia: long-term follow-up. World Neurosurg 2017;102:151–6.

36. Lu VM, Goyal A, Graffeo CS, et al. Glossopharyngeal neuralgia treatment outcomes after nerve section, microvascular decompression, or stereotactic radiosurgery: a systematic review and meta-analysis. World Neurosurg 2018;120: 572–82.e7.

37. Dougherty C. Occipital neuralgia. Curr Pain Headache Rep 2014;18(5):411.

38. Urits I, Schwartz RH, Patel P, et al. A review of the recent findings in minimally invasive treatment options for the management of occipital neuralgia. Neurol Ther 2020;9(2):229–41.

39. Choi I, Jeon SR. Neuralgias of the head: occipital neuralgia. J Korean Med Sci 2016;31(4):479–88.

Posttraumatic Headaches and Postcraniotomy Syndromes

Allison Weyer, MD

KEYWORDS

• Posttraumatic • Postcraniotomy • Hemorrhage • Herniation • Fracture • Injury

KEY POINTS

- Headache is one of the most common sequelae of traumatic brain injury, and imaging is often warranted to evaluate for posttraumatic intracranial abnormalities that may present with headache.
- Many patients experience headache after craniotomy. Imaging identifies postoperative complications and guides management.
- CT and MRI of the brain contribute to the diagnostic evaluation of patients with headache following trauma or craniotomy.
- CT is usually the best initial imaging modality, whereas MRI is more sensitive for particular posttraumatic and postoperative abnormalities.

Abbreviations	
CTA	computed tomography angiography
SDH	subdural hematoma
FLAIR	fluid attenuated inversion recovery
MRI	magnetic resonance imaging
DWI	diffusion weighted imaging
ADC	apparent diffusion coefficient
ICA	internal carotid artery

INTRODUCTION

Disturbance or violation of the intracranial compartment by trauma or surgery may result in headache. The headaches associated with trauma and craniotomy range in severity from mild to severe. The time course of onset also varies from immediate to delayed. Some of the entities discussed have complex clinical presentations with multiple symptoms and signs, of which headache may be one. Several posttraumatic and postcraniotomy pathologies that may manifest with headache are discussed in the following sections with a focus on their imaging appearances.

Division of Neuroradiology, University of Pittsburgh Medical Center, 200 Lothrop Street, South Tower, 2nd Floor, Suite 200, East Wing, Pittsburgh, PA 15213, USA
E-mail address: weyerag2@upmc.edu

Neurol Clin 40 (2022) 609–629
https://doi.org/10.1016/j.ncl.2022.02.003
0733-8619/22/© 2022 Elsevier Inc. All rights reserved.
neurologic.theclinics.com

DISCUSSION
POSTTRAUMATIC HEADACHES

Posttraumatic headache is described in the International Classification of Headache Disorders (ICHD) as a secondary headache that begins within 7 days following trauma or within 7 days after recovering consciousness or the ability to sense and report pain.[1] It is one of the most common sequelae of traumatic brain injury: the 1-year cumulative incidence of new or worsened headache in patients with mild traumatic brain injury (mTBI) has been reported as 91%.[2] Several intracranial traumatic abnormalities are associated with headache, and their imaging features are discussed in detail below.

American College of Radiology Appropriateness Criteria

The American College of Radiology (ACR) publishes Appropriateness Criteria, which are evidence-based guidelines for selecting appropriate diagnostic imaging for various clinical conditions. The Appropriateness Criteria for imaging head trauma are referenced in the following text and provide recommendations for which imaging examination to order in specific contexts. Although specific points are discussed subsequently, it is important to note that noncontrast head CT is usually appropriate for the initial imaging of acute head trauma that is moderate or severe (Glasgow Coma Scale [GCS] 3–12) or penetrating.[3] Noncontrast head CT is also usually appropriate for the initial imaging of mild acute head trauma (GCS 13–15) when imaging is indicated by a clinical decision rule.[3] This is due to the speed and accessibility of CT imaging as well as to the sensitivity of this modality for detecting hemorrhage, herniation, and infarction that may warrant neurosurgical intervention.[4]

Reviewing thin-section reconstructions of a noncontrast head CT in the coronal and sagittal planes improves the detection of intracranial hemorrhage and is recommended when evaluating a patient presenting with acute head trauma.[5,6]

Subdural Hematoma

Subdural hematomas are collections of blood products between the dura and the arachnoid mater that usually result from tears in bridging cortical veins. They do not cross midline but instead track along the falx under the dura. Unlike epidural hematomas, they are not confined by the dural attachments associated with calvarial sutures, and their classic morphology is therefore crescentic (**Fig. 1**).

Acute subdural hematomas are usually hyperdense relative to brain parenchyma on CT and become less dense as the blood products age. Although there are no precise time intervals when blood products demonstrate specific densities, a systematic literature review described mixed and hyperdense subdural hematomas reported after a median time interval of 1 and 2 days, respectively, whereas isodense and hypodense subdural hematomas were reported after 11 and 14 days, respectively.[7] The presence of blood products of different densities within a subdural hematoma is often attributed to acute-on-chronic hemorrhage. However, isodensity or hypodensity does not always indicate older blood. Nonclotted blood will seem hypodense, and this may be observed in the setting of hyperacute hemorrhage (see **Fig. 1; Fig. 2**) or chronic hemorrhage in a patient with coagulopathy. Blood may seem isodense to brain parenchyma if it is subacute, but this appearance can also occur if the patient is anemic or if there is mixing of CSF with acute blood in the setting of an arachnoid tear.

Although MRI is not recommended in the initial imaging of acute head trauma, it may be indicated to evaluate persistent neurologic deficits that are not explained by the initial head CT. Small subdural hematomas are more sensitively detected with MRI than with CT. MRI may also play a role in planning surgical evacuation of subdural

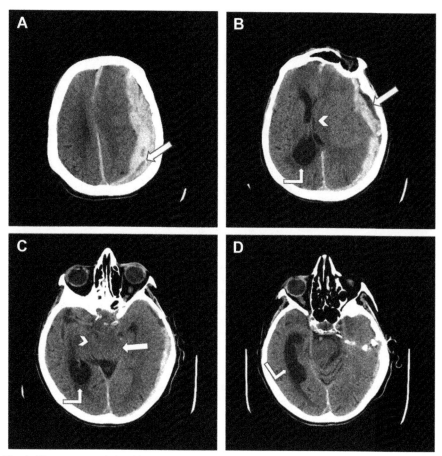

Fig. 1. Hyperacute subdural hematoma in an elderly woman who was found down and last seen well 3 hours prior. (*A*) Axial noncontrast head CT image shows a large crescentic left cerebral convexity SDH that contains low-density hyperacute nonclotted blood products mixed with hyperdense hemorrhage. This is known as the swirl sign (*arrow*). (*B*) Axial non-contrast head CT image at the level of the foramen of Monro again shows hyperacute, mixed-density left SDH (*straight arrow*) with rightward subfalcine herniation (*arrowhead*) and asymmetric dilation of the right lateral ventricle (*angled arrow*) indicating ventricular entrapment. (*C*) Axial noncontrast head CT image at the level of the midbrain demonstrates left uncal herniation (*straight arrow*) as well as partial effacement of the right ambient cistern (*arrowhead*). Entrapment of the right lateral ventricle is also visualized at this level (*angled arrow*). (*D*) Axial noncontrast head CT image demonstrates marked dilation of the temporal and occipital horns of the right lateral ventricle compatible with entrapment (angled *arrow*).

hematomas with subacute or chronic components by demonstrating the presence and location of septations within the hematoma[8,9] (**Fig. 3**). The risk of recurrence of a subdural hematoma following evacuation may also be predicted based on the appearance of blood on T1-weighted and T2-weighted sequences.[10]

Subdural Hygroma

Posttraumatic subdural hygromas are collections of CSF in the subdural compartment, which result from tears of the arachnoid. Because they follow the same density and

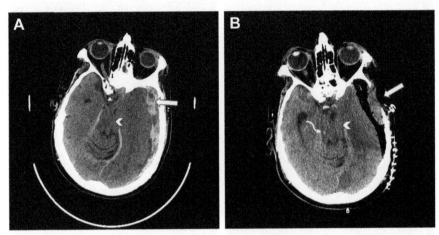

Fig. 2. Hyperacute subdural hematoma with uncal herniation and Duret hemorrhage. (*A*) Axial noncontrast CT image of the head shows the swirl sign of a hyperacute left subdural hematoma (*arrow*) as well as uncal herniation (*arrowhead*). (*B*) Axial noncontrast CT image of the head shows interval left craniectomy for evacuation of the subdural hematoma (*arrow*) with persistent uncal herniation (*arrowhead*) and new punctate hyperdensity in the right dorsal midbrain (curved *arrow*) compatible with acute parenchymal hemorrhage that is known as Duret hemorrhage in the setting of severe uncal herniation.

signal characteristics on CT and MRI as does normal CSF, they may be difficult to distinguish from the normal CSF surrounding the brain, especially in the setting of brain atrophy. However, hygromas will displace the cortical veins away from the calvarium and are often observed in combination with other posttraumatic findings in the brain.

Hygromas tend to appear later following trauma than acute hematomas, with a mean time to appearance of 9 days after injury.[11] However, they may also occur in the first day after injury. Although they should follow the appearance of CSF on all

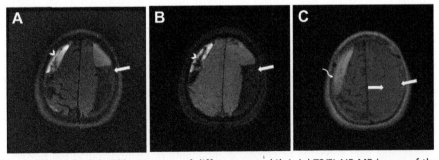

Fig. 3. Bilateral subdural hematomas of different ages. (*A*) Axial T2/FLAIR MR image of the brain shows T2 hypointense blood layering dependently within a chronic left subdural hematoma (*straight arrow*). Linear T2 hypointense structures within a chronic right subdural hematoma (*arrowhead*) represent septations. (*B*) Axial susceptibility-weighted MR image of the brain shows hypointensity associated with the dependent blood products (*straight arrow*) as well as with the septations in the right subdural hematoma (*arrowhead*). (*C*) Axial T1-weighted MR image of the brain shows isointense signal of the more recent left subdural hematoma (*arrow*) and hyperintensity of the subacute blood within the right subdural hematoma (*curved arrow*).

imaging, they may demonstrate transient hyperdensity if the patient recently received intravenous contrast. Dual-energy CT technique can be used to image the brain of a trauma patient who recently received contrast to distinguish between contrast and acute hemorrhage as the cause of hyperdensity within a subdural collection.[12]

Epidural Hematoma

Epidural hematomas are collections of blood products between the inner table of the calvarium and the dura. They are confined by the calvarial sutures because the dura is attached to the calvarium in these locations, and as a result, they tend to have a lenticular or biconvex shape. An epidural hematoma may only cross a suture if a fracture involves the suture.

Epidural hematomas can result from arterial or venous bleeding, but typically they are associated with injury to the middle meningeal artery in the setting of a calvarial fracture (**Figs. 4 and 5**). The presence of an epidural hematoma should prompt a search for a calvarial fracture and vice versa, although they can certainly occur in isolation of each other. Injury to a dural venous sinus may result in a venous epidural hematoma.

As discussed in the section on subdural hematomas, acute blood within an epidural hematoma is hyperdense on CT. However, hyperacute, unclotted blood may seem hypodense and mix with hyperdense hemorrhage, generating a "swirl sign" within an epidural hematoma[13] (shown within subdural hematomas in **Figs. 1 and 2**). This appearance of mixed densities within a hematoma should prompt urgent neurosurgical consultation, as it implies ongoing bleeding and potential rapid expansion of the hematoma. Although MRI is more sensitive for detecting subtle hemorrhage and for determining the age of blood products, it is reserved for evaluation of subacute or chronic head trauma with unexplained neurologic deficits or for follow-up if initial imaging was unremarkable but the patient has a persistent neurologic deficit.[3]

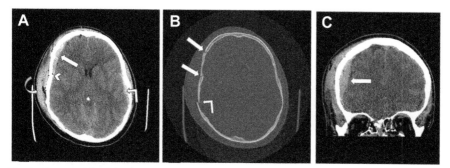

Fig. 4. Acute epidural hematoma in a middle-aged man who was the unhelmeted driver of a motorcycle that collided head-on with a car. (*A*) Axial noncontrast head CT image shows a crescentic acute extra-axial hematoma along the right frontal convexity (*straight arrow*) with a small amount of pneumocephalus (*arrowhead*) as well as soft tissue hemorrhage and gas in the overlying right scalp (*curved arrow*). There is also a contralateral extra-axial hematoma (*angled arrow*). On this image alone, it is difficult to determine whether the hematomas are epidural or subdural. (*B*) Axial noncontrast head CT in bone algorithm reveals multiple acute right calvarial fractures (*straight arrows*) with displacement posteriorly (*angled arrow*). (*C*) Coronal noncontrast head CT shows the classic lentiform, biconvex configuration of the acute EDH along the right frontal convexity (*arrow*).

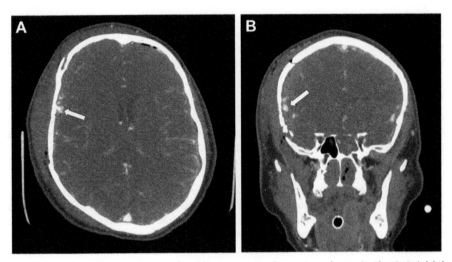

Fig. 5. Active bleeding into the epidural hematoma in the patient shown in **Fig. 4.** Axial (*A*) and coronal (*B*) CT angiographic images of the head show arterial phase contrast extravasation (*arrows*) into the epidural hematoma.

Subarachnoid Hemorrhage

Subarachnoid hemorrhage is located between the arachnoid and pia mater and insinuates within the sulci of the brain. It is generally of smaller volume than subarachnoid hemorrhage caused by aneurysm rupture and tends to be located at or opposite the site of impact (**Fig. 6**). It may also be observed in the basal cisterns, although isolated, cisternal subarachnoid hemorrhage is more often related to ruptured aneurysm and should prompt evaluation for aneurysm. Traumatic subarachnoid hemorrhage may redistribute into the ventricular system, where it may layer dependently or adhere to the ependyma or to the choroid plexus within the ventricles. Intraventricular

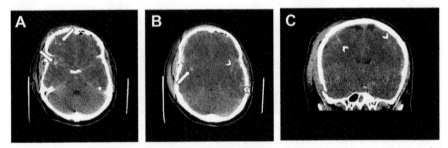

Fig. 6. Brain contusions and subarachnoid hemorrhage in the patient shown in **Fig. 4 and 5.** (*A*) Axial noncontrast head CT image shows multiple small acute parenchymal hemorrhages in the right frontal and anterior temporal lobes (*arrows*) compatible with traumatic contusions. (*B*) Axial noncontrast head CT image at a level superior to that in image *A* shows additional right brain contusion (*arrow*) as well as acute subarachnoid hemorrhage in several left cerebral sulci (*arrowheads*). (*C*) Coronal noncontrast head CT image shows acute subarachnoid hemorrhage in several bilateral cerebral sulci (*arrowheads*). Traumatic subarachnoid hemorrhage tends to be of lower volume than that caused by ruptured aneurysm.

hemorrhage can also arise from a ruptured subependymal vein or via extension from a parenchymal hematoma.

Certain locations of traumatic subarachnoid hemorrhage in the brain are associated with other traumatic brain abnormalities. Hemorrhage in the ambient cisterns or inter-hemispheric fissure on initial head CT has been shown to be a marker of severe diffuse axonal injury (DAI).[14] DAI has also been correlated with intraventricular hemorrhage on initial head CT.[15] Vasospasm is less commonly observed with traumatic subarachnoid hemorrhage than with aneurysmal hemorrhage, although a significant risk for vaso-spasm has been reported in the setting of severe traumatic brain injury.[16] MRI is more sensitive than CT in detecting small volumes of subarachnoid hemorrhage, and MRI performed for short-term follow-up of a patient with persistent neurologic deficit and unremarkable initial head CT may reveal subtle subarachnoid hemorrhage that could not be visualized on CT.

Brain Contusion

Brain contusions are parenchymal "bruises" related to traumatic impact and most often are located in the inferior-anterior frontal and temporal lobes, at coup-contrecoup sites (see **Fig. 6**). Initially, brain contusions may manifest on CT as hypo-dense areas of parenchymal edema with minimal or absent hyperdensity. During the 48 hours following injury, contusions often increase in size and develop progressively hyperdense areas of acute parenchymal hemorrhage. This phenomenon is described as "blossoming" or "blooming" of the contusion.[17] The hyperdense hemorrhage component often then resolves before the edema associated with the contusion. Se-rial imaging is therefore recommended for patients with brain contusions to monitor for progressive mass effect related to the edema, hemorrhage, or both.

The presence of a contusion has also been shown to contribute to the predicted clinical outcome of a patient. Temporal lobe contusions in particular were shown to be associated with a worse functional outcome 6 months following trauma than frontal contusions and extra-axial injuries.[18]

Depending on the age of the contusion, variable degrees of T1 and T2 signal and susceptibility artifact may be present on MRI. MRI is more sensitive than CT for detec-tion of brain contusions, particularly when they are small, located near the calvarium or skull base, or lack hyperdense hemorrhage on CT.[19,20] This contributes to the ACR's determination that noncontrast MRI may be appropriate for short-term follow-up of patients with acute head trauma who have persistent neurologic deficits and normal head CTs.[3] The detection of subtle contusions in these patients, especially those with mild TBI, can assist with determining prognosis.[21]

Fracture

Calvarial and skull base fractures may occur as a result of blunt or penetrating trauma and are frequently associated with intracranial injuries such as epidural hematoma (as discussed above) and brain contusion. Acute fractures are best detected on noncon-trast CT, and some fracture locations are associated with specific additional abnor-malities. Fractures traversing the anterior cranial fossa are often associated with CSF leak,[22] and these patients may report headache features characteristic of intra-cranial hypotension. Imaging findings suggestive of CSF leak may include extra-axial CSF collection or pseudomeningocele, fluid collection in a paranasal sinus, and features of intracranial hypotension such as slumping midbrain and collapsed ventricles (**Fig. 7**). Noncontrast head, face, or temporal bone CT is usually adequate to identify the site of a CSF leak in the setting of head trauma, but if these studies

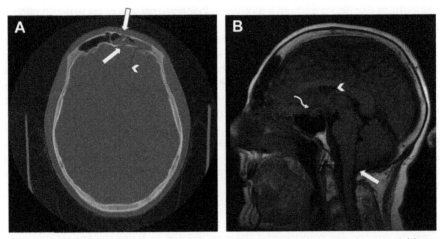

Fig. 7. Acute fractures traversing the left frontal sinus with subsequent intracranial hypotension presumed to relate to CSF leak. (*A*) Axial noncontrast CT image of the head in bone algorithm shows acute displaced fractures disrupting the outer and inner tables of the calvarium at the level of the left frontal sinus (*straight arrows*). A small amount of pneumocephalus is present (*arrowhead*). (*B*) Sagittal T1-weighted MR image of the brain 1 week later shows descent of the cerebellar tonsils into the foramen magnum (*arrow*), collapsed lateral ventricles (*arrowhead*), and effacement of the suprasellar cistern (*curved arrow*), all indicative intracranial hypotension. In the setting of recent fracture involving a paranasal sinus, the cause of the hypotension is most likely a CSF leak.

reveal multiple potential sites of leak, CT cisternography can be used to localize the precise site of CSF leak in order to guide surgical repair.[3,23]

Fractures involving a dural venous sinus or the jugular bulb can cause traumatic venous injury that leads to thrombosis or compression by an extra-axial hematoma.[24] Although findings suggestive of venous sinus injury may be present on noncontrast head CT, such as hyperdensity within a sinus or venous infarct, CT venography is the most useful imaging study to evaluate for suspected acute venous injury[3] (**Fig. 8**).

Long bone or pelvic fractures may rarely result in cerebral fat embolism, in which fat microemboli to the brain cause infarcts and petechial hemorrhage. This entity is best detected with MRI, where it may present with a range of imaging features such as scattered foci of restricted diffusion, areas of confluent T2 hyperintensity, and/or scattered foci of susceptibility artifact primarily in the white matter[25] (**Fig. 9**). The large number of foci of DWI hyperintensity scattered diffusely in the white matter has been described as the "starfield" pattern.[26] Although these patients may experience headache, more severe manifestations of cerebral fat embolism include delirium, seizures, and coma.[27]

Diffuse Axonal Injury

Shearing forces to the white matter can cause DAI. Acceleration–deceleration trauma that may be rotational or translational is associated with DAI and affects both the larger white matter tracts as well as the gray–white matter junction due to the sharp transition between tissues of different densities in this location.[4] MRI is the most sensitive imaging modality to detect DAI and may demonstrate hemorrhagic or nonhemorrhagic white matter lesions (**Fig. 10**). The location of the lesions indicates the severity of the injury per the following grading system: Grade 1 involves the subcortical white matter (at

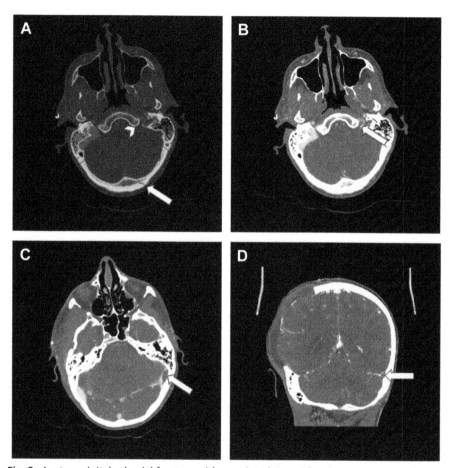

Fig. 8. Acute occipital calvarial fracture with associated sigmoid and transverse sinus thrombosis. (*A*) Axial CTA image of the head in bone algorithm shows acute nondisplaced fractures of the left occipital calvarium (*arrow*) and left aspect of the clivus (*arrowhead*). (*B*) Axial CTA image of the head shows a subocclusive filling defect of the left sigmoid sinus (*arrow*) compatible with thrombus. (*C, D*) Axial (*C*) and coronal (*D*) CTA images of the head show filling defect of the left transverse sinus (*arrows*) with both occlusive (*D*) and subocclusive (*C*) components.

the gray–white matter junction), Grade 2 involves the corpus callosum, and Grade 3 involves the brainstem.[28] DAI lesions restrict diffusion and may demonstrate susceptibility artifact. There may be associated or isolated T2 hyperintense lesions, although these are nonspecific and difficult to attribute to DAI in the absence of signal abnormalities on other sequences. Although both DAI and cerebral fat embolism may demonstrate multifocal susceptibility artifact and restricted diffusion in the white matter, the lesions of cerebral fat embolism tend to be more numerous and diffuse.

Diffusion tensor imaging (DTI) is an advanced imaging technique that has been applied to study patients with mTBI and posttraumatic migraines. Compared with mTBI patients without posttraumatic migraines, migrainous patients had DTI findings suggestive of injury to the corpus callosum and fornix.[29] This imaging tool is not yet used in routine clinical practice, but it has revealed patterns of injury that correlate with posttraumatic headaches.

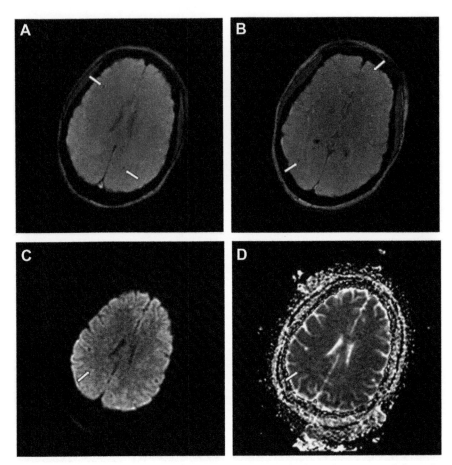

Fig. 9. Cerebral fat embolism in a 26-year-old patient with obtundation several days after sustaining pelvic fractures in a motor vehicle accident. (*A, B*) Axial susceptibility-weighted MR images of the brain show innumerable foci of hypointensity scattered diffusely throughout the white matter (*arrows*) most compatible with petechial hemorrhages related to fat microemboli to the brain. (*C, D*) Axial diffusion-weighted (*C*) and apparent diffusion coefficient (*D*) MR images of the brain show tiny foci of DWI hyperintensity and ADC hypointensity (*arrows*) compatible with restricted diffusion associated with the foci of susceptibility hypointensity. These are compatible with areas of ischemia and have been described as the "starfield" pattern.

Herniation

Mass effect associated with traumatic hemorrhage or edema in the brain may result in herniation, which can then cause secondary infarcts, hemorrhage, or hydrocephalus. Uncal or downward transtentorial herniation (see **Figs. 1 and 2**) may result in ipsilateral third nerve palsy and dilated pupil. The herniating brain can impress on the ipsilateral posterior cerebral artery and result in infarct in that territory. Bilateral or severe unilateral downward transtentorial herniation can also cause hemorrhage in the midbrain, referred to as Duret hemorrhage (see **Fig. 2**). The herniating brain in this setting may compress perforating arteries from the circle of Willis and result in basal ganglia or hypothalamic infarcts.

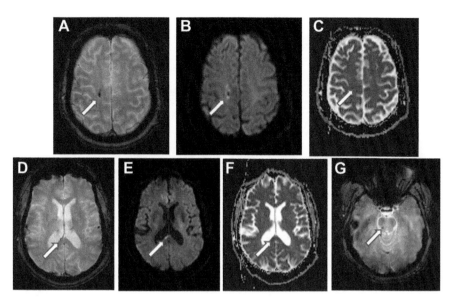

Fig. 10. DAI in a middle-aged man who was the unrestrained passenger in a motor vehicle collision. (*A*) Axial susceptibility-weighted MR image of the brain shows a hypointense focus in the right frontal white matter near the gray–white junction (*arrow*). There is corresponding hyperintensity that surrounds central hypointensity on diffusion-weighted image (*B*) and hypointensity on apparent diffusion coefficient image (*C*) compatible with restricted diffusion (*arrows*). This finding in isolation would indicate grade 1 DAI. (*D*) Axial susceptibility-weighted MR image of the brain in the same patient shows a hypointense focus in the splenium of the corpus callosum with corresponding restricted diffusion (*arrows*) (*E*, *F*). Involvement of the corpus callosum indicates grade 2 DAI. (*G*) Axial susceptibility-weighted MR image of the brain shows a hypointense focus in the dorsal midbrain (*arrow*) which indicates grade 3 DAI.

Subfalcine herniation can cause ipsilateral anterior cerebral artery territory infarction. If the herniating brain obstructs the foramen of Monro, the contralateral lateral ventricle can become dilated: this is referred to as ventricular entrapment (see **Fig. 1**). Cerebellar tonsillar herniation may obstruct the fourth ventricular outlet and cause hydrocephalus. If severe, this type of herniation can impress on the posterior inferior cerebellar artery and result in infarct in that territory. Ascending transtentorial herniation can obstruct the cerebral aqueduct and cause hydrocephalus at that level. The superior cerebellar arteries may be compressed in this setting and cause infarction.

Arterial Injury

Traumatic injury to the middle meningeal artery is discussed above in the section on epidural hematoma (see **Fig. 5**), but there are other arterial injuries that may result in headache. Traumatic injury to the cervical carotid artery more often presents with ipsilateral neck pain, neck hematoma, and possibly signs of infarct or cranial nerve palsy, although a traumatic aneurysm of this artery may result in headache.[30] Traumatic injury of the intracranial internal carotid artery may present with unilateral headache, as can injury to the intradural vertebral artery. CT angiography of the head and neck is usually appropriate to evaluate for arterial injury in patients with head trauma and

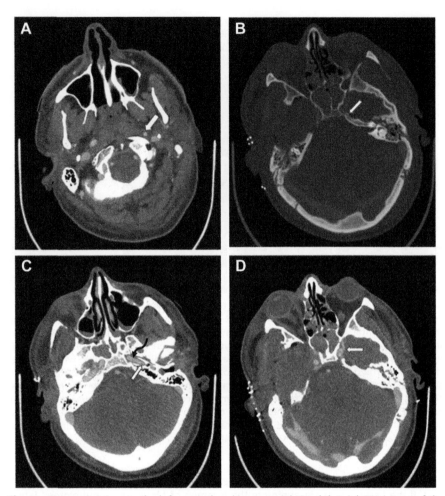

Fig. 11. Traumatic injury to the left cervical and intracranial ICA. (*A*) Axial CTA image of the head shows asymmetric smaller caliber of distal cervical left internal carotid artery relative to the right and slight irregularity (*arrow*) concerning for traumatic injury. (*B*) Axial CTA image of the head in bone algorithm shows an acute nondisplaced fracture involving the left carotid canal (*arrow*). (*C*) Axial CTA image of the head shows eccentric (*arrow*) and equivocal central linear (*black curved arrow*) filling defects in the petrous left ICA concerning for dissection and possible intimal flap. (*D*) Axial CTA image of the head shows asymmetric arterial phase contrast filling of the left cavernous sinus (*arrow*) concerning for traumatic carotid-cavernous fistula.

either clinical risk factors for vascular injury or imaging findings that may indicate vascular injury.[3] Imaging findings may include irregularity and narrowing of the injured artery and/or a linear filling defect compatible with intimal flap (**Fig. 11**). The presence of intracranial hemorrhage or infarct following trauma may prompt CTA, but skull base and cervical spine fractures are particularly concerning and warrant vascular imaging.

Traumatic carotid-cavernous fistula is a specific vascular injury that is associated with skull base fractures, particularly those involving the carotid canal. Damage to the intracranial internal carotid artery can lead to an arteriovenous shunt between the artery and the adjacent cavernous sinus. Symptoms of this fistula include headache, orbital edema, and reduced vision and may present days following the injury or may be delayed and manifest several months later.[31] Noncontrast head CT and CTA may have findings suggestive of this fistula, such as dilation of the ipsilateral superior ophthalmic vein and cavernous sinus or arterial phase contrast filling of these venous structures (see **Fig. 11**). However, digital subtraction angiography is the definitive imaging tool when a traumatic carotid-cavernous fistula is suspected.

POSTCRANIOTOMY SYNDROMES

Although the ICHD classifies headache attributed to craniotomy as a type of posttraumatic headache,[1] some of the mechanisms and imaging features of postcraniotomy headaches are unique from those associated with noniatrogenic trauma. The ICHD describes a headache attributed to craniotomy as one that develops within 7 days after the craniotomy or within 7 days of regaining consciousness or discontinuing medications that impair the ability to sense or report headache.[1] To be attributed to craniotomy, a headache should not be better accounted for by another diagnosis. Postcraniotomy headache is common, with reported incidence of 60% when using the above definition.[32] There is a higher prevalence of headache when the duration of surgery is greater than 4 hours and when a craniectomy is performed rather than craniotomy or cranioplasty.[33] Some of the structural abnormalities and complications of craniotomy and their imaging appearances are discussed below.

Hemorrhage, Edema, and Pneumocephalus

A small amount of extra-axial hemorrhage is expected deep to a craniotomy immediately postoperatively, but if the hematoma is larger than generally observed, increases during serial imaging examinations, and/or causes mass effect (**Fig. 12**), it may

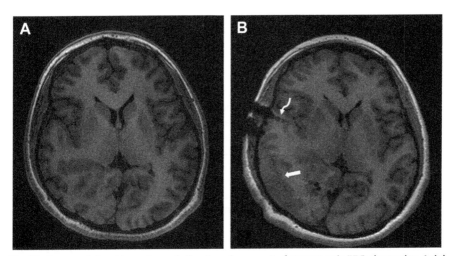

Fig. 12. Large subdural hematoma following placement of stereotactic EEG electrodes. Axial 3D T1-weighted MR images of the brain before (*A*) and following (*B*) placement of intracranial stereotactic EEG electrodes (*curved arrow*) shows a right parietotemporal subdural collection that is isointense to brain and new from the preoperative examination compatible with subdural hematoma. There is a mass effect on the underlying brain, and the hematoma was large enough to warrant subsequent evacuation.

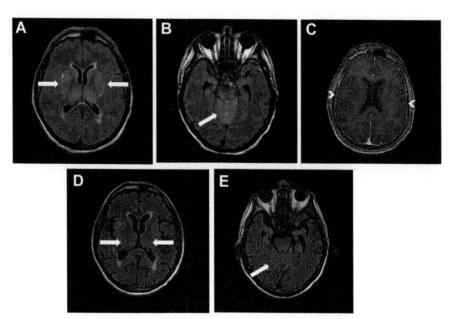

Fig. 13. Postoperative intracranial hypotension in an elderly man presenting with seizure and altered mental status after recent lumbar fusion that was complicated by durotomy. (*A, B*) Axial T2/FLAIR MR images of the brain show symmetric abnormal T2/FLAIR hyperintensity within the bilateral basal ganglia and thalami as well as within the superior cerebellum (*arrows*). (*C*) Axial postcontrast 3D T1-weighted MR image of the brain shows diffuse pachymeningeal enhancement (*arrowheads*) suggestive of intracranial hypotension. (*D, E*) Axial T2/FLAIR MR images of the brain 6 weeks later show resolution of the prior edema within the basal ganglia, thalami, and cerebellum (*arrows*).

become symptomatic and require evacuation to prevent herniation. Noncontrast head CT is the most appropriate examination to initially assess for postoperative hemorrhage, although MRI may detect smaller, more subtle hemorrhage. An extra-axial collection deep to a craniotomy often contains a combination of acute blood and fluid, so its density on CT may be lower than would be expected for purely acute hemorrhage. Extra-axial hematomas after craniotomy are usually extradural and located directly beneath the bone flap, but extradural hematomas may also occur adjacent to the bone flap margins or in a location remote from the flap.[33]

Parenchymal hemorrhage may also be expected postoperatively if the intervention was on the brain parenchyma or required traversal of the brain. For example, resection of an intra-axial tumor or placement of an external ventricular drain may result in a small amount of parenchymal hemorrhage surrounding the resection cavity or along the surgical tract. If the hemorrhage is larger than routinely observed, expands, or exerts significant mass effect, it may become clinically significant and warrant further intervention.

A unique type of parenchymal hemorrhage that may be observed after a craniotomy or even a spinal surgery is remote cerebellar hemorrhage. This occurs distant from the surgical site and is believed to reflect a form of hemorrhagic infarction that results from occlusion of posterior fossa bridging veins when the cerebellum sags in response to low CSF volume/intracranial hypotension.[34]

Intracranial hypotension induced by either an intracranial or spinal operative dural defect can cause low-pressure headaches and manifest on CT or MRI with findings

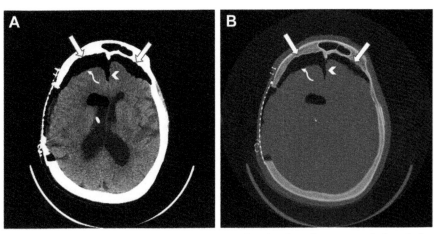

Fig. 14. Tension pneumocephalus in a patient who developed acute confusion 2 days following craniotomy. Axial noncontrast CT images of the head in brain (*A*) and bone (*B*) windows show bifrontal subdural gas (*straight arrows*) tracking into the interhemispheric fissure (*arrowheads*). The right frontal pneumocephalus exerts mass effect on the right frontal lobe (*curved arrows*).

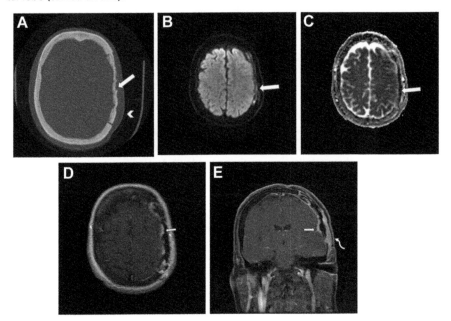

Fig. 15. Infected bone flap in patient with cellulitis of the overlying scalp 1 month after craniotomy. (*A*) Axial noncontrast CT image of the head in bone algorithm shows erosions and lytic changes (*straight arrow*) of the left frontoparietal bone flap with overlying soft tissue swelling (*arrowhead*). (*B, C*) Axial diffusion-weighted (*B*) and apparent diffusion coefficient (*C*) MR images of the head show restricted diffusion involving the bone flap (*straight arrows*). (*D*) Axial postcontrast T1-weighted MR image of the head shows abnormal dural enhancement deep to the craniotomy (*straight arrow*) that is thicker and more irregular than that normally observed after craniotomy. (*E*) Coronal postcontrast T1 fat-saturated MR image of the head shows abnormal dural (*straight arrow*) and soft tissue (*curved arrow*) enhancement concerning for phlegmon.

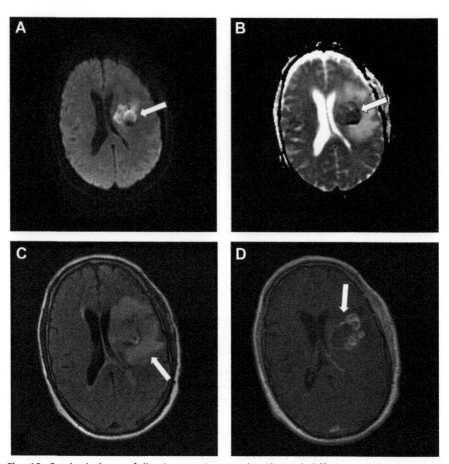

Fig. 16. Cerebral abscess following craniotomy. (*A, B*) Axial diffusion-weighted (*A*) and apparent diffusion coefficient (*B*) MR images of the brain show a collection in the left corona radiata deep to the craniotomy that demonstrates internal restricted diffusion (*arrows*). (*C*) Axial T2/FLAIR MR image of the brain shows confluent T2 hyperintensity surrounding the collection (*arrow*) compatible with vasogenic edema. (*D*) Axial postcontrast T1-weighted MR image of the brain shows peripheral enhancement of the collection (*arrow*). This constellation of imaging features most likely represents abscess.

of slumping brainstem, effacement of the suprasellar cistern, and decreased ventricular caliber as discussed in the section on fracture. However, additional findings of symmetric edema involving the bilateral basal ganglia, thalamus, and/or cerebellum or brainstem have been observed in the setting of postoperative intracranial hypotension[35] (**Fig. 13**).

Pneumocephalus is expected to a slight degree immediately following craniotomy, but when it exerts mass effect on the brain and is associated with neurologic decline, it is considered tension pneumocephalus and becomes a neurosurgical emergency. Imaging findings of this process include gas in the bifrontal subdural compartment, which impresses on and deforms the underlying brain parenchyma (**Fig. 14**). The subdural gas may also track into and widen the interhemispheric fissure.[36]

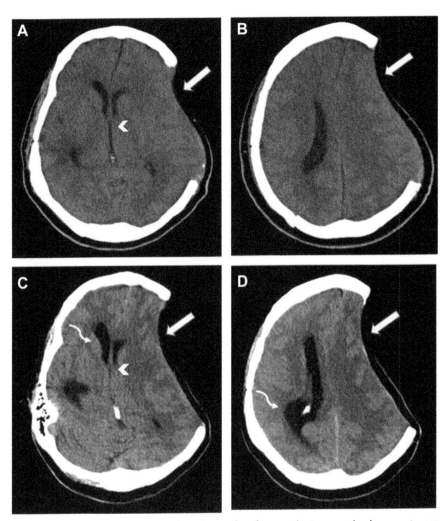

Fig. 17. Trephine syndrome in a patient 3 months after craniectomy and subsequent para-doxical herniation in the same patient following lumbar puncture. (*A, B*) Axial noncontrast CT images of the head demonstrate concave deformity of the left frontal lobe underlying the craniectomy defect (*arrows*). There is slight rightward midline shift at this time (*arrowhead*). (*C, D*) Axial noncontrast CT images of the head in the same patient after lumbar puncture reveal progressed concave deformity of the left frontal lobe (*arrow*) as well as pro-gressed rightward subfalcine herniation (*arrowhead*) and interval dilation of the right lateral ventricle (*curved arrows*) indicating entrapment.

Infection

Postoperative infection may affect the craniotomy bone flap, extra-axial compartment, or brain. Bone flap infection usually manifests a few weeks after surgery and is often preceded by overlying cellulitis. Longer surgeries and repeat craniotomies are associ-ated with a higher rate of bone flap infection, as are surgeries in which the paranasal sinuses are violated. CT and MRI can be useful in the detection of bone flap infection, although the CT findings of osteolysis may also be observed in old, devitalized bone flaps. MRI is therefore more reliable and demonstrates bone marrow edema and enhancement when a bone flap is infected (**Fig. 15**).

The most common extra-axial infection following craniotomy is extradural abscess. The subdural compartment is less frequently involved because postoperative infections often begin in the superficial soft tissues and spread first to the extradural region.[37] CT can be used to detect an extra-axial fluid collection, but MRI is more sensitive for determining whether it is infected. Both extradural abscesses and subdural empyemas demonstrate internal T2 hyperintensity as well as peripheral enhancement. Diffusion restriction of the contents of a rim-enhancing fluid collection generally indicates infection, but this sequence is less reliable in the postoperative setting, in part due to the presence of blood products that can also restrict diffusion.[38] In addition to these false-positive cases of extra-axial infection, false-negative rates of extradural abscess and subdural empyema are higher in postoperative patients: one study demonstrated a 47% false-negative rate for extradural abscess detection on diffusion-weighted imaging of postoperative patients.[38]

Brain or cerebral abscess may occur following craniotomy and demonstrates the same imaging features as extra-axial abscess but is located in the brain parenchyma (**Fig. 16**). In one large retrospective study, the number of patients with intracranial infection who developed a postoperative cerebral abscess was similar to the number of patients who developed a subdural empyema, about 15% of infected patients.[39]

Postcraniectomy

There are two postoperative phenomena unique to patients who have undergone craniectomy. Trephine syndrome or syndrome of the trephined manifests as headaches, seizures, dizziness, and excessive fatigue in the months following craniectomy. Imaging of these patients often reveals a sunken or concave morphology of the skin flap overlying the craniectomy (**Fig. 17**). The symptoms are thought to relate to altered CSF dynamics and reduced cerebral perfusion due to exposure of the intracranial contents to atmospheric pressure.[40] Cranioplasty leads to clinical improvement in some of these patients.

Paradoxical herniation is a rare complication of craniectomy and may be observed in patients with a large craniectomy defect who undergo subsequent CSF drainage via lumbar puncture or ventricular shunting. The decrease in CSF pressure in the setting of brain exposed to the external environment can result in atmospheric pressure overtaking intracranial pressure and causing herniation of the brain away from the craniectomy defect (see **Fig. 17**). Clinical manifestations of this process include depressed level of consciousness and focal neurologic deficits.[40] Paradoxical herniation should be emergently managed by increasing intracranial pressure via clamping of any ventricular catheters and perhaps performing cranioplasty.

SUMMARY

Headache can occur following trauma or surgery to the brain and may be associated with the specific pathologic processes described. In the acute setting following trauma or craniotomy, hemorrhage, edema, and vascular injury are among the causes of headache. Postcraniotomy infection has a more indolent course and delayed presentation. Recognizing the imaging features of these processes allows for prompt diagnosis and management.

CLINICS CARE POINTS

- Noncontrast CT of the brain is usually the best initial imaging tool to evaluate patients with headache following trauma or craniotomy.

- Brain MRI is more sensitive than CT for detecting certain posttraumatic and postoperative abnormalities such as DAI and infection.
- Extra-axial hematomas with mixed density on CT may contain hyperacute, hypodense blood products rather than simply acute on chronic hemorrhage.
- The diagnoses of postoperative tension pneumocephalus and paradoxical herniation should be based on both imaging features and clinical presentation.
- MRI is less reliable in demonstrating extra-axial infection in the postoperative setting than in nonoperative patients, with relatively high false-negative and false-positive rates.

DISCLOSURE

The author has nothing to disclose.

REFERENCES

1. Headache Classification Committee of the International Headache Society (HIS). The International Classification of Headache Disorders, 3rd edition. Cephalalgia 2018;38:1–211.
2. Lucas S, Hoffman JM, Bell KR, et al. A prospective study of prevalence and characterization of headache following mild traumatic brain injury. Cephalalgia 2014; 34:93–102.
3. Shih RY, Burns J, Ajam AA, et al. ACR Appropriateness Criteria Head Trauma. Available at: https://acsearch.acr.org/docs/69481/Narrative/. Am Coll Radiol. Accessed August 20, 2021.
4. Schweitzer AD, Niogi SN, Whitlow CT, et al. Traumatic brain injury: imaging patterns and complications. Radiographics 2019;39:1571–95.
5. Wei SC, Ulmer S, Lev MH, et al. Value of coronal reformations in the CT evaluation of acute head trauma. AJNR Am J Neuroradiol 2010;31:334–9.
6. Zacharia TT, Nguyen DT. Subtle pathology detection with multidetector row coronal and sagittal CT reformations in acute head trauma. Emerg Radiol 2010;17(2): 97–102.
7. Sieswerda-Hoogendoorn T, Postema FAM, Verbaan D, et al. Age determination of subdural hematomas with CT and MRI: a systematic review. Eur J Radiol 2014; 83(7):1257–68.
8. Iliescu IA. Current diagnosis and treatment of chronic subdural hematomas. J Med Life 2015;8(3):278–84.
9. Kolias AG, Chari A, Santarius T, et al. Chronic subdural haematoma: modern management and emerging therapies. Nat Rev Neurol 2014;10(10):570–8.
10. Tsutsumi K, Maeda K, Iijima A, et al. The relationship of preoperative magnetic resonance imaging findings and closed system drainage in the recurrence of chronic subdural hematoma. J Neurosurg 1997;87(6):870–5.
11. Zanini MA, de Lima Resende LA, de Souza Faleiros AT, et al. Traumatic subdural hygromas: proposed pathogenesis based classification. J Trauma 2008;64(3): 705–13.
12. Bodanapally UK, Dreizin D, Issa G, et al. Dual-energy CT in enhancing subdural effusions that masquerade as subdural hematomas: diagnosis with virtual high-monochromatic (190-keV) images. AJNR Am J Neuroradiol 2017;38(10):1946–52.
13. Al-Nashkabandi NA. The swirl sign. Radiology 2001;218(2):433.

14. Mata-Mbemba D, Mugikura S, Nakagawa A, et al. Traumatic midline subarachnoid hemorrhage on initial computed tomography as a marker of severe diffuse axonal injury. J Neurosurg 2018;129(5):1317–24.

15. Mata-Mbemba D, Mugikura S, Nakagawa A, et al. Intraventricular hemorrhage on initial computed tomography as marker of diffuse axonal injury after traumatic brain injury. J Neurotrauma 2015;32(5):359–65.

16. Perrein A, Petry L, Reis A, et al. Cerebral vasospasm after traumatic brain injury: an update. Minerva Anestesiol 2015;81(11):1219–28.

17. Alahmadi H, Vachhrajani S, Cusimano MD. The natural history of brain contusion: an analysis of radiological and clinical progression. J Neurosurg 2010;112(5):1139–45.

18. Yue JK, Winkler EA, Puffer RC, et al. Temporal lobe contusions on computed tomography are associated with impaired 6-month functional recovery after mild traumatic brain injury: a TRACK-TBI study. Neurol Res 2018;40(11):972–81.

19. Paterakis K, Karantanas AH, Komnos A, et al. Outcome of patients with diffuse axonal injury: the significance and prognostic value of MRI in the acute phase. J Trauma 2000;49(6):1071–5.

20. Linsenmaier U, Wirth S, Kanz KG, et al. Imaging minor head injury (MHI) in emergency radiology: MRI highlights additional intracranial findings after measurement of trauma biomarker S-100B in patients with normal CCT. Br J Radiol 2016;89:20150827.

21. Yuh EL, Mukherjee P, Lingsma HF, et al. Magnetic resonance imaging improves 3-month outcome prediction in mild traumatic brain injury. Ann Neurol 2013;73(2):224–35.

22. Baugnon KL, Hudgins PA. Skull base fractures and their complications. Neuroimaging Clin N Am 2014;24(3):439–65, vii-viii.

23. Hiremath SB, Gautam AA, Sasindran V, et al. Cerebrospinal fluid rhinorrhea and otorrhea: a multimodality imaging approach. Diagn Interv Imaging 2019;100(1):3–15.

24. Rischall MA, Boegel KH, Palmer CS, et al. MDCT venographic patterns of dural venous sinus compromise after acute skull fracture. AJR Am J Roentgenol 2016;207(4):852–8.

25. Kuo KH, Pan YJ, Lai YJ, et al. Dynamic MR imaging patterns of cerebral fat embolism: a systematic review with illustrative cases. AJNR Am J Neuroradiol 2014;35(6):1052–7.

26. Parizel PM, Demey HE, Veeckmans G, et al. Early diagnosis of cerebral fat embolism syndrome by diffusion-weighted MRI (starfield pattern). Stroke 2001;32(12):2942–4.

27. Kosova E, Bergmark B, Piazza G. Fat embolism syndrome. Circulation 2015;131(3):317–20.

28. Moen KG, Brezova V, Skandsen T, et al. Traumatic axonal injury: the prognostic value of lesion load in corpus callosum, brain stem, and thalamus in different magnetic resonance imaging sequences. J Neurotrauma 2014;31(17):1486–96.

29. Alhilali LM, Delic J, Fakhran S. Differences in callosal and forniceal diffusion between patients with and without postconcussive migraine. AJNR Am J Neuroradiol 2017;38:691–5.

30. Rutman AM, Vranic JE, Mossa-Basha M. Imaging and management of blunt cerebrovascular injury. Radiographics 2018;38(2):542–63.

31. Shim HS, Kang KJ, Choi HJ, et al. Delayed contralateral traumatic carotid cavernous fistula after craniomaxillofacial fractures. Arch Craniofac Surg 2019;20(1):44–7.

32. Rocha-Filho PA. Post-craniotomy headache: a clinical view with a focus on the persistent form. Headache 2015;55(5):733–8.
33. Sinclair AG, Scoffings DJ. Imaging of the post-operative cranium. Radiographics 2010;30:461–82.
34. Amini A, Osborn AG, McCall TD, et al. Remote cerebellar hemorrhage. AJNR Am J Neuroradiol 2006;27(2):387–90.
35. Hadizadeh DR, Kovacs A, Tschampa H, et al. Postsurgical intracranial hypotension: diagnostic and prognostic imaging findings. AJNR Am J Neuroradiol 2010; 31(1):100–5.
36. Michel SJ. The Mount Fuji sign. Radiology 2004;232(2):449–50.
37. Hlavin ML, Kaminski HJ, Fenstermaker RA, et al. Intracranial suppuration: a modern decade of postoperative subdural empyema and epidural abscess. Neurosurgery 1994;34(6):974–80.
38. Farrell CJ, Hoh BL, Pisculli ML, et al. Limitations of diffusion-weighted imaging in the diagnosis of postoperative infections. Neurosurgery 2008;62(3):577–83.
39. Dashti SR, Baharvahdat H, Spetzler RF, et al. Operative intracranial infection following craniotomy. Neurosurg Focus 2008;24(6):E10.
40. Akins PT, Guppy KH. Sinking skin flaps, paradoxical herniation, and external brain tamponade: a review of decompressive craniectomy management. Neurocrit Care 2008;9(2):269–76.

Role of Computed Tomography and Magnetic Resonance Imaging in the Evaluation of Headache Due to Paranasal Sinus and Teeth Disorder

Ian T. Mark, MD, Christine M. Glastonbury, MBBS*

KEYWORDS

• Facial pain • Headache • Sinusitis • Odontogenic • Dental

KEY POINTS

- In any patient being imaged for headache, attention should be paid to the paranasal sinuses and teeth as a source of symptoms, particularly when the initial brain imaging is normal.
- While frontal, ethmoid, and maxillary sinusitis may be more readily discernible on clinical examination, sphenoid sinusitis patients may not localize well, but present as a deep-seated headache that may feel worse when bending over.
- When unilateral maxillary sinusitis is found, first consider dental disease as the cause ["odontogenic sinusitis"].
- The paranasal sinuses are best evaluated with a dedicated sinus non-enhanced CT protocol which allows coronal and sagittal reformats and facilitates surgical management.
- In patients with a known or suspected sinus infection who develop a severe headache and/or altered mental status, consideration should be given to intracranial complications of sinusitis, and contrast-enhanced CT and/or MRI should be considered for evaluation.

OVERVIEW

For the initial evaluation of patients with headache, CT is typically the first imaging test used. Particularly when no intracranial abnormality is determined, attention should also be paid to the paranasal sinuses and teeth as a source of symptoms. To maximize the value of a head CT examination, bone algorithm images should also be processed then evaluated on bone window settings [for example, window width (W) 2800 and

Department of Radiology & Biomedical Imaging, University of California, San Francisco, Box 0628, 505 Parnassus Avenue, San Francisco, CA 94143, USA
* Corresponding author.
E-mail address: christine.glastonbury@ucsf.edu

Abbreviations	
CT	Computed Tomography
MRI	Magnetic Resonance Imaging
OMC	Ostiomeatal complex
AFIFS	Acute fulminant invasive fungal sinusitis
V1	First, or Ophthalmic, division of the Trigeminal nerve
V2	Second, or Maxillary, division of the Trigeminal nerve
V3	Third, or Mandibular, division of the Trigeminal nerve
SPG	Sphenopalatine ganglion
PPF	Pterygopalatine fossa
TMJ	Temporomandibular joint

window level (L) 600]. This allows evaluation of the calvarium and skull base and importantly for this discussion, of the paranasal sinuses and maxillary dentition. Some head CT examinations might extend inferiorly to include the mandibular teeth also although this is not common.

Detailed imaging of the paranasal sinuses requires thin-slice CT performed in the axial plane with reformat of images in bone algorithm in the sagittal, and coronal planes also. The mucosa of the normal, non-inflamed sinus is not seen on CT and mucosal thickening on non-enhanced CT (NECT) is abnormal, and therefore intravenous contrast is not required to evaluate the mucosa or to categorize it as abnormal.[1] CT can not only evaluate the mucosal thickening or opacification of the individual sinuses, but the spatial resolution of CT allows for examination of the physiologic outflow pathways of mucociliary clearance. Identifying the patency of these outflow tracts helps to plan intervention with functional endoscopic sinus surgery (FESS). These key pathways are the frontal recess, spheno-ethmoidal recess, and the ostiomeatal unit or ostiomeatal complex (OMC). The OMC is a term that encompasses the maxillary sinus ostium, infundibulum, uncinate process, hiatus semilunaris, ethmoid bulla, and middle meatus. This is a common drainage pathway of the frontal sinuses, maxillary sinuses, and anterior ethmoid air cells.

Paranasal sinus development occurs in the first decade of childhood although only the maxillary and ethmoid sinuses are present at birth. Pneumatization of the sphenoid sinuses begins between 4 months and 4 years of age.[2] The frontal sinuses are the last to develop after the age of 5 years.[3] While frontal, ethmoid, and maxillary sinusitis are often more readily discernible on clinical examination, with pain elicited on facial pressure, sphenoid sinusitis patients may not localize well on clinical examination. Sphenoid inflammation may present as a deep-seated headache that may feel worse when bending over. In up to 50% of cases isolated sphenoid sinus inflammatory disease manifests as headaches.[4]

Complications from sphenoid sinus disease can carry significant comorbidities because of the intimate relationship of the paranasal sinuses with critical structures. Multiple cranial nerves are adjacent with the optic nerve superiorly in the optic canal and multiple cavernous sinus cranial nerves, III, IV, and VI, and the internal carotid artery within the cavernous sinus and lateral and superior to the sphenoid sinus. The cranial nerves V1 and V2 course in the cavernous sinus lateral wall. Conventional pneumatization of the sphenoid sinuses means that the sella and pituitary gland along the superior boarder are also critical neighboring structures. Whenever intracranial complications are suspected either a contrast-enhanced CT (CECT) or an MRI are recommended for complete evaluation. Often both are performed to allow surgical planning.

SINUS INFLAMMATION AND "Warning SIGNS"

Sinus inflammatory disease, also known as rhinosinusitis for the concurrent involvement of the nasal cavity, is frequently evident on non-contrast head CT. As an apparently 'incidental' finding on a head CT, sinus opacification should always be described as it may be the true cause of headache symptoms. Most often and as an incidental finding, small fluid density retention cysts may be noted in the paranasal sinus.

Mucosal thickening of the sinus with mild sinus inflammatory disease is seen as linear low density lining the sinus wall. This can progress to moderate, marked, or complete opacification of the paranasal sinuses. Fluid levels or 'frothy' appearing secretions may also be seen, which favors a more acute inflammatory process. The differential for the presence of fluid levels in the paranasal sinus is a denser "blood-level" which indicates recent hemorrhage into the sinus which is most often associated with facial fractures or occurring with epistaxis. Additionally, complete sinus opacification and mucosal thickening greater than 5 mm have been associated with acute sinusitis.[5]

Imaging is generally not recommended for acute sinus inflammation, and only recommended when there is a history of at least 3 months of symptoms and/or there is a concern for orbital or intracranial spread of sinus infection.[6] In this latter situation when, for example, a patient has a significant headache with a clinical concern of subperiosteal or orbital abscess, meningitis, or subdural empyema, then contrast-enhanced head CT should be performed for better sensitivity of detection of such complications. MRI may also be required if there is CT evidence or ongoing clinical concern for intracranial complications.[7]

Several of the findings that are associated with acute sinusitis can be seen in asymptomatic patients, trauma patients, and in the setting of nasal irrigation. In the setting of acute sinusitis, viral (more common) and bacterial sinusitis are difficult to differentiate on imaging. A case series has described using restricted diffusion on MRI diffusion-weighted imaging (DWI) to identify bacteria sinusitis.[8] While this technique could help to suggest the etiology of acute sinusitis without exposing the patient to radiation, MRI in the setting of suspected sinusitis is not indicated as a first-line examination unless there are clinical symptoms concerning for intracranial complications of sinusitis or acute invasive fungal infection.

Acute fulminant invasive fungal sinusitis (AFIFS) is a sinister infection seen in patients with altered immune function from diabetes or low white cell count (eg post-

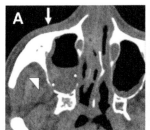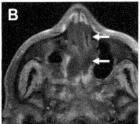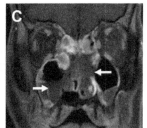

Fig. 1. Acute fulminant invasive fungal sinusitis (AFIFS). Noncontrast CT (*A*) shows mucosal thickening of the right nasal cavity and right maxillary sinus. There is dehiscence of the lateral and medial walls of the right maxillary sinus (*asterisks*), infrequently seen in AFIFS, with inflammatory changes that efface the right premaxillary (*arrow*) and retroantral ((*arrowhead*)) fat pads. Postcontrast T1 weighted axial ((*B*) and coronal (*C*) MRI shows extensive nonenhancing mucosa of the nasal cavities, maxillary sinuses, and ethmoid air cells (*arrows*).

chemotherapy, leukemia) and may present with headache and/or facial pain. If there is any clinical concern for this entity, then contrast-enhanced CT or contrast-enhanced MRI should be performed (**Fig. 1**). AFIFS most often starts at the nasal vestibule and so the earliest imaging findings are of unilateral nasal opacification. As the infection progresses, the fungal elements spread through vessels and results in necrosis of tissues. On imaging, this is first seen as haziness of the peri-sinus fat planes (premaxillary and retroantral), although may also involve orbital fat. Contrast-enhanced imaging best delineates areas of necrosis as areas that have a loss of contrast enhancement. As MRI is more sensitive than CT to contrast enhancement, this is the preferred imaging modality for this diagnosis and for surgical planning, as well as offering excellent detail of orbital and intracranial tissues.

More commonly, non-fungal chronic sinus inflammatory disease most often results in mucoperiosteal thickening and neo-osteogenesis so that the paranasal sinus walls are thickened and hyperdense and there is thickening of the mucosal sinus lining. Secondary fungal colonization may occur in this setting with focal, usually hyperdense on CT, mycetomas which may form round dense balls in the sinuses. On MRI these non-invasive mycetomas usually have low T2 signal intensity and are usually hyperintense on T1 weighted images. Chronic obstruction of a sinus ostium from a benign mass or chronic inflammation, or scarring after surgery or trauma, can result in the expansion of the sinus volume with smooth thinning of the walls, as a mucocele. Ethmoid and frontal mucoceles are most common and frequently present with orbital symptoms from the displacement of the globe, rather than headache. The bone thinning can be so marked as to the wall being almost imperceptible on sinus CT. Frank osseous destruction of the sinus wall, by comparison is concerning for an aggressive process including chronic invasive fungal sinusitis (a less fulminant but still aggressive fungal infection) and granulomatous disease, such as sarcoid, granulomatosis with polyangiitis, and cocaine granulomatosis. These granulomatous processes, however, are chronic inflammatory processes and typically result in areas of soft tissue and bone

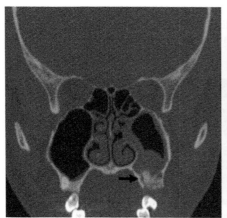 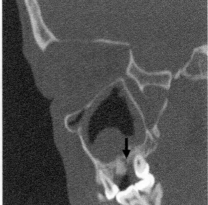

Fig. 2. Odontogenic sinusitis. Coronal and sagittal reformats from a paranasal sinus nonenhanced CT demonstrates unilateral mucosal thickening of the left maxillary sinus. There is extensive dental inflammatory change related to the left maxillary molars with the erosion of the first left maxillary molar and periapical lucency (*arrows*). The palatal root of the tooth extends into the maxillary sinus. There is a more subtle periapical lucency around the roots of the second left maxillary molar.

thickening as well as bone and cartilage destruction. The presence of a soft tissue mass in association with bone destruction should always be most concerning for sino-nasal malignancy, which is most commonly squamous cell carcinoma.

ODONTOGENIC SINUSITIS

When unilateral maxillary sinus inflammatory changes are evident, without inflamma-tion of any of the remaining paranasal sinuses, the first consideration should be dental disease (odontogenic sinusitis) related to the roots of the maxillary molars extending through the maxillary alveolus into the sinus (**Fig. 2**). Focal lucency around the root apex of the tooth represents periodontal or pulpal disease.[9] The second maxillary mo-lars are closest to the inferior maxillary sinus walls, and periapical inflammation from these teeth can extend into the Schneiderian membrane (the membranous lining of the maxillary sinus) and lead to odontogenic sinusitis. Untreated abscesses can also progress to involve the subjacent lamina dura and cortical bone, and manifest as an abscess along the cortex (subperiosteal) or in the nearby soft tissues. This should not be confused with a thin diffuse lucency along the margin of the entire root of the tooth, which is widening of the periodontal ligament.

COMPLICATIONS OF SINUSITIS

The most concerning complications of acute sinusitis are orbital or intracranial exten-sion of infection. Sinus infection can result in extra-axial abscesses in the subdural or epidural space.[10] By definition, an epidural abscess is located between the inner table of the skull and the dura mater. Subdural empyema, by definition, resides in the sub-dural space between the dura mater and the arachnoid mater and has been termed a subdural abscess, cortical abscess, purulent pachymeningitis, phlegmonous meningi-tis, and subdural suppuration.[11] While it would seem most likely that the epidural/sub-dural space immediately deep to the frontal sinuses is the first site of infection from direct intracranial extension, this does not have to be the place whereby infection in-vades. Infection can also seed through valveless diploic veins. Thin subdural and

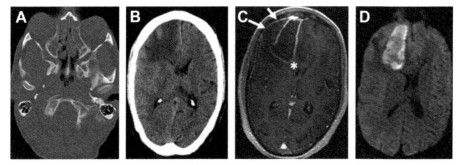

Fig. 3. Intraparenchymal brain abscess from sinusitis. Bone windows on the lowest slice of a head CT showed pansinusitis *(A)*. Further imaging *(B)* demonstrates vasogenic edema in the right frontal lobe with sulcal effacement and mass effect on the frontal horn of the right lateral ventricle. Postcontrast T1 weighted imaging *(C)* shows a peripherally enhancing collection in the right frontal lobe with extensive mass effect and deformity of the right frontal horn *(asterisk)*. Note the dural inflammation with linear enhancement over the right frontal lobe *(arrows)*. Diffusion-weighted imaging *(D)* demonstrates high signal intensity restricted diffusion compatible with an abscess.

epidural collections can be extremely subtle on NECT, although more conspicuous with a contrast-enhanced scan. However, if intracranial involvement is suspected in a patient with sinusitis and headache and/or altered mental status then strong consideration should be given to an MRI. The CT is still useful for the surgeon for surgical planning of sinus drainage. Further intracranial complications can ensure, particularly with subdural empyema, meningitis, cortical venous thrombosis, cavernous sinus thrombophlebitis, or intraparenchymal abscess (**Fig. 3**).

Postgadolinium T1 weighted images and DWI are the 2 most helpful sequences for evaluation of intracranial infection to detect abscesses as well as determine the patency of vascular structures. Peripheral enhancement of an intraparenchymal abscess, leptomeningeal enhancement in meningitis, or dural enhancement in a subdural abscess/epidural empyema reflects inflammation and an immunologic response to the pathogen. Hyperintense DWI (and corresponding low ADC values) localize centrally within the collection, corresponding with the purulent component. Recognizing these imaging findings is vital to the patient outcomes as the intracranial extension of sinus infection carries a morbidity rate of 27% and a mortality rate of 3.3%.[10] Sinus infection can extend superficially to the extracranial tissues as well. For the frontal sinuses, an extracranial abscess goes by the misnomer of Pott puffy tumor (**Fig. 4**), which comprises a subgaleal abscess, subperiosteal abscess, and osteomyelitis.

Acute sinus infection, left untreated can also spread into the orbit. Most frequently this occurs from the ethmoid air cells through natural bony dehiscences in the medial orbital wall, also known as the lamina papyracea, and less often from the frontal sinuses from osteomyelitis. Orbital involvement with sinus infection often begins as a subperiosteal confined abscess, with mass effect on the extraocular muscle cone, but can further progress with infection in the orbital fat and progressive proptosis (**Fig. 5**). Because of the risk for long-term vision loss, these are considered critical situations requiring emergent drainage of the primary sinus infection and intravenous antibiotics.

INNERVATION OF THE SINUSES AND POTENTIAL HEADACHE TREATMENT

The paranasal sinuses are innervated by branches of the trigeminal nerve- V1 (ophthalmic) and V2 (maxillary).[12] Multiple smaller nerves that carry sensory afferent

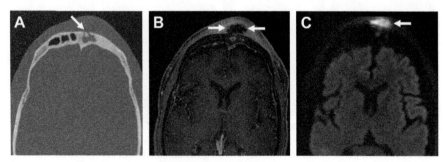

Fig. 4. Pott Puffy Tumor. Nonenhanced CT *(A)* shows opacification of the left frontal sinus with focal dehiscence of the anterior wall *(arrow)*. Contrast-enhanced T1 weighted MR *(B)* shows peripheral enhancement of the opacified left frontal sinus and a focal forehead collection *(arrows)* with extensive inflammatory changes in the surrounding soft tissues. On DWI *(C)*, the peripherally enhancing superficial collection has centrally restricted diffusion consistent with an abscess *(arrow)*.

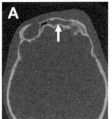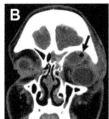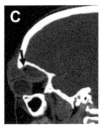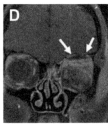

Fig. 5. Left frontal sinusitis with an orbital abscess. Bone window head CT (A) shows left frontal sinus opacification. Coronal (B) and sagittal (C) contrast-enhanced sinus CT images demonstrates an intraorbital, extraconal fluid collection that extends along the orbital roof and results in the marked inferior displacement of the globe. The fluid collection has a small focus of gas (black arrows) from the paranasal sinuses. Coronal contrast-enhanced T1 weighted MR with fat saturation (D) shows hazy enhancement of the orbital fat and the rim-enhancing orbital abscess (white arrows).

fibers from the paranasal sinuses converge on the sphenopalatine ganglion (SPG), also referred to as the pterygopalatine ganglion, nasal ganglion, or Meckel's ganglion.[13] This contains the largest supply of nerves in the head outside of the brain.

Mucosal inflammation leads to a complex response that includes vasodilatation, increased vascular permeability, increased cytokines in nasal lavage fluid, and increased kinin levels that contribute to mucosal hyperresponsiveness.[14] In addition to sinus inflammation leading to pain, mucosal contact points have been implicated as a cause of headaches, although not without controversy. Simply stated, a mucosal contact point is any area within the nasal cavity whereby 2 points meet and remain after the administration of topic decongestant.[15] It has been suggested that the nasal mucosal receptors are stimulated and release substance P, which can lead to vasodilation and hypersecretion.[16] However there are many people with asymptomatic contact points, and also patients who undergo the resection of contact points without the alleviation of symptoms. While this remains controversial, mucosal contact points can be identified on noncontrast CT.

While the exact pathophysiology of headaches related to sinus disease is not well agreed on, interventions to treat the pain are still being explored. Given the anatomic location of the SPG in the pterygopalatine fossa (PPF), nerve blocks have been performed transnasally going through the anterior nasal cavity with the placement of local anesthetic just posterior to the middle turbinate.[17,18] Traditionally, SPG blocks have been performed in the setting of trigeminal neuralgia, chronic migraine headaches, and postherpetic neuralgia. However more recently, SPG blocks have been performed for mucosal headaches presenting as facial pain.[19] The clinical picture of headache related to sinus disease and primary headaches such as migraines or tension-type headaches can be difficult to discern.[20] Imaging can perhaps play a role in these cases when identifying sinus inflammatory disease as a possible etiology, one that could lead to different treatment outside of the traditional oral medication administered for primary headaches.

CORNER SHOTS

Not only can sinus disease, as causative dental disease present as headaches, but temporomandibular joint (TMJ) pain can frequently present with a headache as well.[21] This is important to keep in mind as most studies targeted at the sinuses, whether CT or MRI, generally include the TMJ's within the field of view. Symptoms related to TMJ pain can be localized on physical examination and related to tension headaches, however often they have nonspecific symptoms that are confused for other etiologies. While a dedicated TMJ MRI would include open and closed views to evaluate for appropriate morphology and mobility of the disc, degenerative osseous changes, erosive changes, and effusions can be seen on non-TMJ dedicated imaging.

SUMMARY

Imaging of patients with headaches often occurs with nonlocalizing physical examinations. When no abnormal intracranial findings are observed on brain CT or MR, it is important to evaluate the paranasal sinuses and teeth as potential sources of symptoms. Dedicated cross-sectional imaging can identify disease, localize primary etiologies such as in the case of odontogenic sinusitis, and evaluate for intra and extracranial complications of sinus disease.

DISCLOSURE

The authors have nothing to disclose.

REFERENCES

1. Silberstein SD. Headaches due to nasal and paranasal sinus disease. Neurol Clin 2004;22(1):1–19, v.
2. Fujioka M, Young LW. The sphenoidal sinuses: radiographic patterns of normal development and abnormal findings in infants and children. Radiology 1978; 129(1):133.
3. Adibelli ZH, Songu M, Adibelli H. Paranasal sinus development in children: A magnetic resonance imaging analysis. Am J Rhinol Allergy 2011;25(1):30–5.
4. Nour YA, Al-Madani A, El-Daly A, et al. Isolated sphenoid sinus pathology: spectrum of diagnostic and treatment modalities. Auris Nasus Larynx 2008;35(4): 500–8.
5. Lindbaek M, Johnsen UL, Kaastad E, et al. CT findings in general practice patients with suspected acute sinusitis. Acta Radiol 1996;37(5):708–13.
6. Rosenfeld RM, Piccirillo JF, Chandrasekhar SS, et al. Clinical practice guideline (update): Adult Sinusitis Executive Summary. Otolaryngol Head Neck Surg 2015;152(4):598–609.
7. Kirsch CFE, Bykowski J, Aulino JM, et al. ACR Appropriateness Criteria(®) Sinonasal Disease. J Am Coll Radiol 2017;14(11s):S550–9.
8. Bhatt AA, Donaldson AM, Olomu OU, et al. Can Diffusion-Weighted Imaging Serve as an Imaging Biomarker for Acute Bacterial Rhinosinusitis? Cureus 2020;12(8):e9893.
9. Chapman MN, Nadgir RN, Akman AS, et al. Periapical lucency around the tooth: radiologic evaluation and differential diagnosis. Radiographics 2013;33(1): E15–32.
10. Patel NA, Garber D, Hu S, et al. Systematic review and case report: Intracranial complications of pediatric sinusitis. Int J Pediatr Otorhinolaryngol 2016;86: 200–12.
11. Fernández-de Thomas RJ, De Jesus O. Subdural Empyema. In: StatPearls. Treasure Island (FL). StatPearls Publishing; 2021. Copyright © 2021, StatPearls Publishing LLC.

12. Kirsch CFE. Headache Caused by Sinus Disease. Neuroimaging Clin N Am 2019; 29(2):227–41.
13. Ho KWD, Przkora R, Kumar S. Sphenopalatine ganglion: block, radiofrequency ablation and neurostimulation - a systematic review. J Headache Pain 2017; 18(1):118.
14. Chiarugi A, Camaioni A. Update on the pathophysiology and treatment of rhinogenic headache: focus on the ibuprofen/pseudoephedrine combination. Acta Otorhinolaryngol Ital 2019;39(1):22–7.
15. Harrison L, Jones NS. Intranasal contact points as a cause of facial pain or headache: a systematic review. Clin Otolaryngol 2013;38(1):8–22.
16. Stammberger H, Wolf G. Headaches and sinus disease: the endoscopic approach. Ann Otol Rhinol Laryngol Suppl 1988;134:3–23.
17. Yarnitsky D, Goor-Aryeh I, Bajwa ZH, et al. Wolff Award: Possible parasympathetic contributions to peripheral and central sensitization during migraine. Headache 2003;43(7):704–14.
18. Binfalah M, Alghawi E, Shosha E, et al. Sphenopalatine Ganglion Block for the Treatment of Acute Migraine Headache. Pain Res Treat 2018;2018:2516953.
19. Lee SH, Kim Y, Lim TY. Efficacy of sphenopalatine ganglion block in nasal mucosal headache presenting as facial pain. Cranio 2020;38(2):128–30.
20. Straburzyński M, Gryglas-Dworak A, Nowaczewska M, et al. Etiology of 'Sinus Headache'-Moving the Focus from Rhinology to Neurology. A Systematic Review. Brain Sci 2021;11(1).
21. Reik L Jr, Hale M. The temporomandibular joint pain-dysfunction syndrome: a frequent cause of headache. Headache 1981;21(4):151–6.

Imaging of Painful Ophthalmologic Disorders

Blair A. Winegar, MD

KEYWORDS

- Orbital pain • Optic neuritis • Orbital cellulitis • Idiopathic orbital inflammation
- Orbital compartment syndrome • Thyroid eye disease • Endophthalmitis

KEY POINTS

- Contrast-enhanced computed tomography (CECT) and MRI are invaluable diagnostic tools for the evaluation of painful ophthalmologic disorders.
- CECT is useful in differentiating preseptal cellulitis and orbital cellulitis.
- MRI is helpful in the detection and differentiation of causes of optic neuritis.

INTRODUCTION

Painful ophthalmologic disorders constitute approximately 2% to 3% of primary care and emergency department patient encounters.[1] Many of the typical causative conditions, such as corneal laceration, conjunctivitis, and glaucoma, can be diagnosed with clinical history and physical examination. However, a subset of patients with concerning clinical features (eg, fever, vision loss, dipoplia, proptosis, and so forth) will require cross-sectional imaging with either contrast-enhanced computed tomography (CECT) or MRI. CECT is a first-line imaging for the evaluation of suspected orbital infection. MRI offers better evaluation of the orbital soft tissues, particularly useful in the evaluation of optic neuritis. Using a space-based approach, the discriminating CECT and MRI features of painful ophthalmologic disorders allow for accurate diagnosis and initiation of appropriate treatment.

DISCUSSION
Preseptal Soft Tissues and Lacrimal Apparatus

Preseptal cellulitis
Infection confined to the periorbital tissues anterior to the orbital septum is termed preseptal cellulitis. The orbital septum is a thin fibrous membrane, which is a continuation of the periosteum of the orbital rim and blends with the levator palpebrae superioris tendon in the upper eyelid and tarsal plate in the lower eyelid. The orbital septum

Department of Radiology and Imaging Sciences, University of Utah School of Medicine, 30 North 1900 East, #1A071, Salt Lake City, UT 84132-2140, USA
E-mail address: blair.winegar@hsc.utah.edu

Neurol Clin 40 (2022) 641–660
https://doi.org/10.1016/j.ncl.2022.03.002
0733-8619/22/© 2022 Elsevier Inc. All rights reserved.
neurologic.theclinics.com

acts as a boundary preventing the spread of infection from the preseptal soft tissues into the postseptal orbital soft tissues, a more serious infection termed orbital cellulitis. The preseptal soft tissues may become infected as a result of direct inoculation (minor trauma or insect bite) or from contiguous spread (sinusitis). Imaging, most frequently with CECT, is performed to differentiate preseptal cellulitis from orbital cellulitis.[2] On CECT, inflammatory stranding and swelling are confined to the soft tissues anterior to the expected location of the orbital septum, within the eyelids and periorbital soft tissues anterior to the globe and orbital rim. This infection may be complicated by abscess, a rim-enhancing fluid collection with surrounding inflammation (**Fig. 1**). On MRI, preseptal inflammation shows soft tissue thickening, T1 hypointense reticulations, T2 hyperintensity, and enhancement. A rim-enhancing, internally T2 hyperintense and diffusion restricting fluid collection correlates with preseptal abscess. Imaging may also identify acute sinusitis as the potential causative cause, evidenced by fluid within the frontal or ethmoid air cells with or without osseous wall breach, which is contiguous with the preseptal inflammation.

Keratoconjunctivitis

Keratoconjunctivitis is inflammation involving both the thin lining along the inner eyelids and anterior eye (conjunctivitis) and the cornea (keratitis). These types of inflammation can result from allergies, viral infection, or bacterial infection. Although keratoconjunctivitis is typically a clinical diagnosis, sexually transmitted infection by *Neisseria gonorrhoeae* may result in a severe ulcerative keratoconjunctivitis with subsequent corneal ulceration and potential resultant endophthalmitis, prompting imaging evaluation.[3] On CECT and MRI, keratoconjunctivitis may manifest as thickening and enhancement along the conjunctiva and potential fluid underlying the eyelids, corresponding to chemosis (**Fig. 2**).[4] A decrease of the anterior chamber depth signifies full-thickness corneal ulceration. In this case, MRI is helpful to evaluate for potential superimposed endophthalmitis, described subsequently.

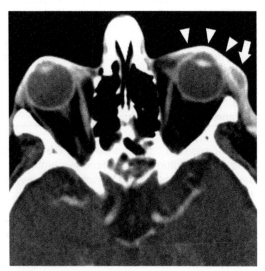

Fig. 1. Preseptal cellulitis. Axial CECT image shows left preseptal soft tissue thickening (*arrowheads*) and rim-enhancing fluid collection (*arrow*) compatible with left preseptal cellulitis and abscess, respectively.

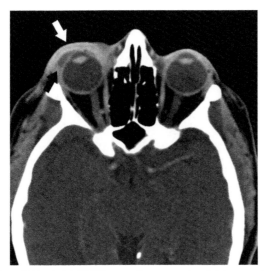

Fig. 2. Keratoconjunctivitis. Axial CECT image demonstrates right preseptal soft tissue thickening, enhancement, and inflammatory stranding (*white arrow*). Fluid underlying the eyelids (*black arrow*) corresponds with chemosis in this case of viral keratoconjunctivitis.

Dacryoadenitis

Lacrimal gland inflammation, termed dacryoadenitis, may result from viral infection, bacterial infection, or systemic inflammatory conditions such as Sjogren syndrome, sarcoidosis, and immunoglobulin G4 (IgG4)-related inflammation. Dacryoadenitis causes painful swelling over the superolateral orbit, pain with eye movements, erythema, and ptosis. Although typically self-limited, systemic disorders often result in recurrent, bilateral dacryoadenitis. CECT and MRI demonstrate enlargement and hyperenhancement of the lacrimal gland with or without adjacent inflammatory stranding (**Fig. 3**).[5] Bacterial dacryoadenitis may be complicated by abscess formation. In cases associated with Sjogren syndrome or IgG4-related inflammation (formerly known as Mikulicz disease), imaging may demonstrate acute or chronic inflammatory changes within the parotid glands.

Acute dacryocystitis

Acute dacryocystitis results from obstruction of the nasolacrimal duct followed by bacterial infection of the lacrimal sac. Nasolacrimal duct obstruction may be congenital or acquired. Patients with acute dacryocystitis present with pain, edema, and erythema adjacent to the medial canthus. Treatment includes antibiotics with subsequent surgical repair of the nasolacrimal duct. On CECT, acute dacryocystitis appears as a rim-enhancing fluid collection in anteromedial orbit at the lacrimal fossa with surrounding inflammatory stranding (**Fig. 4**).[6] Similarly, a rim-enhancing T2 hyperintense fluid collection with adjacent inflammation in the region of the medial canthus will be present on MRI.

Lacrimal gland adenoid cystic carcinoma

Lacrimal gland tumors are rare with a wide variety of pathologies of both epithelial and nonepithelial origins. Epithelial tumors constitute most lacrimal gland tumors, of which approximately 40% to 50% are malignant carcinomas. Of these lacrimal gland carcinomas, adenoid cystic carcinoma is the most common. Most lacrimal tumors result in

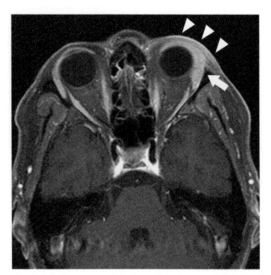

Fig. 3. Dacryoadenitis. Axial T1 postgadolinium fat-saturated image depicts an enlarged and enhancing left lacrimal gland (*arrow*) and adjacent left preseptal soft tissue swelling and enhancement (*arrowheads*) corresponding to acute dacryoadenitis.

localized swelling, globe displacement, diplopia, and ptosis. However, pain is a cardinal sign of adenoid cystic carcinoma.[7] Differentiation of lacrimal gland tumors is difficult on imaging and requires biopsy for definitive diagnosis. On CECT and MRI, adenoid cystic carcinoma will appear as an enhancing mass centered within the lacrimal gland (**Fig. 5**A). On CECT, osseous erosion is the best imaging predictor of

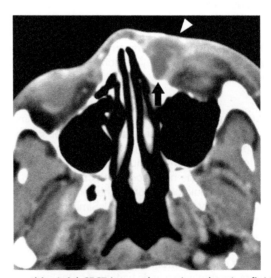

Fig. 4. Acute dacryocystitis. Axial CECT image shows rim-enhancing fluid collection in the left medial canthus (*black arrow*) consistent with a dilated and inflamed lacrimal sac. Adjacent ill-defined fluid and inflammatory stranding within the adjacent left preseptal soft tissues (*arrowhead*) corresponds to early abscess formation in this case of acute dacryocystitis.

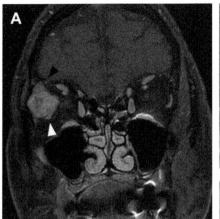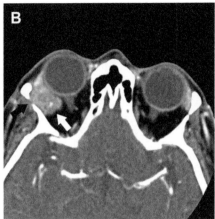

Fig. 5. Lacrimal gland adenoid cystic carcinoma. (*A*) Coronal T1 postgadolinium fat-saturated image displays a right lacrimal gland mass displacing the lateral rectus muscle (*white arrowhead*). A portion of the superior aspect of the lacrimal gland is spared (*black arrowhead*). (*B*) Axial CECT image demonstrates a heterogeneously enhancing mass in the right lacrimal gland (*white arrow*), which results in subtle erosion of the adjacent right lateral orbital wall (*black arrow*), a sign of lacrimal gland epithelial malignancy in this case of adenoid cystic carcinoma.

lacrimal gland carcinoma (**Fig. 5**B).[8] Adenoid cystic carcinoma also has a predilection for perineural tumor spread, which is best evaluated on MRI, as linear contrast enhancement and thickening along the expected course of cranial nerves toward the superior orbital fissure.

Ocular

Uveitis
The uveal tract is the vascular middle layer of the eye divided into anterior (iris and ciliary body) and posterior (choroid) components. Uveitis is typically subdivided into anterior (iris), intermediate (ciliary body and vitreous), posterior (choroid), and panuveitis (all components of the uveal tract) based on the site of inflammation. The potential causes of uveitis are diverse, including infectious and noninfectious conditions.[9] Chorioretinitis defines a subset of posterior uveitis in which both the choroid and retina are inflamed, potentially threatening vision. CECT and MRI findings demonstrate thickening and enhancement of the affected portion of the uveal tract (**Fig. 6**A and B).

Vogt-Koyanagi-Harada (VKH) syndrome is a uveo-meningeal syndrome that results in severe granulomatous panuveitis, vitiligo, aseptic meningitis, and inner ear symptoms (sensorineural hearing loss, tinnitus, and/or vertigo). VKH syndrome is a presumed autoimmune T-cell–mediated disorder that attacks melanin-pigmented tissues found in the retinal pigment epithelium, skin, meninges, and inner ear. On MRI, VKH syndrome demonstrates bilateral uveal tract thickening and enhancement with or without retinal detachment.[10] In addition, pachymeningeal or leptomeningeal thickening and enhancement, signifying associated aseptic meningitis, may be present.

Endophthalmitis
Endophthalmitis refers to inflammation within the ocular cavities, typically as a result of bacterial or fungal infection. Infection may be a result of direct inoculation from open

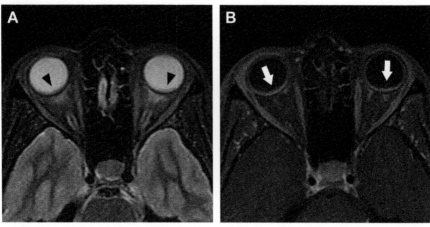

Fig. 6. Uveitis. (*A*) Axial STIR image displays thickening of the bilateral posterior uvea (*black arrowheads*) and mild retrobulbar inflammatory stranding. (*B*) Axial T1 postgadolinium fat-saturated image also displays thickening and enhancement of the bilateral uvea, most pronounced posteriorly (*white arrows*), corresponding to bilateral panuveitis in this patient with Vogt-Koyanagi-Harada Syndrome. STIR, short tau inversion recovery.

globe injury or surgery, termed exogenous endophthalmitis, or from hematogenous spread of infection, termed endogenous endophthalmitis. Endogenous endophthalmitis is less common, accounting for about 2% to 6% of cases, and often misdiagnosed, given lack of predisposing ocular surgery or penetrating trauma.[11] MRI is particularly helpful for the diagnosis of endogenous endophthalmitis, given significant overlap of symptoms with orbital cellulitis. On CECT, endophthalmitis may demonstrate subtle findings, including periocular inflammatory stranding, increased intraocular density, and/or ocular wall thickening and enhancement. MRI is more sensitive for the diagnosis of endophthalmitis with findings including periocular inflammation, ocular wall thickening/enhancement, lack of fluid attenuation inversion recovery (FLAIR) suppression of vitreous, and/or diffusion restricting collection along the posterior ocular walls compatible with purulent material (**Fig. 7**A and B).[12]

Optic Nerve Sheath Complex

Optic neuritis
Optic neuritis is inflammation of the optic nerve resulting in pain with eye movement, vision impairment, relative afferent pupillary defect, and normal to mildly edematous optic disc. Optic neuritis is most often from demyelination in the setting of multiple sclerosis. Optic neuritis constitutes approximately 21% of cases of clinically isolated syndrome, a term designating the first clinical onset of neurologic symptoms that may subsequently develop multiple sclerosis.[13] In cases of optic neuritis as a clinically isolated syndrome, detection of additional intracranial white matter FLAIR hyperintensities that suggest demyelinating plaques places the patient at high risk (83%) for multiple sclerosis.[14] Other demyelinating conditions such as acute disseminated encephalomyelitis, myelin oligodendrocyte glycoprotein (MOG) antibody disease, and neuromyelitis optica (NMO) can result in optic neuritis. Less commonly, optic neuritis may be the result of viral infection (eg, mumps, measles, herpes simplex virus), bacterial infection (eg, Lyme disease, cat-scratch disease, syphilis), and inflammatory conditions (eg, neurosarcoidosis, systemic lupus erythematous).

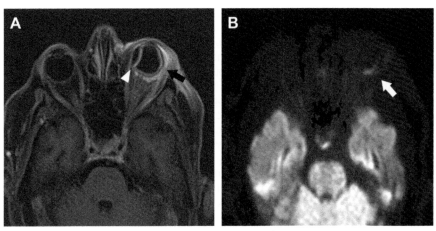

Fig. 7. Endophthalmitis. (*A*) Axial T1 postgadolinium fat-saturated image demonstrates extensive ocular wall enhancement with medial choroidal detachment (*white arrowhead*) and periocular inflammatory enhancement (*black arrow*). (*B*) Axial diffusion trace image shows hyperintensity layering posteriorly within the left globe (*white arrow*) compatible with intraocular purulent material in this case of endogenous endophthalmitis.

On MRI, optic neuritis demonstrates T2 hyperintensity and contrast enhancement within the affected portion of the optic nerve (**Fig. 8**A and B). This portion of the affected nerve may also demonstrate restricted diffusion. Optic neuritis associated with multiple sclerosis typically demonstrates unilateral involvement and only affects a short segment of the optic nerve. In addition to dedicated orbital sequences, whole-brain T2 FLAIR and T1 postcontrast sequences should be obtained to assess for additional hyperintense ± enhancing white matter lesions.

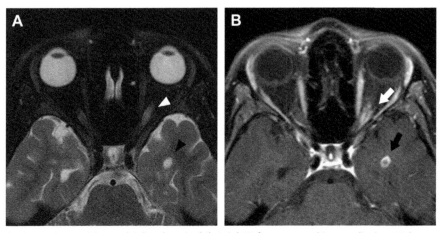

Fig. 8. Optic neuritis—multiple sclerosis. (*A*) Axial T2 fat-saturated image displays T2 hyperintensity within the posterior intraorbital segment of the left optic nerve (*white arrowhead*). A left temporal white matter T2 hyperintensity is also present (*black arrowhead*). (*B*) Axial T1 postgadolinium fat-saturated image shows corresponding enhancement of the left optic nerve (*white arrow*) and ring enhancement of the left temporal white matter lesion (*black arrow*), compatible with left optic neuritis and active demyelination in the left temporal white matter in this case of multiple sclerosis.

NMO is a severe autoimmune disorder characterized by optic neuritis, acute myelitis, and autoantibodies to aquaporin-4, the most abundant water channel protein in the central nervous system. This disease typically results in relapsing episodes of concurrent or successive optic neuritis and acute myelitis. As opposed to MS, NMO more frequently results in bilateral optic neuritis and affects longer portions of the posterior optic nerves and optic chiasm (**Fig. 9**A).[15] The MRI features of the spinal cord also differ, with NMO demonstrating longitudinally extensive transverse myelitis (LETM) evidenced by T2 hyperintensity crossing at least 3 vertebral segment and involving more than 50% of the cross-section of the spinal cord, most commonly in the cervical region (**Fig. 9**B). Contrast enhancement is present during bouts of acute inflammation.

MOG antibody disease is a disorder similar to NMO and recognized as a distinct clinical entity different from multiple sclerosis resulting from autoimmune antibodies to myelin oligodendrocyte glycoprotein expressed in the central nervous system. This disorder most commonly results in optic neuritis and less commonly myelitis. Both monophasic and relapsing patterns may occur, with relapsing disease more frequently affecting the optic nerves.[16] The MRI features of MOG antibody disease differ from multiple sclerosis, with more commonly bilateral optic neuritis, long segment optic nerve involvement, and inflammation extending into the retrobulbar soft tissues adjacent to the optic nerve sheath complex (33% of cases).[17] When compared with NMO, the optic neuritis encountered in MOG antibody disease more commonly affects the anterior segments of the optic nerve, including the optic nerve heads, and rarely the optic chiasm (**Fig. 10**A and B). When encountered, myelitis associated with MOG antibody disease also differs from MS and NMO, with most commonly LETM affecting the thoracic spinal cord.

Optic Perineuritis

Inflammation of the optic nerve sheath is termed optic perineuritis. Most cases are a form of idiopathic orbital inflammation but may be secondary to a variety of systemic diseases such as sarcoidosis, IgG4-related disease, Behcet disease, granulomatosis

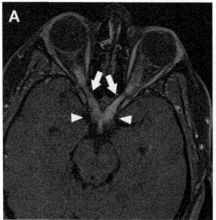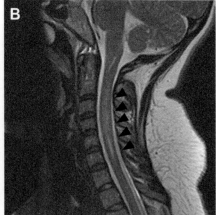

Fig. 9. Optic neuritis—neuromyelitis optica. (*A*) Axial T1 postgadolinium fat-saturated image displays extensive enhancement involving the bilateral posterior optic nerves (*white arrows*) and optic chiasm (*white arrowheads*). (*B*) Sagittal T2 image of the cervical spine shows multisegmental T2 hyperintensity of the cervical spinal cord (*black arrowheads*) compatible with longitudinally extensive transverse myelitis in this case of NMO.

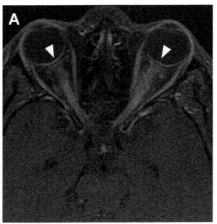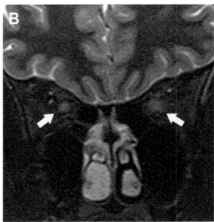

Fig. 10. Optic neuritis—myelin oligodendrocyte glycoprotein antibody disease. (*A*) Axial T1 postgadolinium fat-saturated image demonstrates extensive enhancement of the bilateral optic nerves extending to the optic nerve heads (*arrowheads*). (*B*) Coronal STIR image displays hyperintense signal within the bilateral optic nerves and surrounding perineural inflammation (*arrows*) in this case of MOG antibody disease.

with polyangiitis, and systemic lupus erythematosus or infections (eg, tuberculosis, syphilis, herpes simplex virus, herpes zoster virus). Symptoms of optic perineuritis may mimic optic neuritis, including pain, typically exacerbated by eye movement, and variable degree of vision loss. As opposed to optic neuritis, optic perineuritis is not self-limited and requires corticosteroids for treatment. On MRI, contrast enhancement and inflammation are centered on the optic nerve sheath, resulting in "tram-track" appearance on axial images and "donut" appearance on coronal images (**Fig. 11**A and B).[18]

Extraocular Muscles and Retrobulbar Soft Tissues

Thyroid eye disease

Thyroid eye disease (TED), also known as thyroid-associated ophthalmopathy or Graves ophthalmopathy, refers to the orbital manifestations associated with autoimmune thyroid disease, most commonly Graves disease. In Graves disease, autoantibodies against the thyroid stimulating hormone receptor result in hyperthyroidism and goiter. TED occurs in approximately 50% of patients with Graves disease.[19] The mechanism is not completely understood, but studies suggest autoantibody cross-reactivity and activation of orbital fibroblasts, which then lead to an inflammatory response and glycoaminoglycan deposition, resulting in extraocular muscle expansion and retrobulbar fat accumulation. TED is the most common cause of exophthalmos in adults. In the early active phase of the disease, there is progressive inflammation, swelling, and tissue changes that may result in progressive exophthalmos, pain, and diplopia. Rarely, extraocular muscle enlargement may compress the optic nerve in the orbital apex, requiring urgent surgical decompression.

On CECT, the extraocular muscles seem thickened with relative sparing of the tendinous insertions. There is typically bilateral and symmetric muscle enlargement, often with an order of predilection described by the mnemonic "I'M SLOw," with inferior rectus, medial rectus, superior rectus, lateral rectus, and lastly oblique muscle involvement. Extraocular muscle involvement and prominence of the retrobulbar fat

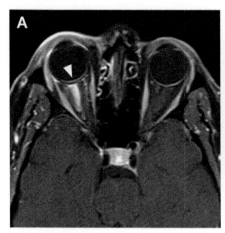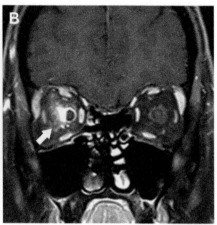

Fig. 11. Optic perineuritis. (*A*) Axial T1 postgadolinium fat-saturated image demonstrates enhancement and inflammatory stranding paralleling the right optic nerve with "tram-track" configuration (*arrowhead*). (*B*) Coronal T1 postgadolinium fat-saturated image shows enhancement and inflammatory stranding surrounding the right optic nerve (*arrow*) giving the "donut" appearance in this case of optic perineuritis.

contribute to exophthalmos. On MRI, T2 and short tau inversion recovery (STIR) hyperintensity within the affected extraocular muscles suggest inflammation within the active phase of disease, whereas low T2 and STIR signal intensity suggest fibrosis within the chronic stable phase disease (**Fig. 12**A and B).[20]

Idiopathic Orbital Inflammation

Idiopathic orbital inflammation (IOI), also known as orbital pseudotumor or nonspecific orbital inflammation, is the most common cause of painful orbital mass in adults. IOI is a poorly understood condition resulting in idiopathic inflammation within the orbit, which may be diffuse or localized. Localized forms can result in dacryoadenitis, myositis, ocular involvement (eg, uveitis, scleritis), optic perineuritis, and orbital apex/cavernous sinus inflammation (eg, Tolosa-Hunt syndrome).[21] CECT and MRI findings demonstrate T2 hyperintensity, contrast enhancement, and surrounding inflammatory stranding of the affected portion of the orbit. Diffusion-weighted imaging may be helpful in differentiating IOI from orbital lymphoma and orbital cellulitis. The myositic form of IOI differs from TED, in that inflammation and thickening of the extra-ocular muscles may involve the tendinous insertions and may affect any extraocular muscle or muscles without specific predilection (**Fig. 13**A–C).[22]

Orbital cellulitis, subperiosteal abscess, and orbital abscess

Orbital cellulitis is infection of the orbital soft tissues posterior to the orbital septum. This infection is most commonly from extension of adjacent acute bacterial sinusitis.[23] Imaging is often obtained to differentiate preseptal cellulitis from orbital cellulitis. The latter is a more serious condition that requires initial intravenous (IV) antibiotics and hospital admission to monitor for potential complications of increase intraorbital pressure and/or optic neuropathy. On CECT, detection of inflammatory stranding in the postseptal soft tissues differentiates orbital cellulitis from preseptal cellulitis (**Fig. 14**). Often, there is opacification in adjacent paranasal sinuses. MRI demonstrates similar findings of inflammatory stranding with T2 hyperintensity and contrast enhancement within the postseptal orbital soft tissues.[24]

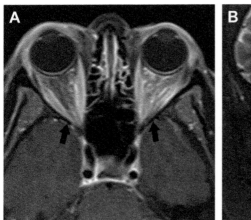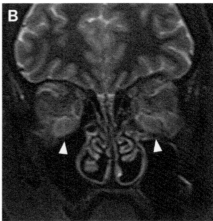

Fig. 12. Thyroid eye disease. (*A*) Axial T1 postgadolinium fat-saturated image shows bilateral thickening and enhancement of the medial and lateral rectus muscles and extensive postseptal inflammatory enhancement (*black arrows*). (*B*) Coronal STIR image demonstrates thickening and hyperintensity of all extraocular muscles, but most pronounced involving the inferior rectus muscles (white *arrowheads*), and extensive inflammatory stranding in this patient with active thyroid eye disease from Grave disease and thyrotoxicosis.

Subperiosteal abscess is a purulent collection that is confined by the periosteum along the orbital wall that develops from an adjacent sinus infection. Subperiosteal abscess is more frequently a complication of acute sinusitis in pediatric patients. Treatment includes IV antibiotics with potential surgical drainage based on multiple factors including patient age, abscess size, probable causative anaerobic bacteria, and clinical factors (eg, optic nerve compromise).[25] On CECT, subperiosteal abscess appears as a dome-shaped rim-enhancing fluid collection with base along the orbital wall, surrounding inflammatory standing and underlying paranasal sinus opacification (**Fig. 15**).[26] Osseous erosions may or may not be present. On MRI, this fluid collection will also demonstrate rim enhancement with internal T2 hyperintensity and restricted diffusion.

Orbital abscess is development of a purulent fluid collection within the orbit not confined to the orbital wall, which is a highly morbid complication of orbital cellulitis. Aside from IV antibiotics, orbital abscesses typically require surgical drainage. On CECT and MRI, orbital abscesses are rim-enhancing fluid collections in the orbit with adjacent inflammation (**Fig. 16**A). MRI demonstrates internal restricted diffusion, which indicates purulent material (**Fig. 16**B).[27]

Acute Invasive Fungal Rhinosinusitis

Acute invasive fungal rhinosinusitis (AIFRS) is a highly morbid, fulminant angioinvasive fungal infection of the sinonasal cavity that can quickly spread to the orbit. AIFRS occurs in the immunocompromised setting, typically patients with poorly controlled diabetes mellitus or absolute neutropenia, from aspergillosis or mucormycosis. Treatment includes correction of immunocompromised state, IV antifungal therapy, aggressive surgical debridement, and potentially orbital exenteration in the setting of orbital involvement.[28] CECT findings of AIFRS with orbital involvement are similar to acute bacterial sinusitis with orbital cellulitis, including sinonasal inflammatory mucosal thickening and postseptal inflammatory stranding. Extension of inflammation

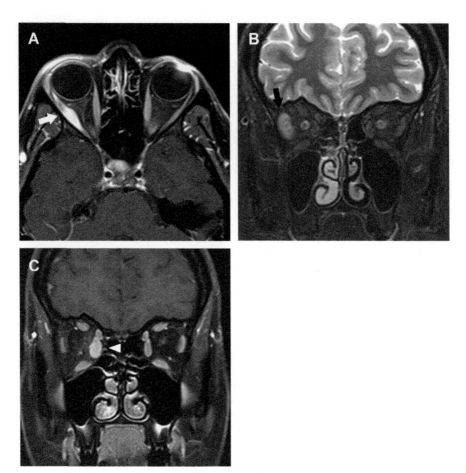

Fig. 13. Idiopathic orbital inflammation. (*A*) Axial T1 postgadolinium fat-saturated image demonstrates thickening and enhancement of the right lateral rectus muscle (*white arrow*). (*B*) Coronal STIR image shows corresponding thickening and hyperintensity within the right lateral rectus muscle (*black arrow*), in this case of myositis from IOI. (C) Six months later, coronal T1 postgadolinium fat-saturated image shows enhancement and thickening of the right medial rectus muscle (*white arrowhead*) and resolution of right lateral rectus muscle inflammation in this patient with relapsing myositis from IOI. IOI, idiopathic orbital inflammation.

beyond the sinonasal cavity into the premaxillary region, retroantral fat, or pterygopalatine fossa are highly specific for AIFRS.[29] Contrast-enhanced MRI is more sensitive and specific compared with CECT for the diagnosis of AIFRS. T1 postcontrast imaging demonstrates lack of contrast enhancement of the devascularized sinonasal mucosa, first described as the "black turbinate sign" (**Fig. 17**A).[30] Orbital involvement may demonstrate T2 hyperintense inflammation, regions of necrosis evidenced by lack of contrast enhancement, and/or ischemic optic neuropathy with optic nerve–restricted diffusion (**Fig. 17**B, C).

Orbital Compartment Syndrome

Orbital compartment syndrome is an ophthalmologic surgical emergency associated with acute increased pressure within the orbit. The increased pressure may be the

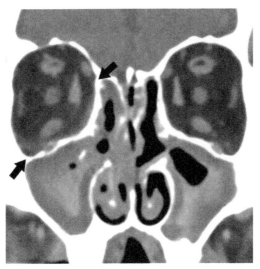

Fig. 14. Orbital cellulitis. Coronal CECT image shows extensive paranasal sinus disease and changes of prior endoscopic sinus surgery with right postseptal inflammatory stranding, most pronounced in the inferior and medial extraconal soft tissues (*black arrows*), in this patient with right orbital cellulitis from sinusitis.

consequence of hematoma (eg, trauma, ruptured orbital venous varix), inflammation (eg, orbital cellulitis, idiopathic orbital inflammation), gas (eg, orbital wall fracture), or expanding mass (eg, orbital venolymphatic malformation). The increased orbital pressure results in progressive painful proptosis, with anterior displacement of the globe

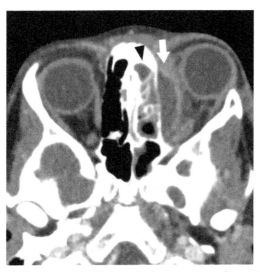

Fig. 15. Subperiosteal abscess. Axial CECT image demonstrates a large rim-enhancing fluid collection (*white arrow*) with base along the left medial orbital wall and surrounding inflammatory stranding, compatible with subperiosteal abscess. There is associated opacification of the adjacent left ethmoid air cells (*black arrowhead*) consistent with inciting ethmoid sinusitis.

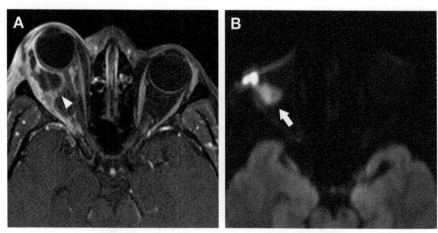

Fig. 16. Orbital abscess. (A) Axial T1 postgadolinium fat-saturated image displays a rim-enhancing fluid collection with adjacent inflammatory stranding in the right retrobulbar soft tissues (*arrowhead*) resulting in exophthalmos. (B) Axial diffusion trace image shows corresponding hyperintensity (*arrow*) consistent with purulent material within this orbital abscess.

limited by tethering to the optic nerve/sheath complex contributing to vision-threatening optic nerve ischemia.[31] On CT and MRI, orbital compartment syndrome is indicated by proptosis with straightened optic nerve/sheath complex and posterior tenting of the globe, resulting in a "guitar pick" appearance **(Fig. 18)**.[32] Imaging is also useful in determining the cause of orbital compartment syndrome to direct appropriate treatment of the underlying condition.

Cavernous Sinus

Cavernous sinus thrombophlebitis

Cavernous sinus thrombophlebitis (CST) is a serious, potentially lethal condition characterized by infectious clot within the cavernous sinuses. CST is caused by extension of infection to the cavernous sinuses from sinusitis, particularly from the adjacent sphenoid sinuses, skull base osteomyelitis, or from spread of medial facial or orbital cellulitis through the valveless veins that communicate with the cavernous sinuses. Infection is frequently bilateral, as infection can spread across venous channels that communicate between the cavernous sinuses; this is one cause of cavernous sinus syndrome, with clinical constellation of ophthalmoplegia (involvement of cranial nerves III, IV, and VI), autonomic dysfunction (Horner syndrome), and facial sensory loss (involvement of cranial nerves V1 and V2).[33] Additional symptoms include severe headache and retroorbital pain, fever, and proptosis.

On CECT, CVT demonstrates nonenhancing filling defects within the cavernous sinuses, which are typically expanded with lateral convex margins **(Fig. 19A)**. Secondary findings include enlargement and potential thrombosis of the superior ophthalmic veins and retrobulbar and extraocular muscle edema from venous engorgement **(Fig. 19B)**. On MRI, similar nonenhancing filling defects demonstrating variable T1 and T2 signal characteristics and potential restricted diffusion are present within the expanded cavernous sinuses with lateral convex margins.[34] MRI is particularly useful in evaluating intracranial complications such as meningitis, subdural empyema, and infarct.

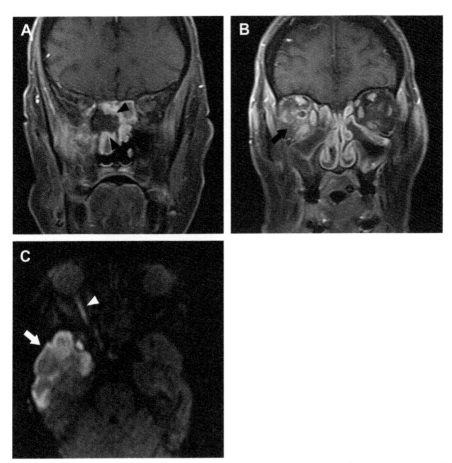

Fig. 17. Acute invasive fungal rhinosinusitis. (*A*) Coronal T1 postgadolinium fat-saturated image demonstrates posterior sinonasal inflammation with region of loss of contrast enhancement (*black arrowhead*). (*B*) Additional coronal T1 postgadolinium fat-saturated image displays inflammatory stranding and enhancement extending into the right orbital apex (*black arrow*). (*C*) Axial diffusion trace image shows restricted diffusion within the right optic nerve (*white arrowhead*), compatible with ischemic optic neuropathy, and large right temporal lobe infarct (*white arrow*) from vascular occlusions resulting from acute invasive fungal rhinosinusitis.

Carotid cavernous fistula

Abnormal communication between the carotid artery and cavernous sinus is termed carotid cavernous fistula (CCF). Barrow and colleagues classified CCF into 4 types based on whether there is direct communication between the internal carotid artery and cavernous sinus (type A) or indirect communication from meningeal branches supplied by the internal carotid artery (type B), external carotid artery (type C), or both (type D).[35] Classic clinical triad of CCF is pulsatile proptosis, chemosis, and orbital bruit. Additional symptoms and signs include orbital/retroorbital pain, diplopia, headache, and vision loss. On CT angiography (CTA) and noncontrast time-of-flight MR angiography (MRA), abnormal early contrast opacification/signal intensity within the enlarged cavernous sinus and superior ophthalmic vein corresponds with CCF

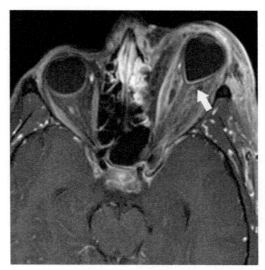

Fig. 18. Orbital compartment syndrome. Axial T1 postgadolinium fat-saturated image shows extensive left preseptal and postseptal inflammation resulting in exophthalmos with posterior tenting of the left globe (*arrow*) in this case of orbital compartment syndrome from severe left orbital cellulitis.

(**Fig. 20**A, B). CTA performs better than MRA at detecting the site of abnormal arteriovenous communication.[36] Conventional digital subtraction angiography is the gold-standard diagnostic imaging examination that can demonstrate the direct or indirect communication between the carotid artery and cavernous sinus and allow for endovascular treatment.

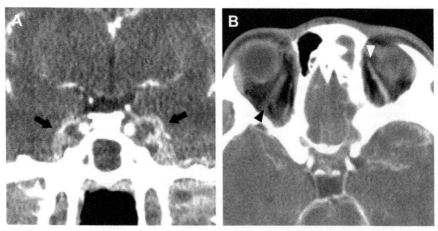

Fig. 19. Cavernous sinus thrombophlebitis. (*A*) Coronal CECT image demonstrates filling defects within the bilateral cavernous sinuses with associated expansion and lateral convexity (*arrows*) and opacification of the sphenoid sinuses, compatible with cavernous sinus thrombophlebitis from adjacent sphenoid sinusitis. (*B*) Axial CECT image shows expansion and nonenhancement of the right superior ophthalmic vein (*black arrowhead*), in comparison to normal enhancing left superior ophthalmic vein (*white arrowhead*), in keeping with extension of thrombophlebitis into the right superior ophthalmic vein.

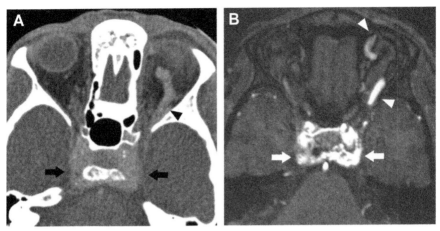

Fig. 20. Carotid cavernous fistula. (*A*) Axial CECT image displays expansion and lateral convexity of the cavernous sinuses (*black arrows*) and enlarged, contrast-opacified left superior ophthalmic vein (*black arrowhead*). (*B*) Axial noncontrast 3-dimensional time-of-flight MRA image shows abnormal hyperintense signal within the expanded cavernous sinuses (*white arrows*) and left superior ophthalmic vein (*white arrowheads*), confirming arterialized flow in the cavernous sinuses and left superior ophthalmic vein consistent with carotid cavernous fistula.

Tolosa-Hunt syndrome

Tolosa-Hunt syndrome is a rare disorder caused by idiopathic inflammation of the cavernous sinus, resulting in unilateral retro-orbital headache and painful ophthalmoplegia. Tolosa-Hunt syndrome is a diagnosis of exclusion and therefore requires a diagnostic workup to exclude other conditions that may result in cavernous sinus

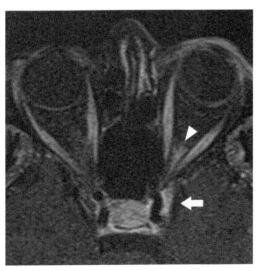

Fig. 21. Tolosa-Hunt syndrome. Axial T1 postgadolinium fat-saturated image demonstrates abnormal enhancing soft tissue in the left orbital apex (*arrowhead*) and cavernous sinus (*arrow*) in this patient with painful ophthalmoplegia consistent with Tolosa-Hunt syndrome.

syndrome. Treatment with corticosteroids results in a dramatic and prompt symptom improvement. Most cases lack residual deficits, but approximately 50% of patients may have recurrence.[37] On MRI, inflammation within the cavernous sinus results in soft tissue thickening and enhancement of the affected cavernous sinus, which may extend into the adjacent superior orbital fissure or orbital apex (**Fig. 21**).[38] CECT may show similar findings of enlarged and enhancing cavernous sinus but is less sensitive to detect the abnormality.

SUMMARY

Cross-sectional imaging is an invaluable tool in the evaluation of painful ophthalmologic disorders. CECT is particularly useful in the assessment of orbital infections and differentiating preseptal cellulitis from orbital cellulitis. MRI offers better evaluation of the orbital soft tissues, crucial for the diagnosis of ocular and optic nerve disease entities.

CLINICS CARE POINTS

- CECT is a first-line imaging to differentiate preseptal cellulitis and orbital cellulitis.
- MRI offers better evaluation of the orbital soft tissues and essential for evaluation of optic neuritis.
- Contrast-enhanced MRI is more sensitive than CT for the detection of acute invasive fungal rhinosinusitis.
- CTA or MRA should be performed in patients with suspected carotid cavernous fistula.

DISCLOSURE

The author has nothing to disclose.

REFERENCES

1. Pflipsen M, Massaquoi M, Wolf S. Evaluation of the Painful Eye. Am Fam Physician 2016;93(12):991–8.
2. Mathew AV, Craig E, Al-Mahmoud R, et al. Paediatric post-septal and pre-septal cellulitis: 10 years' experience at a tertiary-level children's hospital. Br J Radiol 2014;87(1033):20130503.
3. Ullman S, Roussel TJ, Forster RK. Gonococcal keratoconjunctivitis. Surv Ophthalmol 1987;32(3):199–208.
4. Horton JC, Miller S. Magnetic Resonance Imaging in Epidemic Adenoviral Keratoconjunctivitis. JAMA Ophthalmol 2015;133(8):960–1.
5. Ferreira TA, Saraiva P, Genders SW, et al. CT and MR imaging of orbital inflammation. Neuroradiology 2018;60(12):1253–66.
6. Raslan OA, Ozturk A, Pham N, et al. A comprehensive review of cross-sectional imaging of the nasolacrimal drainage apparatus: what radiologists need to know. AJR Am J Roentgenol 2019;213(6):1331–40.
7. von Holstein SL, Coupland SE, Briscoe D, et al. Epithelial tumours of the lacrimal gland: a clinical, histopathological, surgical and oncological survey. Acta Ophthalmol 2013;91(3):195–206.
8. Qin W, Chong R, Huang X, et al. Adenoid cystic carcinoma of the lacrimal gland: CT and MRI findings. Eur J Ophthalmol 2012;22(3):316–9.

9. Krishna U, Ajanaku D, Denniston AK, et al. Uveitis: a sight-threatening disease which can impact all systems. Postgrad Med J 2017;93(1106):766–73.

10. Lohman BD, Gustafson CA, McKinney AM, et al. MR imaging of Vogt-Koyanagi-Harada syndrome with leptomeningeal enhancement. AJNR Am J Neuroradiol 2011;32(9):E169–71.

11. Jackson TL, Eykyn SJ, Graham EM, et al. Endogenous bacterial endophthalmitis: a 17-year prospective series and review of 267 reported cases. Surv Ophthalmol 2003;48(4):403–23.

12. Radhakrishnan R, Cornelius R, Cunnane MB, et al. MR imaging findings of endophthalmitis. Neuroradiol J 2016;29(2):122–9.

13. Efendi H. Clinically isolated syndromes: clinical characteristics, differential diagnosis, and management. Noro Psikiyatr Ars 2015;52(Suppl 1):S1–11.

14. O'Riordan JI, Thompson AJ, Kingsley DP, et al. The prognostic value of brain MRI in clinically isolated syndromes of the CNS. A 10-year follow-up. Brain 1998; 121(Pt 3):495–503.

15. Kim HJ, Paul F, Lana-Peixoto MA, et al. MRI characteristics of neuromyelitis optica spectrum disorder: an international update. Neurology 2015;84(11):1165–73.

16. Wynford-Thomas R, Jacob A, Tomassini V. Neurological update: MOG antibody disease. J Neurol 2019;266(5):1280–6.

17. Denève M, Biotti D, Patsoura S, et al. MRI features of demyelinating disease associated with anti-MOG antibodies in adults. J Neuroradiol 2019;46(5):312–8.

18. Purvin V, Kawasaki A, Jacobson DM. Optic perineuritis: clinical and radiographic features. Arch Ophthalmol 2001;119(9):1299–306.

19. Bahn RS. Graves' ophthalmopathy. N Engl J Med 2010;362(8):726–38.

20. Kahaly GJ. Imaging in thyroid-associated orbitopathy. Eur J Endocrinol 2001; 145(2):107–18.

21. Yuen SJ, Rubin PA. Idiopathic orbital inflammation: distribution, clinical features, and treatment outcome. Arch Ophthalmol 2003;121(4):491–9.

22. LeBedis CA, Sakai O. Nontraumatic orbital conditions: diagnosis with CT and MR imaging in the emergent setting. Radiographics 2008;28(6):1741–53.

23. Lee S, Yen MT. Management of preseptal and orbital cellulitis. Saudi J Ophthalmol 2011;25(1):21–9.

24. Winegar BA, Gutierrez JE. Imaging of Orbital Trauma and Emergent Nontraumatic Conditions. Neuroimaging Clin N Am 2015;25(3):439–56.

25. Garcia GH, Harris GJ. Criteria for nonsurgical management of subperiosteal abscess of the orbit: analysis of outcomes 1988-1998. Ophthalmology 2000;107(8): 1454–6.

26. Nguyen VD, Singh AK, Altmeyer WB, et al. Demystifying orbital emergencies: a pictorial review. Radiographics 2017;37(3):947–62.

27. Sepahdari AR, Aakalu VK, Kapur R, et al. MRI of orbital cellulitis and orbital abscess: the role of diffusion-weighted imaging. AJR Am J Roentgenol 2009;193(3): W244–50.

28. Kalin-Hajdu E, Hirabayashi KE, Vagefi MR, et al. Invasive fungal sinusitis: treatment of the orbit. Curr Opin Ophthalmol 2017;28(5):522–33.

29. Silverman CS, Mancuso AA. Periantral soft-tissue infiltration and its relevance to the early detection of invasive fungal sinusitis: CT and MR findings. AJNR Am J Neuroradiol 1998;19(2):321–5.

30. Safder S, Carpenter JS, Roberts TD, et al. The "Black Turbinate" sign: An early MR imaging finding of nasal mucormycosis. AJNR Am J Neuroradiol 2010;31(4): 771–4.

31. McCallum E, Keren S, Lapira M, et al. Orbital compartment syndrome: an update with review of the literature. Clin Ophthalmol 2019;13:2189–94.
32. Dalley RW, Robertson WD, Rootman J. Globe tenting: a sign of increased orbital tension. AJNR Am J Neuroradiol 1989;10(1):181–6.
33. Lee JH, Lee HK, Park JK, et al. Cavernous sinus syndrome: clinical features and differential diagnosis with MR imaging. AJR Am J Roentgenol 2003;181(2): 583–90.
34. Mahalingam HV, Mani SE, Patel B, et al. Imaging spectrum of cavernous sinus lesions with histopathologic correlation. Radiographics 2019;39(3):795–819.
35. Barrow DL, Spector RH, Braun IF, et al. Classification and treatment of spontaneous carotid-cavernous sinus fistulas. J Neurosurg 1985;62(2):248–56.
36. Chen CC, Chang PC, Shy CG, et al. CT angiography and MR angiography in the evaluation of carotid cavernous sinus fistula prior to embolization: a comparison of techniques. AJNR Am J Neuroradiol 2005;26(9):2349–56.
37. Kline LB, Hoyt WF. The Tolosa-Hunt syndrome. J Neurol Neurosurg Psychiatr 2001;71(5):577–82.
38. Schuknecht B, Sturm V, Huisman TA, et al. Tolosa-Hunt syndrome: MR imaging features in 15 patients with 20 episodes of painful ophthalmoplegia. Eur J Radiol 2009;69(3):445–53.

Role of MRI and CT in the Evaluation of Headache in Pregnancy and the Postpartum Period

Carlos Zamora, MD, PhD[a],*, Mauricio Castillo, MD[b]

KEYWORDS

• Pregnancy • Postpartum • Headaches • MRI • CT

KEY POINTS

- Head CT is the imaging modality of choice in the acute setting and is sensitive for detecting conditions that may necessitate urgent care.
- MRI is appropriate in patients with (1) new-onset headache and optic disc edema or (2) new/progressive headaches and subacute head trauma, headache related to activity or positional, neurologic deficits, malignancy, immunocompromised status, pregnancy, or age older than 50.
- MRI is the most appropriate modality in patients with trigeminal autonomic headaches or chronic headaches with new features or increasing frequency.
- Routine screening for pregnancy is not currently recommended before the intravenous administration of iodinated contrast media for CT.
- MRI gadolinium-based contrast agents should be avoided in pregnancy and restricted to those situations where they are considered critical for diagnosis.

BACKGROUND

Pregnancy is accompanied by substantial physiologic changes and is an established risk factor for secondary headaches.[1] Among pregnant women presenting with acute headaches, one study found that 35% of them had a secondary headache, and the majority presented in the third trimester.[2] Headaches are also common in the postpartum period where they occur in 30% to 40% of patients.[1] Most secondary headaches are due to hypertensive disorders, namely preeclampsia-eclampsia, posterior reversible

[a] Division of Neuroradiology, Department of Radiology, University of North Carolina School of Medicine, CB 7510, 3320 Old Infirmary, Chapel Hill, NC 27599-7510, USA; [b] Division of Neuroradiology, Department of Radiology, University of North Carolina School of Medicine, CB 7510, 3326 Old Infirmary, Chapel Hill, NC 27599-7510, USA
* Corresponding author.
E-mail address: carlos_zamora@med.unc.edu

Neurol Clin 40 (2022) 661–677
https://doi.org/10.1016/j.ncl.2022.02.010   neurologic.theclinics.com
0733-8619/22/© 2022 Elsevier Inc. All rights reserved.

encephalopathy syndrome (PRES), and acute arterial hypertension. Other relevant causes include reversible cerebral vasoconstriction syndrome (RCVS), pituitary apoplexy, and cerebral venous thrombosis. Some of these conditions can be life-threatening and need to be diagnosed and managed promptly. Additionally, imaging of pregnant patients warrants special considerations regarding any potential effects of ionizing radiation and intravenous contrast agents on the fetus. In this article, we review general recommendations for imaging the pregnant patient and discuss the imaging findings of common causes of headaches in pregnancy and the postpartum period.

DISCUSSION
Guidelines for Imaging the Pregnant Patient

Radiation considerations

The potential adverse sequelae of radiation on living tissue have been classified into deterministic and stochastic effects. Deterministic effects are directly related to the radiation dose and have a threshold below which they do not occur, their hallmark being tissue damage. In contrast, stochastic effects occur by chance and do not have a defined threshold. Although the risk of stochastic effects increases with the radiation dose, their severity does not (eg, cancer and hereditary effects).[3] Because there is no "safe level" of ionizing radiation, any study must consider the risk versus benefit as well as the standard of care for a given clinical situation.

Fetal studies have shown that deterministic radiation effects vary by gestational age and that organogenesis is the period of highest susceptibility (between weeks 2 and 7). Potential deterministic effects have been observed following doses between 50 and 100 mGy, with possible malformations linked to doses more than 100 mGy during the period of organogenesis. No adverse effects have been observed with doses less than 50 mGy. A routine head CT, the modality likely to be used during the acute workup of a headache, carries with it a dose of 1.6 mSv (1 mSv = dose produced by exposure to 1 mGy of radiation). This is equivalent to approximately 7 months of natural background ionizing radiation and well below the thresholds for deterministic effects mentioned above.[4] According to practice parameters from the American College of Radiology (ACR) and Society of Pediatric Radiology, diagnostic X-ray examinations that do not directly expose the gravid uterus do not require verification of pregnancy status.[5] Therefore, pregnancy is not a contraindication for routine head CT when clinically appropriate. Effective radiation doses associated with brain CT perfusion are variable and usually severalfold that of routine head CT.

Use of contrast agents

There is scant information regarding the use of iodinated contrast media (ICM) and gadolinium-based contrast agents (GBCAs) during pregnancy, and the potential effects on the fetus are not entirely known. Both ICM and GBCAs cross the placenta, enter the fetus, and are subsequently excreted in the urine and amniotic fluid. Contrast material in the amniotic fluid is then swallowed by the fetus starting a process of recirculation; however, this is poorly understood.[6] A small amount of contrast material is absorbed through the gastrointestinal tract, enters the bloodstream, and is excreted in the urine.[7] Some contrast material is probably also sent back to the maternal circulation via the placenta.[8] This process of recirculation introduces a particular situation in the fetus who may be exposed to a contrast agent for a prolonged time.

In vivo tests in animals have not shown a teratogenic effect with low osmolar ICM, although there are no well-controlled human trials. There are rare reports of transient congenital hypothyroidism after amniofetography using lipid-soluble ICM; however, this procedure is no longer performed. There have been no reports of congenital hypothyroidism with the water-soluble ICM that are currently used.[9] The ACR does not currently recommend routine screening for pregnancy before the intravenous administration of ICM. Most ICM are classified as category B by the Food and Drug Administration (FDA), and their use should not be withheld in pregnant or lactating women when necessary for diagnostic purposes.[10,11]

In contrast, GBCAs are classified as FDA category C. Gadolinium is a heavy metal that is toxic in its free form and needs to be chelated to a ligand to be administered safely. It is now known that some dechelation of gadolinium does occur *in vivo* after intravenous injection of GBCAs and is dependent on several factors including the chemical stability of the compound. Animal studies have shown teratogenic effects after high and repeated doses of GBCAs; however, there are no well-controlled human studies. Retrospective studies of pregnant women who inadvertently received GBCAs during pregnancy fail to show a teratogenic effect. A large population-based cohort study found that administration of GBCAs during pregnancy was associated with stillbirth and neonatal death, as well as a range of inflammatory, rheumatologic, and infiltrative skin conditions.[12] That study, however, had substantial methodological limitations. Currently, due to the uncertain but possible risk associated with GBCAs, their use in pregnancy should be restricted to situations where they are considered critical for diagnosis.[10] If the administration of GBCAs is necessary, macrocyclic agents (gadobutrol, gadoteridol, and gadoterate meglumine) are preferred due to their higher chemical stability and lower risk for dechelation.

Computed tomography

Noncontrast head CT is the imaging modality of choice in any acute setting due to its speed and sensitivity for the detection of hemorrhage, herniation, significant mass effect, and hydrocephalus. In patients with sudden onset, severe headache, or "worst headache of life," noncontrast head CT is the first-line modality and should be performed regardless of pregnancy status. MR angiography (MRA) is preferred over CT angiography (CTA) and may follow noncontrast head CT in patients with suspected aneurysmal hemorrhage (ie, sudden onset severe headaches and 2 or more first-degree family members with a history of aneurysmal subarachnoid hemorrhage [SAH]).[13] MRI is the modality of choice for further characterization of headaches and is recommended for certain situations as described below. CT with contrast usually does not play a role in the evaluation of headaches but may be performed in patients who are unable to undergo MRI (eg, severe claustrophobia, MRI incompatible devices, and so forth).

Magnetic resonance imaging

MRI is the modality of choice for a comprehensive evaluation of headaches due to its higher contrast and spatial resolution compared with CT. MRI excels at soft tissue characterization and offers several advanced sequences that may aid in refining the diagnosis. MRI is as sensitive as CT in the detection of acute intracranial hemorrhage if Fluid-attenuated inversion recovery (FLAIR) and SWI or T2*/GRE sequences are included.[14] However, due to the high sensitivity of CT, MRI is usually not indicated as an initial study in the setting of "worst headache of life."[13] MRI is appropriate in patients with new-onset headache and optic disc edema, as well as in patients with new or progressively worsening headaches and any of the following "red flags": subacute head trauma, headache related to activity, positional headaches, neurologic deficits, known or suspected malignancy, immunocompromised status, current pregnancy, or age older than 50.[13] In these situations, however, noncontrast head CT may be performed as initial evaluation in the acute setting avoiding the need for MRI.

MRI is also the most appropriate initial imaging modality to evaluate patients with trigeminal autonomic headaches or patients with chronic headaches who present with new features or increasing frequency. Outside of the "red flags" mentioned above, no imaging is currently recommended for patients with new headaches that are consistent with classic migraines or tension-type headaches and an otherwise normal neurologic examination. Finally, imaging is not indicated in patients who have chronic headaches without new features or neurologic deficits.[13]

Causes of Headache

Cerebral venous thrombosis

Pregnancy is accompanied by a physiologic hypercoagulable state due to an increase in several prothrombotic factors and a decrease in protein S, which is an anticoagulant.[15] The risk for venous thromboembolism in pregnant women is increased severalfold relative to the general population and is substantially higher in the postpartum period.[15,16] Additionally, the risk for pregnancy-related cerebral venous thrombosis is higher in patients with hypertension, infection, excessive vomiting, increased age, and cesarean section.[17] Headache is seen in 89% of patients with cerebral venous thrombosis and is by far the most common presentation. Other clinical manifestations include papilledema, mental status changes, paresis, and seizures, among others.[18]

Noncontrast head CT is highly specific but has only moderate sensitivity for the detection of cerebral venous thrombosis.[19] The cortical veins and/or dural sinuses may show increased attenuation and can have an expansile appearance (**Fig. 1**). This should not be confused with the increased venous attenuation that can be seen in healthy patients who have a high normal hematocrit level. In patients with venous thrombosis, there may be areas of parenchymal hypodensity if there is associated venous ischemia. CT or MR venography show filling defects corresponding to the thrombosed vessels. On MRI, there is loss of the expected vascular signal void, and there can be signal dropout with blooming on SWI sequences and/or restricted diffusion depending on the stage of the thrombus (see **Fig. 1**). MRI is highly accurate for the detection of venous ischemia and associated hemorrhage.[20,21]

Aneurysmal subarachnoid hemorrhage

The mortality associated with SAH is high for both mother and fetus. However, whether there is an increased risk of aneurysmal rupture during pregnancy, labor, or the postpartum period remains controversial.[22,23] Patients with aneurysmal SAH typically present with sudden-onset severe headaches that are frequently described as the "worst headache of life." Noncontrast head CT is the initial modality of choice and is highly sensitive for the detection of acute SAH, although its sensitivity decreases over time.[24] Hemorrhage tends to be more abundant surrounding the source and is more pronounced, for instance, along the anterior interhemispheric fissure for anterior communicating aneurysms and interpeduncular cistern for basilar tip aneurysms (**Fig. 2**). MRI is as sensitive as head CT in the acute setting if both FLAIR and SWI or T2*/GRE sequences are included. Demonstration of the aneurysm requires intravenous contrast for CTA but may be done without contrast on MRI using time-of-flight technique angiography. CTA and MRI may also have a role in patients who develop vasospasm and delayed cerebral ischemia. The gold standard for the evaluation of aneurysms is digital subtraction catheter angiography, which allows access to those that are amenable to endovascular treatment.

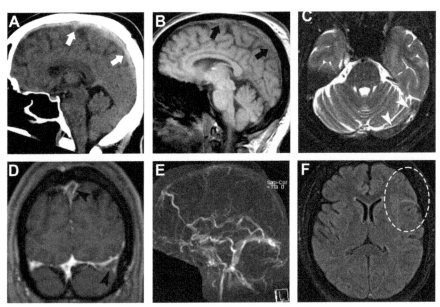

Fig. 1. Cerebral venous thrombosis. Sagittal noncontrast CT reformat (*A*) demonstrates increased attenuation along the superior sagittal sinus consistent with thrombus (*white arrows*). Sagittal noncontrast T1-weighted image on MRI (*B*) shows corresponding hyperintensity (*black arrows*). Axial T2-weighted image (*C*) shows lack of the normal signal void in the left transverse sinus (*white arrowheads*). Coronal postcontrast T1-weighted image (*D*) shows filling defects within the superior sagittal sinus and left transverse sinus (*black arrowheads*). A 3D reconstruction from the time-of-flight MRA (*E*) demonstrates absence of the superior sagittal and left transverse sinuses. On FLAIR (*F*) there increased signal along left frontal sulci (oval) because of SAH.

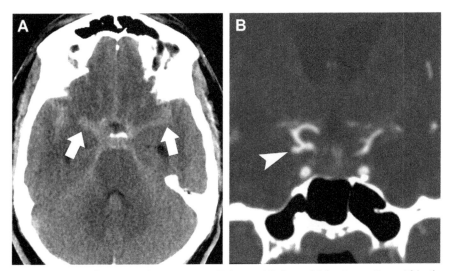

Fig. 2. Aneurysmal SAH. Axial noncontrast CT image (*A*) shows high attenuation within the basal cisterns and sylvian fissures (*white arrows*) due to extensive SAH. Coronal reconstruction from CTA (*B*) shows a small aneurysm at the right supraclinoid internal carotid artery (*white arrowhead*).

Arteriovenous malformations

Rupture of an arteriovenous malformation (AVM) is another important cause of intra-cranial hemorrhage during pregnancy and is associated with high mortality.[25] Earlier studies differ on whether there is an increased risk of AVM rupture during pregnancy or the postpartum period.[22] AVMs can occur anywhere but most of them are supra-tentorial.[26] The pattern of hemorrhage varies according to location and may be intra-parenchymal, intraventricular, and/or subarachnoid (**Fig. 3**). Noncontrast head CT is highly sensitive to detect acute hemorrhage and on rare occasions may demonstrate enlarged, serpiginous, and hyperdense vessels in patients with sufficiently large AVMs. However, visualization of an AVM requires CTA or MRI with MRA, which can delineate the vascular nidus, enlarged arterial feeders, and draining veins. T2-weighted MRI sequences may show a tangle of vessels with signal voids due to rapid blood flow and lesions show contrast enhancement (**Fig. 4**). Patients with AVMs can develop aneurysms within the nidus (intranidal) or along arterial feeders (flow-related) that are associated with SAH.[27] AVMs with exclusive deep drainage or a single drain-ing vein are associated with an increased risk for hemorrhage.[28] Arterial spin labeling perfusion may be helpful to identify arteriovenous shunting in small AVMs, which may be difficult to visualize otherwise.[29] Catheter angiography is the best-suited modality to delineate the AVM architecture and hemodynamics and allows for embolization of amenable lesions.

Posterior reversible encephalopathy syndrome, preeclampsia, and eclampsia

Patients with PRES can present with headaches, visual disturbances, altered mental status, focal neurologic deficits, and seizures. The pathophysiology is not completely understood. One proposed mechanism involves acute hypertension exceeding the limits of cerebral autoregulation and leading to hyperperfusion, breakdown of the blood–brain barrier, and extravasation of blood products and fluid. An alternative model postulates that severe hypertension results in vasospasm, ischemia, and breakdown of the blood–brain barrier. Another competing theory is that PRES is caused primarily by endothelial dysfunction, which is supported by the fact that 30% of patients do not have hypertension significant enough to cause failed

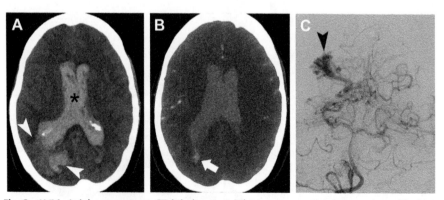

Fig. 3. AVM. Axial noncontrast CT (*A*) shows a right temporoparietal parenchymal hemor-rhage (*white arrowheads*) with extensive intraventricular hemorrhage (*asterisk*). On CTA (*B*), there is a small irregular focus of enhancement superior to the parenchymal hemor-rhage corresponding to an AVM (*white arrow*). Frontal view digital subtraction angiog-raphy (*C*) demonstrates the nidus (*arrowhead*) with small intranidal aneurysms and feeders from the right posterior cerebral artery.

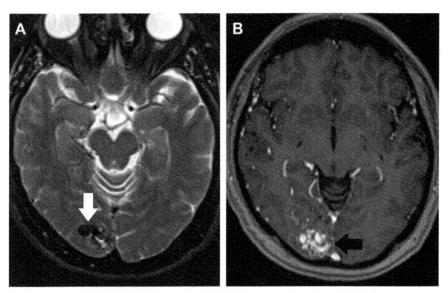

Fig. 4. AVM. Axial T2-weighted sequence (*A*) (different patient than **Fig. 3**) demonstrates a tangle of vessels with signal voids in the right occipital lobe consistent with an AVM (*white arrow*). The lesion shows avid enhancement on the postcontrast T1-weighted image (*B*) (*black arrow*).

autoregulation.[30] Patients with preeclampsia-eclampsia have been found to have elevated levels of endothelial inflammatory markers and lower blood pressures than other reported cases of PRES.[31–33] Also, pregnant women are at increased risk of hypoalbuminemia, which may play a role in the development of edema by reducing the colloid osmotic pressure.[34] Eclampsia, similar to PRES, can present with seizures, and it is uncertain whether these entities are part of the same spectrum. RCVS is thought to share a similar mechanism with PRES and will be described below. Other triggers of PRES include impaired renal function, transplantation, sepsis, autoimmune disease, and cytotoxic agents.[35]

CT may demonstrate subcortical white matter hypodensities with a typical posterior distribution; however, its sensitivity is low.[36] MRI shows bilateral and symmetric vasogenic edema primarily involving the parietal and occipital lobes and along the superior frontal sulci (**Fig. 5**).[37] Leptomeningeal or cortical enhancement and microhemorrhage are common, and some patients can have small amounts of SAH (**Fig. 6**).[38] Rarely, PRES may be associated with small foci of restricted diffusion indicating cytotoxic edema.[39] Atypical forms can be seen primarily affecting the brainstem, cerebellum, thalamus, and basal ganglia without significant cortical/subcortical involvement.[40]

Reversible cerebral vasoconstriction syndrome
Headaches are universal in patients with RCVS, and these are frequently severe, recurrent, and thunderclap-like.[41] Like PRES, the pathophysiology is unknown but thought to be related to dysregulation of vascular tone. Several conditions have been associated with RCVS, including postpartum state, preeclampsia-eclampsia, and several vasoconstrictive drugs, among others. However, epidemiologic data are lacking, and a definite causal relationship has not been established. Initial imaging on patients with RCVS is frequently normal, particularly on CT. However, 81% of patients eventually develop brain lesions, which are best seen on MRI, most commonly

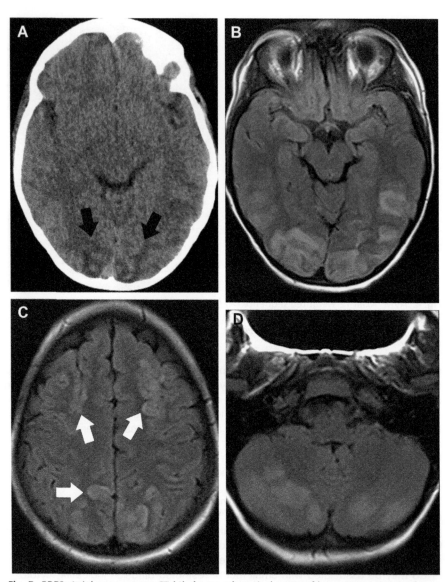

Fig. 5. PRES. Axial noncontrast CT (*A*) shows subcortical areas of low attenuation in the occipital lobes bilaterally (*black arrows*). Axial FLAIR images (*B–D*) demonstrate cortical and subcortical signal abnormalities along the posterior cerebrum and frontal lobes (*white arrows*) as well as cerebellum.

infarction, small volume convexity SAH, intraparenchymal hemorrhage, or edema in a PRES-like distribution.[41] Areas of ischemia are commonly watershed as opposed to defined vascular territories.[41,42] Angiographic imaging shows areas of severe stenosis and dilatation, sometimes with a beaded appearance (**Fig. 7**). Although CTA or MRA show arterial abnormalities in 80% of patients, these may be difficult to visualize, and catheter digital subtraction angiography is the gold standard.[43] The arterial abnormalities in RCVS may mimic primary central nervous system (CNS) angiitis; however, the latter has a more insidious onset and is not associated with watershed infarcts or

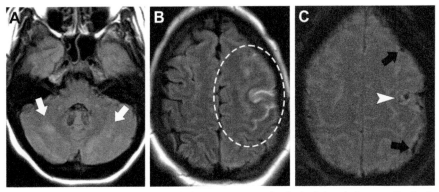

Fig. 6. PRES. Axial FLAIR images (*A, B*) demonstrate patchy foci of signal abnormality in the cerebellum (*white arrows*). There is increased signal along left frontal convexity due to SAH (oval). SWI sequence (*C*) shows corresponding signal loss along the sulci (*black arrows*) as well as small cortical hemorrhages (*arrowhead*).

PRES-like edema.[41] Additionally, RCVS is characterized by a lack of inflammatory markers on cerebrospinal fluid (CSF), and the angiographic findings are usually reversible.[42–44] In the past, postpartum RCVS was known as "postpartum vasculopathy."

Carotid and vertebral artery dissection

Pregnancy has been associated with an increased risk for cervical artery dissection, particularly in the postpartum period.[45] Presumed mechanisms include physiologic increases in cardiac output and blood volume throughout pregnancy, as well as hormonal changes leading to decreased vascular elasticity.[46,47] Headache is the earliest manifestation in 47% of patients and may rarely be the only symptom.[48,49] Stroke is the most severe complication, but it is rare after a first spontaneous dissection. Recurrent dissections are uncommon without other predisposing factors.[50] Spontaneous dissections most commonly involve the vertebral arteries followed by the internal carotid arteries.[48] Vertebral artery dissections most commonly occur at points of potential mechanical stress: as the vessel enters the C6 foramen transversarium, at the level of the C1 vascular loop, and as it pierces the dura at the skull base.[51–53] Dissections of the internal carotid artery most commonly develop at mobile vascular segments. They typically occur 2 to 3 cm above the bifurcation (from where they may extend intracranially), before the vessel enters the skull base, and at the supraclinoid segment.[54,55] CTA is highly accurate in diagnosing arterial dissections. MRA is also appropriate and GBCAs can be avoided in pregnancy using the time-of-flight technique. Because proximal internal carotid dissections frequently spare the carotid bulb, they produce a characteristic "flame-shaped" appearance in the acute phase. Imaging findings include irregular narrowing of the vessel with or without dilatation. An intimal flap or double lumen is a reliable sign; however, it is not present in every case and is rarely seen in vertebral dissections.[49] On MRI, cervical arterial dissections may be accompanied by a T1-hyperintense crescent representing intramural hemorrhage (**Fig. 8**). Dissections can also be complicated by pseudoaneurysm formation and intraluminal thrombus, which increases the risk for stroke.[56]

Pituitary infarction (Sheehan syndrome)

Pregnancy is normally accompanied by a substantial increase in the size of the anterior pituitary gland.[57] This is a highly vascularized organ, and its larger size during pregnancy is thought to render it more prone to ischemia.[58] Also, a small sella turcica

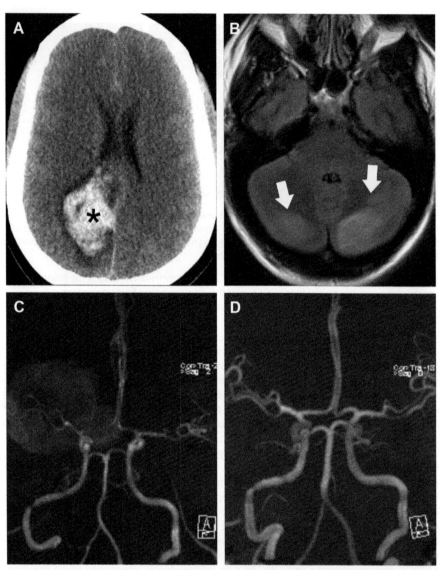

Fig. 7. RCVS. Axial noncontrast CT (*A*) shows a large hemorrhage in the medial right parietal lobe (*asterisk*). Axial FLAIR (*B*) shows areas of edema in the cerebellum in a PRES-like pattern (*white arrows*). Coronal 3D reformat from time-of-flight MRA (*C*) demonstrates multifocal stenoses in the anterior and posterior circulation, which resolved on follow several weeks later (*D*).

has been proposed as a predisposing factor.[59] Pituitary infarction is usually seen in the postpartum period after massive hemorrhage that results in hypotension, although occasionally there is no apparent trigger.[58] Patients with Sheehan syndrome can present with headaches, visual disturbance, failed lactation, and varying degrees of hypopituitarism.[59] MRI demonstrates an enlarged pituitary gland with areas of hypoenhancement because of necrosis.[60] The gland decreases in size over time and follow-up MRI frequently shows a flattened gland with an "empty sella" (**Fig. 9**).

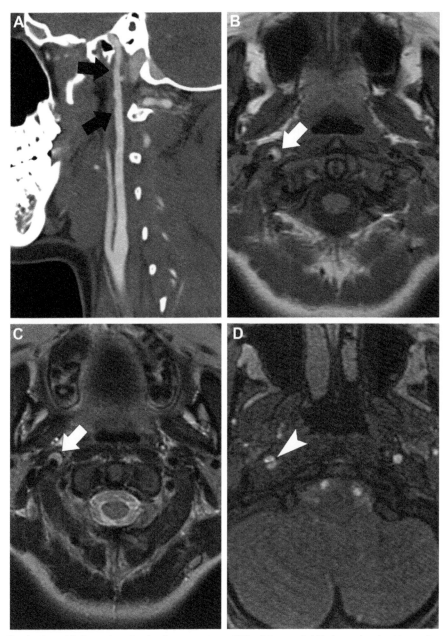

Fig. 8. Carotid dissection. Sagittal postcontrast CTA of the neck (*A*) shows luminal irregularity involving the distal internal carotid artery (*black arrows*). Axial noncontrast T1 (*B*) and T2 (*C*) demonstrate a crescent of increased signal along the periphery of the right internal carotid artery in keeping with intramural thrombus (*white arrows*). Axial time-of-flight MRA more distally (*D*) shows an intimal flap across the vessel (white *arrowhead*).

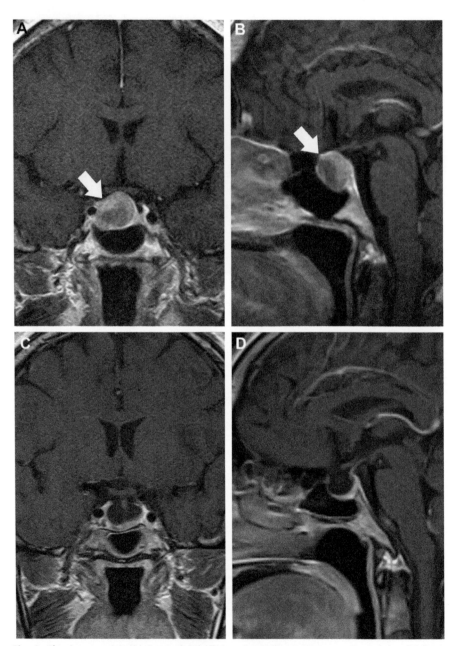

Fig. 9. Sheehan syndrome. Coronal (*A*) and sagittal (*B*) postcontrast T1-weighted images demonstrate an enlarged pituitary gland with central hypoenhancement (*white arrows*). Follow-up 6 months later (*C, D*) shows interval decrease in the size of the gland resulting in a flattened appearance and an "empty sella."

Postdural puncture headache

Seventy-one percent of women undergo neuraxial analgesia during labor in the form of epidural or spinal (ie, intrathecal) blockades.[61] Headaches are a common

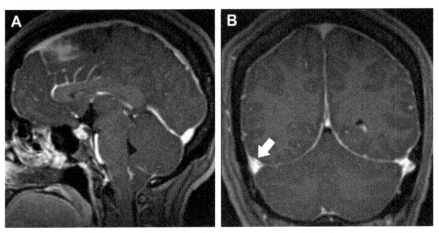

Fig. 10. Intracranial hypotension. Sagittal postcontrast T1-weighted sequence (*A*) shows cerebellar and brainstem sagging with crowding of the posterior fossa and decreased distance between the pons and mammillary bodies. The pituitary gland is engorged. Coronal postcontrast T1-weighted sequence (*B*) shows engorgement of the dural sinuses with a rounded appearance. There is also mild thickening of the dura.

complication of intrathecal access and thought to be secondary to CSF leak leading to intracranial hypotension. They may also occur as a complication of epidural catheter insertion.[62] Incidence is varied and has been reported in up to 11% of patients who underwent lumbar puncture with standard (ie, nontraumatic) needles and 88% of patients in whom there was inadvertent dural puncture during epidural anesthesia.[63,64] The cause of headaches is not entirely understood. Several mechanisms have been proposed, including venous distention, brainstem sagging, and possible traction of cranial nerves or meningeal membranes.[65] Headaches associated with postdural puncture are postural: they are exacerbated in the upright position and relieved when lying flat. Some of the characteristic imaging findings are a reflection of the Monro-Kelly doctrine, which dictates that fluid drawn from the rigid intracranial compartment must be accompanied by an equivalent replacement of volume.[66] In intracranial hypotension, loss of CSF is compensated by distention of dural venous sinuses and plexuses, dural thickening, and engorgement of the pituitary gland, which is normally highly vascularized. Patients may also present with subdural effusions and less commonly subdural hematomas. Most patients have some degree of brainstem sagging and inferior displacement of the cerebellar tonsils; however, the absence of these findings does not preclude the diagnosis.[67] Displacement of the brainstem can be accompanied by flattening of the pons against the clivus, decreased pontomesencephalic angle, and decreased pontomamillary distance (**Fig. 10**).[68] Patients can rarely present with uncal herniation.[69]

SUMMARY

Headaches are common during pregnancy and in the postpartum period and, in some cases, may be the manifestation of a serious underlying condition. Although imaging is not indicated in patients with typical primary headaches who have a normal neurologic examination, further workup is warranted in the presence of certain "red flags," as discussed above. CT is usually accurate in identifying conditions that necessitate urgent care, and MRI is generally warranted for further characterization. In this article, we have reviewed the role of CT and MRI and relevant imaging features of the most common conditions associated with headaches in this population.

CLINICS CARE POINTS

- Pregnancy status is not a contraindication for routine head CT when clinically appropriate.
- Head CT is the modality of choice in the acute setting and is sensitive for detecting conditions that may necessitate urgent care.
- MRI is appropriate in patients with (1) new-onset headache and optic disc edema or (2) new/progressive headaches and subacute head trauma, headache related to activity or positional, neurologic deficits, malignancy, immunocompromised status, pregnancy, or age older than 50 years.
- MRI is the most appropriate modality in patients with trigeminal autonomic headaches or chronic headaches with new features or increasing frequency.
- Routine screening for pregnancy is not currently recommended before the intravenous administration of ICM.
- GBCAs are generally avoided in pregnancy and should be restricted to those situations where they are considered critical for diagnosis.

DISCLOSURE

No relevant disclosures.

REFERENCES

1. Negro A, Delaruelle Z, Ivanova TA, et al. Headache and pregnancy: a systematic review. J Headache Pain 2017;18(1):106.
2. Robbins MS, Farmakidis C, Dayal AK, et al. Acute headache diagnosis in pregnant women: a hospital-based study. Neurology 2015;85(12):1024–30.
3. Wunderle K, Gill AS. Radiation-related injuries and their management: an update. Semin Intervent Radiol 2015;32(2):156–62.
4. Patient safety - radiation dose in X-ray and CT exams. Radiological Society of North America (RSNA); 2019. Available at: https://www.radiologyinfo.org/en/info/safety-xray. Accessed September 18, 2021.
5. ACR–SPR Practice parameter for imaging pregnant or potentially pregnant adolescents and women with ionizing radiation. 2018.
6. Muhler MR, Clement O, Salomon LJ, et al. Maternofetal pharmacokinetics of a gadolinium chelate contrast agent in mice. Radiology 2011;258(2):455–60.
7. Tremblay E, Therasse E, Thomassin-Naggara I, et al. Quality initiatives: guidelines for use of medical imaging during pregnancy and lactation. Radiographics 2012;32(3):897–911.
8. Oh KY, Roberts VH, Schabel MC, et al. Gadolinium chelate contrast material in pregnancy: fetal biodistribution in the nonhuman primate. Radiology 2015;276(1):110–8.
9. Bourjeily G, Chalhoub M, Phornphutkul C, et al. Neonatal thyroid function: effect of a single exposure to iodinated contrast medium in utero. Radiology 2010;256(3):744–50.
10. ACR manual on contrast media. Am Coll Radiol 2021.

11. Puac P, Rodriguez A, Vallejo C, et al. Safety of contrast material use during pregnancy and lactation. Magn Reson Imaging Clin N Am 2017;25(4):787–97.
12. Ray JG, Vermeulen MJ, Bharatha A, et al. Association between MRI exposure during pregnancy and fetal and childhood outcomes. JAMA 2016;316(9):952–61.
13. ACR Appropriateness Criteria® — Headache. Am Coll Radiol 2019.
14. Chalela JA, Kidwell CS, Nentwich LM, et al. Magnetic resonance imaging and computed tomography in emergency assessment of patients with suspected acute stroke: a prospective comparison. Lancet 2007;369(9558):293–8.
15. James AH. Venous thromboembolism in pregnancy. Arterioscler Thromb Vasc Biol 2009;29(3):326–31.
16. James AH, Jamison MG, Brancazio LR, et al. Venous thromboembolism during pregnancy and the postpartum period: incidence, risk factors, and mortality. Am J Obstet Gynecol 2006;194(5):1311–5.
17. Lanska DJ, Kryscio RJ. Risk factors for peripartum and postpartum stroke and intracranial venous thrombosis. Stroke 2000;31(6):1274–82.
18. Ferro JM, Canhao P, Stam J, et al. Prognosis of cerebral vein and dural sinus thrombosis: results of the International Study on Cerebral Vein and Dural Sinus Thrombosis (ISCVT). Stroke 2004;35(3):664–70.
19. Buyck PJ, Zuurbier SM, Garcia-Esperon C, et al. Diagnostic accuracy of noncontrast CT imaging markers in cerebral venous thrombosis. Neurology 2019;92(8): e841–51.
20. Sadigh G, Mullins ME, Saindane AM. Diagnostic performance of MRI sequences for evaluation of dural venous sinus thrombosis. AJR Am J Roentgenol 2016; 206(6):1298–306.
21. Patel D, Machnowska M, Symons S, et al. Diagnostic performance of routine brain MRI sequences for dural venous sinus thrombosis. AJNR Am J Neuroradiol 2016;37(11):2026–32.
22. Tiel Groenestege AT, Rinkel GJ, van der Bom JG, et al. The risk of aneurysmal subarachnoid hemorrhage during pregnancy, delivery, and the puerperium in the Utrecht population: case-crossover study and standardized incidence ratio estimation. Stroke 2009;40(4):1148–51.
23. Porras JL, Yang W, Philadelphia E, et al. Hemorrhage risk of brain arteriovenous malformations during pregnancy and puerperium in a North American Cohort. Stroke 2017;48(6):1507–13.
24. van Gijn J, van Dongen KJ. The time course of aneurysmal haemorrhage on computed tomograms. Neuroradiology 1982;23(3):153–6.
25. Dias MS, Sekhar LN. Intracranial hemorrhage from aneurysms and arteriovenous malformations during pregnancy and the puerperium. Neurosurgery 1990;27(6): 855–65 [discussion: 865-856].
26. Pekmezci M, Nelson J, Su H, et al. Morphometric characterization of brain arteriovenous malformations for clinical and radiological studies to identify silent intralesional microhemorrhages. Clin Neuropathol 2016;35(3):114–21.
27. Hung AL, Yang W, Jiang B, et al. The effect of flow-related aneurysms on hemorrhagic risk of intracranial arteriovenous malformations. Neurosurgery 2019;85(4): 466–75.
28. Alexander MD, Cooke DL, Nelson J, et al. Association between Venous Angioarchitectural Features of Sporadic Brain Arteriovenous Malformations and Intracranial Hemorrhage. AJNR Am J Neuroradiology 2015;36(5):949–52.
29. Hodel J, Leclerc X, Kalsoum E, et al. Intracranial arteriovenous shunting: detection with arterial spin-labeling and susceptibility-weighted imaging combined. AJNR Am J Neuroradiology 2017;38(1):71–6.

30. Fischer M, Schmutzhard E. Posterior reversible encephalopathy syndrome. J Neurol 2017;264(8):1608–16.

31. Savvidou MD, Hingorani AD, Tsikas D, et al. Endothelial dysfunction and raised plasma concentrations of asymmetric dimethylarginine in pregnant women who subsequently develop pre-eclampsia. Lancet 2003;361(9368):1511–7.

32. Wagner SJ, Acquah LA, Lindell EP, et al. Posterior reversible encephalopathy syndrome and eclampsia: pressing the case for more aggressive blood pressure control. Mayo Clin Proc 2011;86(9):851–6.

33. Schwartz RB, Feske SK, Polak JF, et al. Preeclampsia-eclampsia: clinical and neuroradiographic correlates and insights into the pathogenesis of hypertensive encephalopathy. Radiology 2000;217(2):371–6.

34. Nakamura Y, Sugino M, Tsukahara A, et al. Posterior reversible encephalopathy syndrome with extensive cytotoxic edema after blood transfusion: a case report and literature review. BMC Neurol 2018;18(1):190.

35. Hinduja A. Posterior reversible encephalopathy syndrome: clinical features and outcome. Front Neurol 2020;11:71.

36. Dandoy CE, Linscott LL, Davies SM, et al. Clinical utility of computed tomography and magnetic resonance imaging for diagnosis of posterior reversible encephalopathy syndrome after stem cell transplantation in children and adolescents. Biol Blood Marrow Transplant 2015;21(11):2028–32.

37. Anderson RC, Patel V, Sheikh-Bahaei N, et al. Posterior reversible encephalopathy syndrome (PRES): pathophysiology and neuro-imaging. Front Neurol 2020;11:463.

38. McKinney AM, Sarikaya B, Gustafson C, et al. Detection of microhemorrhage in posterior reversible encephalopathy syndrome using susceptibility-weighted imaging. AJNR Am J Neuroradiology 2012;33(5):896–903.

39. Saad AF, Chaudhari R, Wintermark M. Imaging of atypical and complicated posterior reversible encephalopathy syndrome. Front Neurol 2019;10:964.

40. McKinney AM, Jagadeesan BD, Truwit CL. Central-variant posterior reversible encephalopathy syndrome: brainstem or basal ganglia involvement lacking cortical or subcortical cerebral edema. AJR Am J Roentgenol 2013;201(3):631–8.

41. Singhal AB, Hajj-Ali RA, Topcuoglu MA, et al. Reversible cerebral vasoconstriction syndromes: analysis of 139 cases. Arch Neurol 2011;68(8):1005–12.

42. Miller TR, Shivashankar R, Mossa-Basha M, et al. Reversible Cerebral vasoconstriction syndrome, part 2: diagnostic work-up, imaging evaluation, and differential diagnosis. AJNR Am J Neuroradiology 2015;36(9):1580–8.

43. Burton TM, Bushnell CD. Reversible cerebral vasoconstriction syndrome. Stroke 2019;50(8):2253–8.

44. de Boysson H, Parienti JJ, Mawet J, et al. Primary angiitis of the CNS and reversible cerebral vasoconstriction syndrome: a comparative study. Neurology 2018; 91(16):e1468–78.

45. Salehi Omran S, Parikh NS, Poisson S, et al. Association between pregnancy and cervical artery dissection. Ann Neurol 2020;88(3):596–602.

46. Sanghavi M, Rutherford JD. Cardiovascular physiology of pregnancy. Circulation 2014;130(12):1003–8.

47. Karkkainen H, Saarelainen H, Valtonen P, et al. Carotid artery elasticity decreases during pregnancy - the Cardiovascular Risk in Young Finns study. BMC Pregnancy Childbirth 2014;14:98.

48. Arnold M, Cumurciuc R, Stapf C, et al. Pain as the only symptom of cervical artery dissection. J Neurol Neurosurg Psychiatry 2006;77(9):1021–4.

49. Rodallec MH, Marteau V, Gerber S, et al. Craniocervical arterial dissection: spectrum of imaging findings and differential diagnosis. Radiographics 2008;28(6): 1711–28.

50. Touze E, Gauvrit JY, Moulin T, et al. Risk of stroke and recurrent dissection after a cervical artery dissection: a multicenter study. Neurology 2003;61(10):1347–51.

51. Sasaki O, Ogawa H, Koike T, et al. A clinicopathological study of dissecting aneurysms of the intracranial vertebral artery. J Neurosurg 1991;75(6):874–82.

52. Arnold M, Bousser MG, Fahrni G, et al. Vertebral artery dissection: presenting findings and predictors of outcome. Stroke 2006;37(10):2499–503.

53. Bartels E. Dissection of the extracranial vertebral artery: clinical findings and early noninvasive diagnosis in 24 patients. J Neuroimaging 2006;16(1):24–33.

54. Fusco MR, Harrigan MR. Cerebrovascular dissections–a review part I: Spontaneous dissections. Neurosurgery 2011;68(1):242–57 [discussion: 257.

55. Petro GR, Witwer GA, Cacayorin ED, et al. Spontaneous dissection of the cervical internal carotid artery: correlation of arteriography, CT, and pathology. AJR Am J Roentgenol 1987;148(2):393–8.

56. Wu Y, Wu F, Liu Y, et al. High-resolution magnetic resonance imaging of cervicocranial artery dissection: imaging features associated with stroke. Stroke 2019; 50(11):3101–7.

57. Foyouzi N, Frisbaek Y, Norwitz ER. Pituitary gland and pregnancy. Obstet Gynecol Clin North Am 2004;31(4):873–92, xi.

58. Kelestimur F. Sheehan's syndrome. Pituitary 2003;6(4):181–8.

59. Karaca Z, Laway BA, Dokmetas HS, et al. Sheehan syndrome. Nat Rev Dis Primers 2016;2:16092.

60. Kaplun J, Fratila C, Ferenczi A, et al. Sequential pituitary MR imaging in Sheehan syndrome: report of 2 cases. AJNR Am J Neuroradiology 2008;29(5):941–3.

61. Butwick AJ, Wong CA, Guo N. Maternal body mass index and use of labor neuraxial analgesia: a population-based retrospective cohort study. Anesthesiology 2018;129(3):448–58.

62. Kuntz KM, Kokmen E, Stevens JC, et al. Post-lumbar puncture headaches: experience in 501 consecutive procedures. Neurology 1992;42(10):1884–7.

63. Nath S, Koziarz A, Badhiwala JH, et al. Atraumatic versus conventional lumbar puncture needles: a systematic review and meta-analysis. Lancet 2018; 391(10126):1197–204.

64. Sprigge JS, Harper SJ. Accidental dural puncture and post dural puncture headache in obstetric anaesthesia: presentation and management: a 23-year survey in a district general hospital. Anaesthesia 2008;63(1):36–43.

65. Lay CM. Low cerebrospinal fluid pressure headache. Curr Treat Options Neurol 2002;4(5):357–63.

66. Mokri B. The Monro-Kellie hypothesis: applications in CSF volume depletion. Neurology 2001;56(12):1746–8.

67. Urbach H. Intracranial hypotension: clinical presentation, imaging findings, and imaging-guided therapy. Curr Opin Neurol 2014;27(4):414–24.

68. Capizzano AA, Lai L, Kim J, et al. Atypical Presentations of Intracranial Hypotension: Comparison with Classic Spontaneous Intracranial Hypotension. AJNR Am J Neuroradiology 2016;37(7):1256–61.

69. Savoiardo M, Minati L, Farina L, et al. Spontaneous intracranial hypotension with deep brain swelling. Brain 2007;130(Pt 7):1884–93.

Neuroimaging in Pediatric Headache

Aline Camargo, MD, Sangam Kanekar, MD, DNB*

KEYWORDS

- Pediatric headache • ACR Appropriateness Criteria • MRI • Migraine
- Intracranial hypertension and hypotension

KEY POINTS

- Both AAN and ACR do not recommend neuroimaging for patients with primary headache.
- The main goal of the clinical examination and history is to identify the associated "red flags" which will favor subjecting the patient to neuroimaging.
- The decision to order an imaging study for a child with headache should involve risk stratification based on clinical history and physical examination so the benefits of neuroimaging outweigh the risks of radiation exposure from CT or potential sedation for MRI.

Abbreviations	
EPI	echo planar imaging (EPI)
DTI.	Diffusion tensor imaging (DTI)
PPTH	Replace it with PTH
TBI	traumatic brain injury (TBI)
PTCS	pseudotumor cerebri syndrome
DWI	Diffusion weighted imaging (DWI)
ADC	Apparent diffusion coefficient (ADC)

INTRODUCTION

Headache is a major health condition in the United States in both adult and pediatric population. It represents one of the most common disorders in childhood and leads to nearly half a million visits to the physician's office or emergency department every year.[1] According to a systematic review, the prevalence of headache in children is 58.4%.[2] It is rare before the age of 4 years, with increasing frequency throughout the childhood with a peak around 13 years.[3–5] Literature estimates that 75% of children will report significant headache by the age of 15 years.[6] It is important to highlight, however, that the actual incidence of headache in the pediatric population

Radiology Research, Division of Neuroradiology, Penn State Health, Penn State College of Medicine, Mail Code H066 500 University Drive, Hershey, PA 17033, USA
* Corresponding author.
E-mail address: skanekar@pennstatehealth.psu.edu

Neurol Clin 40 (2022) 679–698
https://doi.org/10.1016/j.ncl.2022.02.007
0733-8619/22/© 2022 Elsevier Inc. All rights reserved.

neurologic.theclinics.com

might be underestimated, given only a percentage of cases seek medical attention. There is a significant economic burden associated with pediatric headache, making the clinical examination and judicious use of imaging vitally important.

Headaches are classified as either primary or secondary. Primary headaches result from the headache condition itself, whereas secondary headache is a result of another underlying condition. Primary headache disorders are the most common cause of recurrent headache in the pediatric population, which include migraine, tension-type headache, mixed-type headaches, and numerous less common primary headache disorders. Migraine among this is the most prevalent, followed by tension-type headache.[7] Secondary headache causes may range from infection, trauma to neoplasm, which most of the time is associated with some "red flags" on examination that prompts the physician to subject the patient for further evaluation including neuroimaging.

CLINICAL EVALUATION

The first step in the evaluation of a child or adolescent with a complaint of headache is to determine whether the headache is primary or secondary (**Table 1**). This process includes a detailed clinical history and relevant clinical examinations.[8] History focuses to establish the presence of exacerbating symptoms such as caffeine intake, stress, exercise, or sleep deprivation, as that can suggest migraine or tension-type headache. In addition, the presence of recent head trauma, fever, or other symptoms related to systemic disease may lead to a screening for secondary etiologies.[9] The temporal pattern can offer a significant guidance. Usually, acute or chronic progressive headaches suggest a secondary etiology, whereas an episodic or chronic nonprogressive headache may indicate a primary disorder.[10] The family history, including the history of primary headache disorders, brain tumors, vascular disorders, and autoimmune diseases, helps in differentiating and narrowing the causes of headache.[9] As part of the evaluation process in patients with headache, a thorough general and neurologic examination should also be performed, including, but not limited to, palpation for sinus or temporomandibular joint tenderness, assessment for meningeal signs, as well as examination of the cranial nerves and the optic discs.[7,9]

The main goal of the clinical examination and history is to identify the associated "red flags" which will favor the neuroimaging (**Table 2**). Some of the red flags on examination include abnormal neurologic examination; atypical presentation, including vertigo, intractable vomiting, or headache waking the child from sleep; a recent headache of less than 6 months' duration; no family history of migraine or primary headaches; occipital headache; change in type of headache; subacute onset and progressive headache severity; a new-onset headache in a child with

Table 1	
Primary and secondary headache	
Primary Headache	**Secondary Headache**
Migraine	Posttraumatic headache
Tension-type headache	Chiari malformation and headache
Mixed-type headaches	Neoplasm and hydrocephalus
Trigeminal autonomic cephalalgias	Idiopathic intracranial hypertension
	Febrile headache
	Vascular headache
	Sinus- and mastoid-related headache

Table 2	
"Red flags" on clinical history and physical examination	
Recent onset of severe headache	Papilledema
Sudden onset of headache (first or worst ever)	Visual field defects
Change of the headache pattern	Cranial nerve dysfunction
History of neurologic dysfunction	Increased head circumference
Worsening of headache with cough or Valsalva maneuver	Abnormal ocular movements, Pathologic pupillary responses
Seizures or fever	Focal neurologic deficit or meningismus
Nocturnal or early morning headaches	Asymmetric motor function
Occipital headache	Abnormal cerebellar function
Age < 6 y	
Systemic symptoms or illness (SLE, SCD, substance abuse)	

Abbreviations: SCD, Sickle cell disease; SLE, Systemic lupus erythematosus.

immunosuppression; first or worst headache; systemic symptoms and signs; and a headache associated with confusion, mental status changes, or focal neurologic complaints.[11,12] For pediatric headache, Gofshteyn and Stephenson and colleagues[5] gave a "SNOOOPPPPY" mnemonic for identifying these red flags: Systemic symptoms or illness (eg, fever, altered level of consciousness, anticoagulation therapy, pregnancy, cancer, or HIV infection), Neurologic signs or symptoms (eg, papilledema, asymmetric cranial nerve function, asymmetric motor function, abnormal cerebellar function, new seizure, or focal findings at examination), Onset recently or suddenly (thunderclap headache), Occipital localization of pain, Precipitated by Valsalva maneuver, Positional, Progressive, Parent (ie, lack of family history), and Years (ie, age < 6 years). Good physical examination and detailed history is proven to avoid subjecting the child to neuroimaging either with computed tomography (CT) or MRI, in turn avoiding the unnecessary radiation and sedation. A normal neurologic examination has been demonstrated to correlate with the absence of relevant intracranial processes, with the following 2 important limitations: (1) interindividual variation with regard to clinical experience and diagnostic accuracy; and (2) fluctuating neurologic symptoms in the initial stages of an intracranial disease.

INDICATIONS FOR NEUROIMAGING

The decision to order an imaging study for a child with headache should involve risk stratification based on the clinical history and physical examination so the benefits of neuroimaging outweigh the risks of radiation exposure from CT or potential sedation for MRI. The American Academy of Neurology (AAN) practice parameter[13] does not recommend routine neuroimaging in patients with recurrent headache, in child with no red flags, and a normal neurologic examination. Neuroimaging and further evaluation is suggested in all the conditions mentioned earlier with red flags.

According to ACR Appropriateness Criteria,[14] MRI is classified as "usually appropriate" for the following indications among pediatric patients: sudden severe headache, headache attributed to infection, headache attributed to remote trauma, and initial imaging for investigation of secondary headache. Per ACR, CT of the head without contrast is classified as "usually appropriate" only for sudden severe headache (thunderclap headache), because the etiology might be related to a ruptured aneurysm or arteriovenous malformation (AVM) as CT is very sensitive in detecting acute subarachnoid hemorrhage (SAH).[13–15] Both AAN and ACR do not recommend neuroimaging for patients with primary headache.[13,14]

Literature, however, has shown a high number of imaging studies performed in children and adolescents with headache, despite the evidence of low diagnostic yield of imaging.[1,16–18] The reasons for such high requests might be justified by families' requests as well as by the fear of missing a serious intracranial pathology, especially if the differentiation of primary versus secondary headache is challenging and stress inducing.[14] Though neuroimaging is, negative or do not show any significant intracranial abnormality on majority of the patient with headache, a small percentage of significant and even life-threatening disorders may be manifest clinically as isolated headache. This physician's dilemma led to many pediatric patients undergo costly cross-sectional imaging, such as CT and MRI. It has been reported that 14% to 28% of pediatric patients with headache who undergo neuroimaging have an abnormal finding. However, most of those abnormalities correspond to incidental benign findings of no clinical significance, such as pineal cyst, focal areas of gliosis, and other unspecific white matter (WM) abnormalities, and therefore, do not lead to the etiology of headache or change in management.[19,20]

CT is usually suboptimal for the evaluation of intracranial masses and infection. In addition, it also exposes the pediatric patient to radiation, increasing the risk of malignancy later in life.[21,22] Therefore, the high and unnecessary use of CT for pediatric patients should be addressed so its use is limited to reserved cases, such as trauma. MRI, although the preferred neuroimaging for children and adolescents due to lack of radiation exposure, should also be used with caution to avoid unnecessary sedation or general anesthesia as well as inappropriate use of resources. Today large number of the institutions have used highly ultrafast MRI brain protocols (eg, GOBrain 5 mts protocol on Siemens magnet), which may be completed within 5 to 6 mts reducing the need for sedation or anesthesia. There is ongoing effort to use the EPI techniques to bring the pediatric MRI brain scan time as low as 1 to 2 mts. At the authors' institution, ultrafast MRI brain protocols are routinely used for evaluation of hydrocephalus, in patients with headache, and all in-house pediatric patients.

CLASSIFICATION OF TYPES OF HEADACHE
Primary Headaches

Primary pediatric headache disorders include migraine, tension-type headache, trigeminal autonomic cephalalgias, among other less common conditions.[9] Clinically, the diagnosis of primary headache is usually accomplished by using the criteria of the International Headache Society (IHS).[7] Differentiating the type of primary headache during the first office visit may be very challenging for the physician. However, detail clinical history from the patient and/or the parents/caretakers and elaborate clinical examination is of vital importance to avoid the over investigation of the child.

Migraine is the most common type of headache in the pediatric population with an estimated prevalence of 7.7%.[2] The diagnosis can be challenging as the presentation may differ from the one observed in adults, which is thought to be related to differences in myelination, plasticity, and synaptic formation.[9] Clinicians should also inquiry family about behavioral changes, such as photophobia, as those may be one of the few clues that the child has migraine.[5] Besides photophobia, other specific features indicative of migraine include phonophobia, osmophobia, presence of gastrointestinal symptoms, improvement of headache after sleeping, and worsening with physical activity.[5] It is more often bilateral, differently from adults, who usually have a unilateral pain.[7] Occipital headache is an unusual presentation for migraine in children and, therefore, calls for diagnostic caution.[7] Visual symptoms are the most common type of aura in children, similar to adults. However, unlike adult patients, the visual aura in children and adolescents has a higher likelihood of being bilateral and crossing the visual fields. The attacks can be as short as 2 hours in children, as opposed to the ones in adults that last at least 4 hours without treatment.[7,8]

Tension-type headache is the second most common primary headache in pediatric patients. It is usually bilateral, diffuse, mild to moderate in intensity, and less disabling. Differently from migraine, it does not appear to differ from adult patients.[8]

On MRI examination, WM hyperintensities (WMH) on fluid-attenuated inversion recovery (FLAIR)/T2-weighted images have been well recognized in migraine[23] (**Fig. 1**). These WMH are thought to be due to demyelination and axonal injury. On DTI imaging,[24] studies have shown decreases in mean diffusivity (MD), radial diffusivity (RD), and axial diffusivity (AD) in the WM tracts located in the brainstem, thalamus, and fronto-temporo-occipital lobes, bilaterally without WMH, suggesting WM tract disruption. Similar findings were also noted in the optic tract and optic radiations.

Recent MR studies have also documented gray matter abnormality particularly in the periaqueductal gray matter, which is thought to be a migraine generator.[25] In patient with migraine, the diameter of the pons is found to be significantly greater, supporting the brainstem migraine generator theory.[26] These patients also showed significantly less gray matter density in the frontal and temporal lobes as compared with the age-matched controls. Furthermore, it has been documented that migraine patients have significantly less gray matter density and decreased cortical volume in the frontal and temporal lobes.[27,28] Migraine association with cognitive impairment and dementia is thought to be due to changes in these lobes and therefore preventing or limiting migraine in pediatrics becomes critically important. MR perfusion imaging techniques such as dynamic susceptibility contrast or arterial spin labeling have demonstrated transient hypoperfusion contralateral to the side of aura.[29,30]

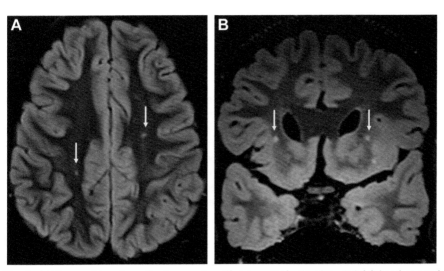

Fig. 1. A 14-year-old male patient presents with trigeminal migraine. Axial (*A*)and coronal (*B*) FLAIR images show few scattered punctate hyperintensities (*arrows*) in the cerebral white matter bilaterally.

Secondary Headaches

According to the International Headache Society, secondary headaches can be attributed to head and/or neck trauma, cranial or cervical vascular disorder, nonvascular intracranial disorder, substance use, infection, a disorder of homeostasis, or psychiatric disorder.[7] Secondary headaches are common in younger children and the majority of cases have benign etiologies. In the setting of acute headache, the most common cause is infection, ranging from viral upper respiratory illness to acute meningitis.[31] We discuss in detail the etiologies of secondary headache in the pediatric population as well as the role of neuroimaging for such patients.

Posttraumatic headache

A posttraumatic headache (PTH) is defined as a secondary headache that occurs after injury or trauma to the head and/or neck. It can present within 7 days after injury, 7 days after regaining consciousness, or 7 days after recovering the ability to report pain.[7] If symptoms continue past 3 months, it is classified as persistent PTH.

Clinically, PTH presents very similar to primary headache disorders often resembling migraines. Symptoms might include headache-associated nausea/vomiting, photo/phonophobia, and worsening pain with activity or tension-type headaches with a nonpulsating characteristic and neither photophobia nor phonophobia. The alterations of brain structure and neurometabolic pathways, which occur in patients after traumatic brain injury, is thought to be the cause of the symptoms in PTH.

Neuroimaging plays an important role in the setting of head injury for diagnosis and management. CT is considered the first-line imaging modality for suspected acute intracranial injury.[32] However, neither CT nor MRI is recommended routinely for the evaluation of subacute or chronic PTH.[14,32,33] Imaging, mostly MRI is warranted when "red flags" such as increasing severity or frequency, occipital location, awakening from sleep because of headache, or morning headache with vomiting is present.

Susceptibility imaging on MRI is very sensitive in documenting hemosiderin deposition in the intra-axial and extra-axial compartments of the brain. Parenchyma may show multiple microhemorrhages or macrohemorrhages in the supra or infratentorial brain parenchyma. In addition, there may be changes of superficial hemosiderosis, deposition of hemosiderin over the cortical sulci. FLAIR images are very sensitive in demonstrating the encephalomalacia and gliotic changes in the brain (**Fig. 2**). MRI imaging in PPTH may reveal a decrease in the thickness, area, and/or volume measurements of the affected brain parenchyma (35,36). Voxel-based morphometry has shown decreased gray matter density in the anterior cingulate cortex and dorsolateral prefrontal cortex in patients with PTH 3 months post-TBI. In addition, studies have also found decreased cortical thickness in patients with PPTH and compared with healthy controls in several areas (left and right superior frontal, caudal middle frontal, and precentral, right supramarginal, right superior and inferior parietal, right precuneus region).[34,35] MR spectroscopy and perfusion studies have also shown derangements in the neurometabolite concentrations (decreased NAA/creatinine and increased choline/creatinine ratios) and decreased cerebral blood flow in patients with PTH.[36,37]

Chiari malformation and headache

The Chiari I deformity is a condition characterized by at least 5 mm downward displacement of the cerebellar tonsils through the foramen magnum.[38] The estimated prevalence of Chiari I malformation in the pediatric population is approximately 1%.[39] A prior study, however, found that as many as 3.6% of normal children involved in their study had a Chiari I malformation.[40] The most common symptom is headache, with

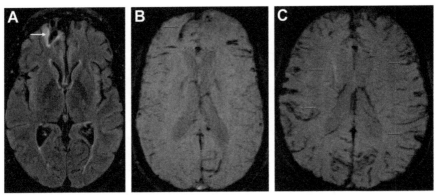

Fig. 2. A 16-year-old male patient presents persistent posttrauma headache following a motor vehicular accident. Axial FLAIR image shows area of encephalomalacia in the right frontal lobe anteriorly (*yellow arrow*), sequela of prior hemorrhagic contusion. Axial susceptibility-weighted imaging (SWI) images show hemosiderin deposition within the right frontal lobe encephalomalacia and over the superficial convexity sulci, superficial siderosis (*red arrows*).

additional clinical manifestations including scoliosis in children older than 3 years and abnormal oropharyngeal function in children younger than 3 years, such as cough, dysphagia, abnormal vocal cord movement, and aspiration.[38,40]

The headache in Chiari I malformation is reported to be occipital or suboccipital and worsened by cough, Valsalva maneuver, or physical activity. It usually occurs in children older than 3 years and the frequency increases with age.[38,39] According to literature, the frequency of headache in adults with Chiari I malformation ranges from 30% to 80% and 15% to 75% in children.[38]

There is an incidental coexistence between Chiari I malformation and primary headache, such as migraine and tension-type headache.[39] The etiology of the headache, either primary or secondary to Chiari I deformity, is crucial for treatment plan (surgical vs nonsurgical management). Potentially, such differentiation might be guided by imaging, because it has been reported an increased likelihood of developing secondary headache when the tonsillar ectopia exceeds 13 mm, and when there is a lesser degree of ectopia associated with narrowing of the cerebrospinal fluid (CSF) space posterior to the cerebellar tonsils, resulting in syringomyelia.[40]

MRI of the brain and cervical spine without contrast is recommended in suspected patients with Chiari malformation. It is not uncommon to find the tonsillar herniation (Chiari I Malformation) as an incidental finding when the child is evaluated for other conditions.[41,42] To measure the degree of tonsillar herniation, a line is drawn from opisthion to basion (**Fig. 3**). A perpendicular measurement from the caudal tip of the cerebellar tonsil to the opisthion-basion line gives the extent of tonsillar herniation. Any measurement of cerebellar ectopia less than 5 mm is of no clinical significance; however, there are exceptions to this rule. Secondary radiologic features which help in diagnosing a Chiari I malformation include a pointed appearance of the cerebellar tonsils, compression of the cerebellar cistern (demonstrated by effacement of vallecula and cisterna magna), retroflexion of the odontoid process, compression of the fourth ventricle, and syringohydromyelia.[42] At our institution, we routinely performed whole spine T2 sagittal and axial images through the entire cord and CSF flow examination when a tonsillar herniation is documented on the MRI brain examination.

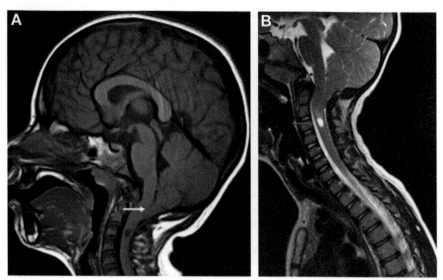

Fig. 3. An 11-year-old male patient presented with occipital headache, worsening with cough. Chiari malformation with cervical syrinx. Sagittal T1-weighted image (WI) shows 11 mm tonsillar herniation below the opisthion to basion line (*yellow arrow*). Sagittal T2 WI shows focal syrinx in the cervical cord at C3 level (*red arrow*).

It is very important to differentiate between Chiari I malformation and CSF leak, as both can cause downward displacement of the cerebellar tonsils. A patient with CSF leak presents with intracranial hypotension. The main symptom of intracranial hypotension is an orthostatic headache that worsens in an upright position, on coughing, laughing, and the Valsalva maneuver. The most important MRI finding is a characteristic diffuse pachymeningeal enhancement. Other findings include sagging of the brain, pituitary enlargement, subdural fluid collections, posterior lobe pituitary hematomas, diffuse dural enhancement of the spinal canal, spinal epidural fluid collection, distension of the spinal epidural venous plexus, and abnormal intensity around the root sleeves[43,44] (**Fig. 4**). To confirm the diagnosis of intracranial hypotension, at least 1 of the following signs must be present: low CSF pressure, evidence of CSF leakage (on CT myelography, conventional myelography, or radionuclide cisternography), or diffuse pachymeningeal enhancement on brain MRI imaging.

Neoplasm and hydrocephalus

Hydrocephalus can be divided into congenital and acquired. Aqueduct stenosis is the most common etiology for congenital hydrocephalus. Acquired hydrocephalus may be secondary to obstructive processes, mainly from neoplasms, or infection that affects ventricular outflow.[45]

Central nervous system neoplasms (malignant and nonmalignant) symptoms vary depending on the location of the tumor and patient's age. These symptoms may be secondary to invasion or mass effect of adjacent structures, and/or result of increased intracranial pressure due to obstruction of CSF flow.[14,46] Headache is the most common manifestation of CNS tumors, which is thought to be due to intracranial hypertension (ICH). ICH headache has been classically described as occurring in the early morning headache and often relieved by vomiting. A review of headache patterns in children with CNS tumors found that 61% of pediatric patients (43/71) had nocturnal

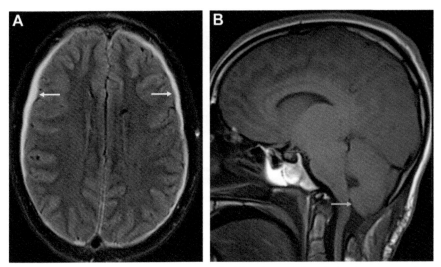

Fig. 4. A 19-year-old female patient presented with orthostatic headache that worsens in an upright position. Intracranial hypotension. Axial T2 image shows bilateral hyperintense subdural fluid collections (*yellow arrows*). Sagittal T1-WI shows sagging of the midbrain (*red arrow*) with mild tonsillar decent (*green arrow*).

or early morning headache. However, 18% (13/71) had continuous headache and 21% (15/71) had daytime or evening headache.[47] Therefore, the absence of classic morning headache should not dissuade the diagnosis of ICH.

Literature suggests that nearly all children diagnosed with a brain tumor have a neurologic sign, papilledema, or other symptoms, in association with headache, reinforcing the importance of recognizing red flags that may lead to further investigation. Neurologic symptoms include gait disturbance, abnormal reflexes, cranial nerve abnormalities, altered sensation, poor coordination, seizures, and visual disturbances, such as double or blurred vision.[14,46] Additional symptoms include unfused cranial sutures in infants, macrocephaly, nausea, and vomiting. Torticollis has also been described as a symptom of CNS tumors and it should be approached with concern for posterior fossa tumor and spinal cord tumor in patients with sudden onset nontraumatic torticollis, particularly when associated with a neurologic sign and/or in younger children.[46]

Precontrast and postcontrast MRI is the modality of choice for patients with increased intracranial pressure and suspicion for intracranial neoplasm.[22] In addition to the diagnostic role of MRI in patients with CNS tumor, this study modality also offers important information related to tumor staging, such as the presence of leptomeningeal spread in patients with medulloblastoma, atypical teratoid/rhabdoid tumors, ependymomas, germinomas, and high-grade astrocytomas (**Fig. 5**). MRI spectroscopy is also used to evaluate metabolite concentrations to help in the differentiation neoplasm from its mimics and yet times characterization of intracranial tumor.[48]

Idiopathic intracranial hypertension (pseudotumor cerebri syndrome)

Idiopathic intracranial hypertension (IIH) is a complex condition that commonly presents with headache and visual disturbances.[49,50] IIH presents with symptoms and signs of ICH, with normal brain parenchyma, without underlying space-occupying neoplasm, ventriculomegaly, or infection on imaging. Early diagnosis and treatment

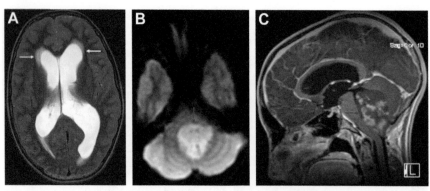

Fig. 5. A 4-year-old male child with a clinical history of early morning occipital headache and relieved by vomiting. Medulloblastoma with hydrocephalus. Axial T2 image shows moderate dilation of the lateral ventricles with periventricular seepage (*yellow arrows*), suggestive of obstructive hydrocephalus. Axial DWI and postcontrast sagittal T1-WIs show mass within the fourth ventricle, which shows restricted diffusion (*red arrow*) and enhancement on the postcontrast scan.

of this condition is of utmost importance because it has the potential of irreversible vision loss from papilledema. In the absence of an underlying cause, the term IIH is preferred. Secondary IIH refers to patients with cerebral venous abnormalities, such as thrombosis/stenosis, due to medications toxicity, such as vitamin A and lithium, or medical disorders such as endocrinopathies.[49,50] Differently from adults, where the typical patient with IIH is an obese female of child-bearing age, in young children, there is an equal distribution between males and females and obesity becomes a risk factor only beyond age 12 years.[50,51]

The most common symptoms among pediatric patients include headache, papilledema, abducens (CN VI) palsy, nausea, vomiting, and transient visual obscurations. Headache in children with PTCS is more likely to involve the neck and shoulders. The classic high-pressure headache triad of daily headache, worsening with Valsalva, and diffuse nonpulsating pain is found in less than half of children with IIH.[49,50] According to a 2013 review of diagnostic criteria for PTCS in adults and children, both papilledema and elevated CSF pressure are required for the diagnosis of definite IIH. Patients with elevated opening pressure with abducens palsy or specific imaging findings may be given the diagnosis of IIH without papilledema.[50]

Neuroimaging, MRI of the brain with and without contrast, is the modality of choice in a suspected case of IIH. MRI usually reveals normal brain parenchyma without hydrocephalus, mass, or any other structural lesion or abnormal meningeal enhancement.[14] From highest to lowest specificity, according to Görkem and colleagues,[52] specific PTCS imaging findings include posterior globe flattening, intraocular protrusion of the optic nerve, horizontal nerve sheath tortuosity, decreased pituitary gland size/empty sella, and optic nerve sheath enlargement (**Fig. 6**). Thin T2 axial and coronal sections through the orbits are recommended to better evaluate the optic sheath and nerves. Transverse sinus stenosis has been reported as one of the causes of the IIH and therefore along with MRI brain, MR-Venogram is recommended. Contrast-enhanced MR angiography (MRA) in combination with a 3D T1-MPRAGE is very sensitive in identifying the venous pathology. Bilateral sinus stenosis is pathognomonic for this disease. Stenosis is most commonly found at the transition from the transverse sinus to the sigmoid sinus; however, it may be also seen along the course of the

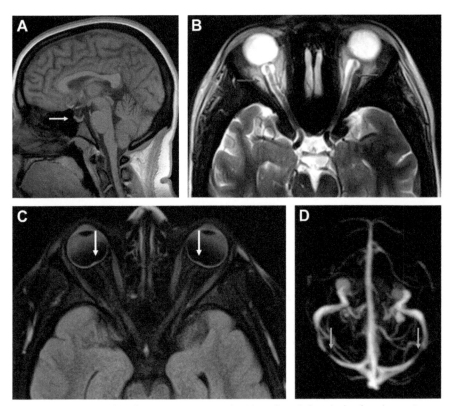

Fig. 6. A 16-year-old female patient presented with a chronic headache for almost 2 years and blurry vision for 1 week. Idiopathic intracranial hypertension. Sagittal T1-WI shows empty sella (*yellow arrow*), axial T2 and FLAIR images through orbit show posterior globe flattening, intraocular protrusion of the optic nerve (*white arrows*), and horizontal nerve sheath tortuosity (*red arrows*). MR-Venogram shows stenosis (*green arrows*) at the transition of the transverse sinus to the sigmoid sinus.

transverse sinus and in the distal sigmoid sinus above the confluence of sinuses. In addition, there may be the presence of enlarged occipital emissary veins.

Febrile headache

The triad of headache, fever, and nausea/vomiting in pediatric patients is highly suggestive of headache attributed to infection. The likelihood is even higher when there is associated lethargy, focal neural deficits, or convulsion.[7] The temporal course of febrile headaches is usually affected by the offending pathogen, host's immune system, and ability to provide adequate treatment.[9] In the setting of meningitis and meningoencephalitis, the clinical presentation includes neurologic deficits, altered mental status, encephalopathy, holocranial/nuchal headache, neck stiffness, and photosensitivity.[9]

MRI of the brain with and without contrast is recommended for patients with headache and suspicion for meningitis, encephalitis, and brain abscess or suspicion for an extracranial or intracranial spread of infection, such as sinusitis or mastoiditis.[7,14] Even though imaging is commonly performed, CSF gives the specific diagnosis in most cases.[7]

Herpes simplex encephalitis, including types 1 and 2, is the most common cause of fatal sporadic necrotizing viral encephalitis.[53] Type 1 herpes simplex virus (HSV) usually involves the temporal and frontal lobes in adults and older children. Type 2 HSV usually occurs in neonates and presents with diffuse brain involvement. MRI findings for meningoencephalitis may include vasogenic edema, cytotoxic edema, demonstrated on diffusion-weighted imaging, meningeal enhancement, focal, multifocal, or confluent T2 hyperintense lesions as well as parenchymal enhancement and, less commonly, intracranial hemorrhage and hydrocephalus[7,14,54] (**Fig. 7**). It is important to highlight, however, that the classic limbic distribution of HSV-1 may not always be present, and that extratemporal involvement is not uncommon.[14,54] Enterovirus encephalitis might involve the brain stem and spinal cord, whereas basal ganglia and thalamus involvement is more common with West Nile virus or Japanese encephalitis. The location of abnormal findings on imaging might help guide which encephalitis pathogen is involved; however, it is often nonspecific and inaccurate.[54] Although the number of cases of varicella-zoster encephalitis has decreased over the past decades due to immunization, it should still be considered in the appropriate clinical setting. It has been reported that 30% of the cases are under 15 years, usually in immunocompetent patients, and might cause brain infarction due to varicella-zoster vasculopathy.[53]

Extra-axial infection, such as subdural or epidural empyema, can also present with headache, and MRI is particularly helpful for demonstrating the extra-axial fluid collection with restricted diffusion on diffusion-weighted imaging (**Fig. 8**). It has been reported that subdural empyema is usually a result of direct spread of sinusitis or otitis media in older children, whereas in infants, it is usually a complication of purulent meningitis.[14] Although the role of CT is poor in diagnosing encephalitis or meningitis, it is helpful in the assessment of sinusitis and mastoiditis.[54] In the setting of mastoiditis or sphenoid sinusitis, a CT or MR-Venogram is recommended if there is clinical suspicion for venous sinus thrombosis, given the increased risk at this group of patients.[14]

In the setting of headache attributed to systemic infection without associated meningitis or meningoencephalitis, such as influenza, there is no indication for neuroimaging. Noting, however, that symptoms of viral meningitis may resemble those of flu.[14] Headache can also be due to COVID-19, although it occurs less commonly in children when compared with adults. Encephalitis secondary to COVID-19 has also been reported both in children and adults.[55,56] However, literature is still very scarce on this topic and more studies are needed to better elucidate such entity.

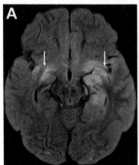 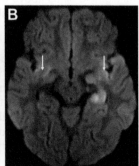 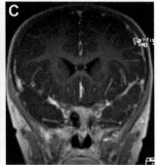

Fig. 7. A 10-year-old female patient presented to emergency room (ER) with a history of acute headache, fever, and nausea for 2 days. Herpes encephalitis. Axial FLAIR and DWI images show bilateral hyperintensity (*white arrows*) and restricted diffusion (*yellow arrows*) in the bilateral medial temporal lobes, and insular cortex. Postcontrast T1-WI shows leptomeningeal enhancement (*red arrows*) on the left Sylvian fissure and over the left frontal convexities.

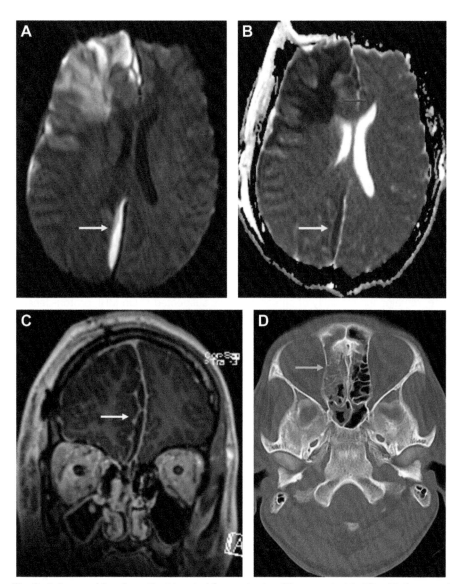

Fig. 8. A 6-year-old male patient treated for acute sinusitis presented to ER with fever and seizure and mild symptoms of delirium. Cerebritis, subdural empyema with sinusitis. Axial DWI and ADC images show a large area of restricted diffusion in the right frontal lobe (*red arrow*) and subdural empyema along the falx (*yellow arrow*). Postcontrast coronal T1-WI shows peripheral enhancement of the subdural empyema (*white arrow*). Axial CT of the patient shows near-complete opacification of the right frontal and ethmoid air cells (*green arrow*).

Vascular disorders

Although less common in the pediatric population, vascular disorders may also represent a cause of secondary headache in children.

Intracranial arterial aneurysms account for at least 10% to 15% of hemorrhagic strokes during the first two decades of life. The most common nontraumatic etiology for SAH in children is aneurysmal rupture.[9,57] In addition to headache, SAH may present with altered mentation, seizures, paresis, fever, cranial nerve palsies, and coma. As against adults, the proportion of total aneurysms found in the posterior circulation is twice as high in pediatric patients. In young children, a greater proportion of aneurysms develop distal to the circle of Willis.

Similar to adults, there are a variety of etiologies for aneurysms in children, including idiopathic, posttraumatic, vasculopathic, excessive hemodynamic stress, oncotic, and infectious/inflammatory. Conditions associated with increased risk for aneurysms in children include coarctation of the aorta, polycystic renal disease, fibromuscular dysplasia, tuberous sclerosis, Ehlers-Danlos syndrome, and Marfan syndrome.[57]

It has been reported an increased likelihood of recurrent headache and migraine in pediatric patients with sickle cell disease. However, sudden thunderclap headache in such pediatric population, as well as in patients with thalassemia minor and glucose-6-phosphatase deficiency, should be approached with high suspicion for SAH, given the higher incidence of intracranial aneurysms also noted among those patients.[14,57,58] Severe acute headache in patients who have a first-degree relative with a history of vascular abnormality should also be screened for SAH.[14]

CT of the head without contrast is very sensitive in the detection of SAH, and, therefore, remains the modality of choice if SAH is suspected.[14] On MRI, proton-density-weighted imaging, susceptibility-weighted imaging/gradient-recalled echo imaging, and T2-weighted FLAIR imaging increase the sensitivity for acute SAH.[59] In addition, CT angiography (CTA)/MRA is commonly used to diagnose the underlying aneurysm or vascular malformation. Surgical and endovascular intervention remains the definitive treatment of cerebral aneurysms in children.

Headache tend to be ipsilateral to certain vascular abnormalities such as AVMs, dural arteriovenous fistulas (AVFs), and cavernous fistulas.[9] Literature reports that children with brain AVMs are more likely to present with hemorrhage than adults; however, they are less likely to have a subsequent hemorrhage after the initial presentation when compared with adult patients. A smaller AVM nidus, infratentorial nidus location, and exclusively deep venous drainage predict an increased risk of presentation with hemorrhage in the pediatric population.[60,61] Dural AVFs are rare intracranial arteriovenous shunts and may present with headache associated with tinnitus in children.[9,62]

CT/CTA and/or MR/MRA are often performed in ruptured AVMs to evaluate the location and the size of the hematoma (**Fig. 9**). Digital subtraction angiography (DSA) is important to characterize vascular anomalies detected on CTA or MRA, and to investigate intraparenchymal hemorrhage without clear etiology on initial imaging, given its higher sensitivity for intracranial shunts because of its higher spatial and temporal resolutions.[14,63] DSA has a better capability than any other neuroimaging modality to define the AVM size, location, feeding vessels, draining veins, location of the nidus, and the presence of any associated vascular lesions.

Cerebral venous thrombosis (CVT) can occur at any age, although it is more common in neonates and young adults (20–40 years old). Diagnosis is difficult because the clinical manifestations of CVT are nonspecific, such as headache, seizures, decreased level of consciousness, and focal neurologic deficits. Predisposing factors in the pediatric age group include infection, hematological disorders, trauma, and tumors. Venous infarction may lead to parenchyma edema to venous infarction and intracranial hemorrhage. Noncontrast CT shows hyperattenuation in the occluded sinus (cord sign).[64] CT venography shows triangular area of contrast enhancement that surrounds a hypoattenuating thrombus, called "empty delta" sign.[64,65] The empty

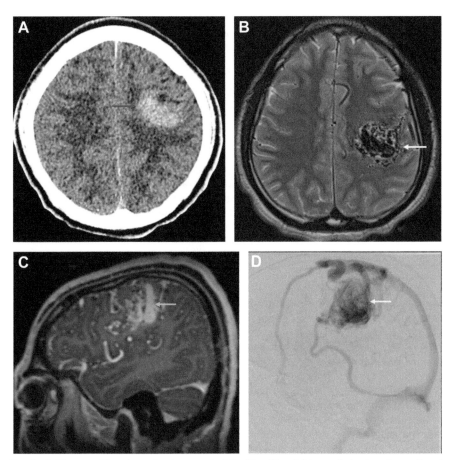

Fig. 9. A 11-year-old male patient presented to ER with a history of single seizure, headache, and right-sided weakness. Arteriovenous malformation with bleed. Axial CT scan of the brain shows acute bleed in the left frontal lobe (*red arrow*). Axial T2 and postcontrast sagittal T1-WIs show large AVM in the left frontal lobe with nidus (*white arrow*) and large draining vein (*green arrow*). The lateral view of the digital angiogram confirms the large AVM (*yellow arrow*) with venous drainage into the superior sagittal sinus.

delta sign is seen in 29% to 35% of cases and may be absent in the acute phases of the process, in which the thrombus is hyperattenuating. MR brain followed by contrast-enhanced MR venography (MRV) and 3D contrast-enhanced gradient-recalled-echo T1-weighted MRI are very sensitive in demonstrating parenchymal changes and venous thrombosis.[66] MRV is recommended for patients at increased risk for CVT, such as children with acute mastoiditis and patients with hypercoagulability conditions, who present with headache (**Fig. 10**).

Sinus and mastoid headache

The diagnosis of uncomplicated acute sinusitis should be made based on the clinical history and physical examination, without the necessity of an imaging study. According to ACR appropriateness Criteria, CT of the paranasal sinuses without contrast is "usually appropriate" for children with persistent sinusitis, who have worsening and

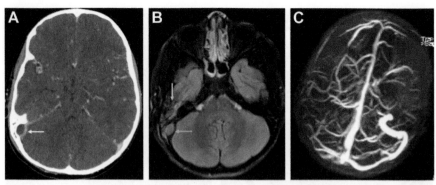

Fig. 10. A 20-year-old female patient presented with a history of fever, seizure, headache, and vertigo. Acute right mastoiditis with sigmoid sinus thrombosis. Contrast-enhanced axial CT scan shows right sigmoid sinus thrombosis with peripheral enhancement (*delta sign-white arrow*). Axial FLAIR image shows sigmoid sinus thrombosis (*green arrow*) with near-complete opacification of the right mastoid air cells (*orange arrow*). MR venogram shows thrombosis (*red arrows*) of the distal transverse and entire sigmoid sinuses.

severe symptoms, or who are not responding to treatment. Recurrent and chronic sinusitis as well as imaging for surgical planning are accepted indications for CT without contrast.[14,67]

CT or MRI of the head and paranasal sinuses with intravenous contrast is recommended when there is clinical concern for invasive fungal sinusitis or complications secondary to orbital/intracranial spread.[67,68] As mentioned earlier, patients with acute sinusitis and, more commonly, mastoiditis are at increased risk for venous sinus thrombosis and, therefore, MRV or CTV of the head may be appropriate in the appropriate clinical setting. Such studies should always be performed as complementary examinations to standard CT or MRI of the head and sinuses with contrast, as potential complications might be missed if CTV or MRV is performed alone.[67]

CLINICS CARE POINTS

- The significant economic burden is associated with pediatric and adult headaches, making the clinical examination and judicious use of imaging vitally important.
- Primary headache disorders are the most common cause of recurrent headaches in the pediatric population, and both AAN and ACR do not recommend neuroimaging for patients with primary headaches.

REFERENCES

1. Sheridan DC, Meckler GD, Spiro DM, et al. Diagnostic testing and treatment of pediatric headache in the emergency department. J Pediatr 2013;163:1634–7.
2. Abu-Arafeh IS, Razak S, Sivaraman B, et al. Prevalence of headache and migraine in children and adolescents: A systematic review of population-based studies. Developmental Med Child Neurol 2010;52(12):1088–97.
3. Fearon P, Hotopf M. Relation between headache in childhood and physical and psychiatric symptoms in adulthood: national birth cohort study. BMJ 2001;322:1145.

4. Straube A, Heinen F, Ebinger F, et al. Headache in school children: prevalence and risk factors. Dtsch Arztebl Int 2013;110:811–8.
5. Gofshteyn JS, Stephenson DJ. Diagnosis and management of childhood headache. Curr Probl Pediatr Adolesc Health Care 2016;46:36–51.
6. Bille B. Migraine and tension-type headache in children and adolescents. Cephalalgia 1996;16:78.
7. Headache Classification Committee of the International Headache Society (IHS) The International Classification of Headache Disorders. Cephalalgia. 3rd edition 2018;38(1):1–211.
8. Hershey AD. Pediatric headache. Continuum (Minneap Minn) 2015;21(4): 1132–45.
9. Kelly M, Strelzik J, Langdon R, et al. Pediatric headache: overview. Curr Opin Pediatr 2018;30(6):748–54.
10. Blume HK. Childhood headache: a brief review. Pediatr Ann 2017;46:e155–65.
11. Trofimova A, Vey BL, Mullins ME, et al. Imaging of children with nontraumatic headaches. AJR Am J Roentgenol 2018;210(1):8–17.
12. Kabbouche MA, Cleves C. Evaluation and management of children and adolescents presenting with an acute setting. Semin Pediatr Neurol 2010;17:105–8.
13. Lewis DW, Ashwal S, Dahl G, et al. Practice parameter: evaluation of children and adolescents with recurrent headaches. Report of the Quality Standards Subcommittee of the American Academy of Neurology and the Practice Committee of the Child Neurology Society. Neurology 2002;59:490–8.
14. Hayes LL, Palasis S, Bartel TB, et al. ACR appropriateness criteria® Headache–child. J Am Coll Radiol 2018;15(5):S78–90.
15. Mortimer AM, Bradley MD, Stoodley NG, et al. Thunderclap headache: diagnostic considerations and neuroimaging features. Clin Radiol 2013;68:e101–13.
16. Cain MR, Arkilo D, Linabery AM, et al. Emergency department use of neuroimaging in children and adolescents presenting with headache. The J Pediatr 2018; 201:196–201.
17. Gandhi R, Lewis EC, Evans JW, et al. Investigating the necessity of computed tomographic scans in children with headaches: a retrospective review. CJEM 2015;17:148–53.
18. Tsze DS, Ochs JB, Gonzalez AE, et al. Red flag findings in children with headaches: prevalence and association with emergency department neuroimaging. Cephalalgia 2019;39(2):185–96.
19. Rho YI, Chung HJ, Suh ES, et al. The role of neuroimaging in children and adolescents with recurrent headaches—Multicenter study. Head- ache 2011;51: 403–8.
20. Schwedt TJ, Guo Y, Rothner AD. Benign imaging abnormalities in children and adolescents with headache. Headache 2006;46:387–98.
21. Trottier ED, Bailey B, Lucas N, et al. Diagnosis of migraine in the pediatric emergency department. Pediatr Neurol 2013;49:40–5.
22. Pearce MS, Salotti JA, Little MP. Radiation exposure from CT scans in childhood and subsequent risk of leukaemia and brain tumours: a retrospective cohort study. Pediatr Radiol 2013;43:517–8.
23. Webb ME, Amoozegar F, Harris AD. Magnetic Resonance Imaging in Pediatric Migraine. Can J Neurol Sci 2019;46(6):653–65.
24. Messina R, Rocca MA, Colombo B, et al. White matter microstructure abnormalities in pediatric migraine patients. Cephalalgia Int J Headache 2015;35(14): 1278–86.

25. Rocca MA, Ceccarelli A, Falini A, et al. Brain gray matter changes in migraine patients with T2-visible lesions: a 3-T MRI study. Stroke 2006;37(7):1765–70.
26. Hämäläinen ML, Autti T, Salonen O, et al. Brain MRI in children with migraine: a controlled morphometric study. Cephalalgia Int J Headache 1996;16(8):541–4.
27. Dai Z, Zhong J, Xiao P, et al. Gray matter correlates of migraine and gender effect: a meta-analysis of voxel-based morphometry studies. Neuroscience 2015; 299:88–96.
28. Kim JH, Suh S-I, Seol HY, et al. Regional grey matter changes in patients with migraine: a voxel-based morphometry study. Cephalalgia Int J Headache 2008;28(6):598–604.
29. Masuzaki M, Utsunomiya H, Yasumoto S, et al. A case of hemiplegic migraine in childhood: transient unilateral hyperperfusion revealed by perfusion MR imaging and MR angiography. AJNR Am J Neuroradiol 2001;22(9):1795–7.
30. Bosemani T, Burton VJ, Felling RJ, et al. Pediatric hemiplegic migraine: role of multiple MRI techniques in evaluation of reversible hypoperfusion. Cephalalgia Int J Headache 2014;34(4):311–5.
31. Nallasamy K, Singhi SC, Singhi P. Approach to headache in emergency department. Indian J Pediatr 2012;79:376–80.
32. Expert Panel on Pediatric Imaging, Ryan ME, Pruthi S, Desai NK, et al. ACR Appropriateness Criteria® Head Trauma-Child. J Am Coll Radiol 2020;17(5S): S125–37.
33. Doll E, Gong P, Sowell M, et al. Post-traumatic Headache in Children and Adolescents. Curr Pain Headache Rep 2021;25(8):51.
34. Schwedt TJ, Chong CD, Peplinski J, et al. Persistent post-traumatic headache vs. migraine: an MRI study demonstrating differences in brain structure. J Headache Pain 2017;18(1):87.
35. Obermann M, Nebel K, Schumann C, et al. Gray matter changes related to chronic posttraumatic headache. Neurology 2009;73(12):978–83.
36. Sarmento E, Moreira P, Brito C, et al. Proton spectroscopy in patients with post-traumatic headache attributed to mild head injury. Headache 2009;49(9): 1345–52.
37. Maugans TA, Farley C, Altaye M, et al. Pediatric sports-related concussion produces cerebral blood flow alterations. Pediatrics 2012;129(1):28–37.
38. Victorio MC, Khoury CK. Headache and Chiari I malformation in children and adolescents. Semin Pediatr Neurol 2016;23(1):35–9.
39. Toldo I, Tangari M, Mardari R, et al. Headache in children with chiari I malformation. Headache 2014;54:899–908.
40. Heiss JD, Argersinger DP. Epidemiology of Chiari I malformation. InThe Chiari malformations 2020 (pp. 263-274). Springer, Cham (Switzerland).
41. Kanekar S, Kaneda H, Shively A. Malformations of dorsal induction. Semin Ultrasound CT MR 2011;32(3):189–99.
42. Milhorat T, Chou M, Trinidad E, et al. Chiari I malformation redefined: Clinical and radiographic findings for 364 symptomatic patients. Neurosurgery 1999;44: 1005–17.
43. Spears RC. Low-pressure/spinal fluid leak headache. Curr pain headache Rep 2014;18(6):425.
44. Green MW. Secondary headache. Continuum (Minneap Minn) 2012;33:783–95.
45. Kahle KT, Kulkarni AV, Limbrick DD Jr, et al. Hydrocephalus in children. Lancet 2016;387(10020):788–99.
46. Lau C, Teo WY. Clinical manifestations and diagnosis of central nervous system tumors in children. Uptodate. Accessed October 26, 2021.

47. Wilne SH, Ferris RC, Nathwani A, et al. The presenting features of brain tumours: a review of 200 cases. Arch Dis Child 2006;91(6):502–6.

48. Panigrahy A, Krieger MD, Gonzalez-Gomez I, et al. Quantitative short echo time 1H-MR spectroscopy of untreated pediatric brain tumors: preoperative diagnosis and characterization. AJNR Am J Neuroradiol 2006;27(3):560–72.

49. Barmherzig R, Szperka CL. Pseudotumor cerebri syndrome in children. Curr pain headache Rep 2019;23(8):1–9.

50. Friedman DI, Liu GT, Digre KB. Revised diagnostic criteria for the pseudotumor cerebri syndrome in adults and children. Neurology 2013;81(13):1159–65.

51. Sheldon CA, Paley GL, Xiao R, et al. Pediatric idiopathic intracranial hypertension: age, gender, and anthropometric features at diagnosis in a large, retrospective multisite cohort. Ophthalmology 2016;123(11):2424–31.

52. Görkem SB, Doğanay S, Canpolat M, et al. MR imaging findings in children with pseudotumor cerebri and comparison with healthy controls. Childs Nerv Syst 2015;31(3):373–80.

53. Jayaraman K, Rangasami R, Chandrasekharan A. Magnetic resonance imaging findings in viral encephalitis: a pictorial essay. J neurosciences Rural Pract 2018;9(04):556–60.

54. Bykowski J, Kruk P, Gold JJ, et al. Acute pediatric encephalitis neuroimaging: single-institution series as part of the California encephalitis project. Pediatr Neurol 2015;52:606–14.

55. CDC COVID-19 Response Team. Coronavirus disease 2019 in children e United States, February 12-April 2, 2020. MMWR Morb Mortal Wkly Rep 2020;69: 422e426.

56. McAbee GN, Brosgol Y, Pavlakis S, et al. Encephalitis associated with COVID-19 infection in an 11-year-old child. Pediatr Neurol 2020;109:94.

57. Levy ML, Levy DM, Manna B. Pediatric cerebral aneurysm. StatPearls; 2021.

58. Kossorotoff M, Brousse V, Grevent D, et al. Cerebral haemorrhagic risk in children with sickle-cell disease. Developmental Med Child Neurol 2015;57(2):187–93.

59. Agrawal M, Modi N, Sinha VD. Neurological outcome in patients of traumatic subarachnoid haemorrhage: a study of prognostic factors and role of MRI. IJNT 2014;11:10–6.

60. Ellis MJ, Armstrong D, Vachhrajani S, et al. Angioarchitectural features associated with hemorrhagic presentation in pediatric cerebral arteriovenous malformations. J Neurointerv Surg 2013;5:191–5.

61. Fullerton HJ, Achrol AS, Johnston SC, et al. Long-term hemorrhage risk in children versus adults with brain arteriovenous malformations. Stroke 2005;36: 2099–104.

62. Geibprasert S, Pongpech S, Jiarakongmun P, et al. Radiologic assessment of brain arteriovenous malformations: what clinicians need to know. Radiographics 2010;30(2):483–501.

63. Sporns PB, Psychogios MN, Fullerton HJ, et al. Neuroimaging of Pediatric Intracerebral Hemorrhage. J Clin Med 2020;9(5):1518.

64. Teasdale E. Cerebral venous thrombosis: making the most of imaging. J R Soc Med 2000;93(5):234–7.

65. Walecki J, Mruk B, Nawrocka-Laskus E, et al. Neuroimaging of cerebral venous thrombosis (CVT): old dilemma and the new diagnostic methods. Pol J Radiol 2015;80:368–73.

66. Liang L, Korogi Y, Sugahara T, et al. Evaluation of the intracranial dural sinuses with a 3D contrast-enhanced MP-RAGE sequence: prospective comparison

with 2DTOF MR venography and digital subtraction angiography. AJNR Am J Neuroradiol 2001;22(3):481–92.

67. Tekes A, Palasis S, Durand DJ, et al. ACR Appropriateness Criteria® Sinusitis-Child. J Am Coll Radiol 2018;15(11S):S403–12.

68. Pfeifer CM. Paranasal sinus CT is of variable value in patients with pediatric cancer with neutropenic fever. Am J Neuroradiology 2019;40(4):E19.

Printed and bound by CPI Group (UK) Ltd, Croydon, CR0 4YY

03/10/2024

01040474-0005